Geriatric Oncology

Editors

ARATI V. RAO
HARVEY JAY COHEN

CLINICS IN
GERIATRIC MEDICINE

www.geriatric.theclinics.com

February 2016 • Volume 32 • Number 1

ELSEVIER

1600 John F. Kennedy Boulevard • Suite 1800 • Philadelphia, Pennsylvania, 19103-2899

http://www.theclinics.com

CLINICS IN GERIATRIC MEDICINE Volume 32, Number 1
February 2016 ISSN 0749–0690, ISBN-13: 978-0-323-41688-7

Editor: Jessica McCool
Developmental Editor: Colleen Viola

Clinics in Geriatric Medicine (ISSN 0749-0690) is published quarterly by Elsevier Inc., 360 Park Avenue South, New York, NY 10010-1710. Months of issue are February, May, August, and November. Business and Editorial Offices: 1600 John F. Kennedy Blvd., Suite 1800, Philadelphia, PA 191023-2899. Periodicals postage paid at New York, NY, and additional mailing offices. Subscription prices are $265.00 per year (US individuals), $557.00 per year (US institutions), $100.00 per year (US student/resident), $370.00 per year (Canadian individuals), $706.00 per year (Canadian institutions), $195.00 per year (Canadian student/resident), $390.00 per year (international individuals), $706.00 per year (international institutions), and $195.00 per year (international student/resident). Foreign air speed delivery is included in all *Clinics* subscription prices. All prices are subject to change without notice. POSTMASTER: Send address changes to *Clinics in Geriatric Medicine,* Elsevier Health Sciences Division, Subscription Customer Service, 3251 Riverport Lane, Maryland Heights, MO 63043. **Telephone: 1-800-654-2452 (U.S. and Canada); 314-447-8871 (outside U.S. and Canada). Fax: 314-447-8029. E-mail:** journalscustomerservice-usa@elsevier.com **(for print support) or** journalsonlinesupport-usa@elsevier.com **(for online support).**

Reprints. For copies of 100 or more, of articles in this publication, please contact the Commercial Reprints Department, Elsevier Inc., 360 Park Avenue South, New York, New York 10010-1710. Tel.: 212-633-3874; Fax: 212-633-3820, E-mail: reprints@elsevier.com.

Clinics in Geriatric Medicine is covered in *MEDLINE/PubMed (Index Medicus), EMBASE/Excerpta Medica, Current Contents/Clinical Medicine (CC/CM),* and the *Cumulative Index to Nursing & Allied Health Literature.*

Contributors

EDITORS

ARATI V. RAO, MD
Associate Professor of Medicine, Division of Hematologic Malignancies and Cell Therapy, Division of Geriatrics, Duke University Medical Center, Durham, North Carolina

HARVEY JAY COHEN, MD
Walter Kempner Professor of Medicine, Director, Center for the Study of Aging, Duke University Medical Center, Durham, North Carolina

AUTHORS

SYED ALI AKBAR, MBBS
Fellow, Department of Medicine, Upstate Medical University, Syracuse, New York

KOSHY ALEXANDER, MD
Geriatrics, Memorial Sloan-Kettering Cancer Center; Department of Medicine, Weill Cornell Medical College, New York, New York

ANDREW J. ARMSTRONG, MD, ScM, FACP
Associate Professor of Medicine and Surgery; Associate Director for Clinical Research in Genitourinary Oncology; Divisions of Medical Oncology and Urology, Duke Cancer Institute, Duke University Medical Center, Durham, North Carolina

JEANNE CARTER, PhD
Department of Medicine, Memorial Sloan Kettering Cancer Center, New York, New York

SELINA CHOW, MD
Clinical Associate, Sections of Geriatrics and Palliative Medicine and Hematology/Oncology, Department of Medicine, University of Chicago, Chicago, Illinois

WILLIAM DALE, MD, PhD
Associate Professor, Sections of Geriatrics and Palliative Medicine and Hematology/Oncology, Department of Medicine, University of Chicago, Chicago, Illinois

NIENKE A. DE GLAS, MD, PhD
Department of Internal Medicine, Tergooi Hospitals, Hilversum, The Netherlands

NAJAM UD DIN, MBBS
Fellow, Department of Medicine, Upstate Medical University, Syracuse, New York

AJEET GAJRA, MD, FACP
Associate Professor of Medicine, Upstate Cancer Center, Upstate Medical University, Syracuse, New York

JESSICA GOLDBERG, MSN, AGPCNP-BC
Palliative Medicine, Memorial Sloan Kettering Cancer Center, New York, New York

EMILY J. GUERARD, MD
Division of Hematology and Oncology, Department of Medicine, University of North Carolina at Chapel Hill, Chapel Hill, North Carolina

MITCHELL T. HEFLIN, MD, MHS
Associate Professor of Medicine and Geriatrics, Center for the Study of Aging and Human Development, Duke University Medical Center, Duke University, Durham, North Carolina

JOLEEN M. HUBBARD, MD
Assistant Professor, Department of Oncology, Mayo Clinic, Rochester, Minnesota

ARTI HURRIA, MD
Department of Medical Oncology, City of Hope Comprehensive Cancer Center, Duarte, California

MEGHAN KARUTURI, MD
Department of Breast Medical Oncology, MD Anderson Cancer Center, Houston, Texas

HEIDI D. KLEPIN, MD, MS
Section on Hematology and Oncology, Department of Internal Medicine, Wake Forest School of Medicine, Winston-Salem, North Carolina

BEATRIZ KORC-GRODZICKI, MD, PhD
Geriatrics, Memorial Sloan Kettering Cancer Center; Department of Medicine, Weill Cornell Medical College, New York, New York

DANENG LI, MD
Department of Medical Oncology, City of Hope Comprehensive Cancer Center, Duarte, California

STUART M. LICHTMAN, MD
Professor of Medicine, Weill Cornell Medical College; Department of Medicine, Memorial Sloan Kettering Cancer Center, New York, New York

JUDD W. MOUL, MD, FACS
James H. Semans, MD Professor of Surgery; Director, Duke Prostate Center, Division of Urologic Surgery, Duke University Medical Center, Durham, North Carolina

HYMAN MUSS, MD
Lineberger Comprehensive Cancer Center and Department of Medicine, University of North Carolina, Chapel Hill, North Carolina

SALEHA SAJID, MD
Advanced Fellow, Sections of Geriatrics and Palliative Medicine and Hematology/Oncology, Department of Medicine, University of Chicago, Chicago, Illinois

ARMIN SHAHROKNI, MD, MPH
Department of Medicine, Memorial Sloan Kettering Cancer Center, New York, New York

KAE JACK TAY, MBBS, MRCS(Ed), MCI, FAMS (Urology)
Society of Urologic Oncology Fellow, Division of Urologic Surgery, Duke University Medical Center, Durham, North Carolina

SASCHA A. TUCHMAN, MD
Division of Cellular Therapy and Hematologic Malignancies, Duke Cancer Institute, Durham, North Carolina

NOAM VANDERWALDE, MD
Department of Radiation Oncology, University of Tennessee West Cancer Center, Memphis, Tennessee

SARAH WALL, MD
Clinical Fellow, Hematology and Oncology, The Ohio State University Comprehensive Cancer Center, Columbus, Ohio

SARAH A. WINGFIELD, MD
Advanced Fellow, Geriatric Medicine, Duke University Medical Center, Durham, North Carolina

JENNIFER A. WOYACH, MD
Assistant Professor of Medicine, The Ohio State University Comprehensive Cancer Center, Columbus, Ohio

ABRAHAM J. WU, MD
Department of Medicine, Memorial Sloan Kettering Cancer Center, New York, New York

Contents

Cancer is a disease of aging as older adults are much more likely to develop cancer compared with their younger counterparts. Understanding the biology of cancer and aging remains complex, and numerous theories regarding the relationship between the two have been proposed. Cancer treatment decisions in older patients are particularly challenging, because the evidence is scarce and the risk of toxicity increases with age. Determination of biologic age is essential due to heterogeneity of functional status, comorbidity, and physiologic reserves between patients of the same chronologic age.

Cancer screening is an important tool for reducing morbidity and mortality in the elderly. In this article, performance characteristics of commonly used screening tests for colorectal, lung, prostate, breast, and cervical cancers are discussed. Guidelines are emphasized and key issues to consider in screening older adults are highlighted.

Older adults with cancer require a geriatrics approach to treatment. Such an approach targets appropriate treatments based on physiologic, not chronologic, age. Patients older than 65 years of age constitute the largest group of patients with cancer, making them the most expensive group of patients with cancer, especially with the advent of expensive new treatments with minimal impact on overall survival. Geriatric assessment, combined with targeted inventions, can optimize the value propositions in caring for older patients with cancer. Over the past 20 years, geriatric oncology care models have emerged applying these care principles in clinical practice.

Older patients with cancer are best served by a multidisciplinary approach with palliative care (PC) playing an integral role. PC focuses on symptom control irrespective of its cause and should not be associated only with terminal care. It provides an additional layer of support in the care of patients with cancer with an emphasis on quality of life. This article discusses the evaluation and management of pain and other common nonpain symptoms that occur in elderly patients with cancer, as well as end-of-life care.

With earlier cancer diagnosis among older patients with cancer, the possibility of curing cancer increases. However, cancer treatment may have a long-lasting impact on older cancer survivors. It is vital to screen, diagnose, and properly manage the long-term toxicities of cancer treatment in order to maintain the quality of life of older cancer survivors.

Lung cancer disproportionately affects the elderly. Aging is typically associated with higher risk of comorbidity, declines in physical, organ, and cognitive function, and diminished social support. Hence the management of a disease as complex and potentially lethal as lung cancer in this population is challenging. Despite most patients with lung cancer being elderly, most high-level evidence has been derived from studies that included younger patients and only a minority of the fit elderly. This article reviews the literature on the care of older adults with lung cancer. The evolving role of geriatric assessment in lung cancer is discussed.

Treatment for colorectal cancer should not be based on age alone. Pooled analyses from clinical trials show that fit older adults are able to tolerate treatment well with similar efficacy as younger adults. When an older adult is considered for treatment, the clinical encounter must evaluate for deficits in physical and cognitive function and assess comorbidities, medications, and the degree of social support, all which have may affect tolerance of treatment. Based on the degree of fitness of the patient, multiple alternatives to aggressive treatment regimens and strategies exist to minimize toxicity and preserve quality of life during treatment.

The impact of localized prostate cancer in the elderly depends on disease aggressiveness and life expectancy. In men with localized prostate cancer, those with low-risk disease or a shorter life expectancy should be managed expectantly, whereas those with long life expectancy or more aggressive disease may benefit from curative treatment. Comorbidity and quality-of-life concerns are key considerations during the selection of therapeutic modalities in the elderly in localized and metastatic settings. A variety of new agents have changed the therapeutic landscape in castrate-resistant prostate cancer, but their benefits need to be considered alongside their side effects and cost.

Breast cancer is the mostly commonly diagnosed cancer in women both in the United States and worldwide. Although advanced age at diagnosis is associated with more favorable tumor biology, mortality rates are comparatively higher in older adults, possibly attributed to advanced stage at presentation. There are minimal specific treatment-based guidelines in elderly patients with cancer, mostly attributable to their limited inclusion on clinical trials. In addition to the existing evidence from clinical trials and retrospective studies, practitioners need to take into consideration functional status, social support, patient preference, presence of comorbidities, and life expectancy when selecting optimal treatment.

Myelodysplastic syndromes (MDS) and acute myeloid leukemia (AML) are hematologic diseases that frequently affect older adults. Treatment is challenging. Management of older adults with MDS and AML needs to be individualized, accounting for both the heterogeneity of disease biology and patient characteristics, which can influence life expectancy and treatment tolerance. Clinical trials accounting for the heterogeneity of tumor biology and physiologic changes of aging are needed to define optimal standards of care. This article highlights key evidence related to the management of older adults with MDS and AML and highlights future directions for research.

Chronic lymphocytic leukemia affects less than 1% of US adults but is the most common leukemia, and it primarily affects older patients. Non-Hodgkin lymphomas are the seventh most common cancers in the United States and also primarily affect older patients. In general, older patients should be treated differently than their younger, fitter counterparts. Fitness level and comorbidities should be taken into account when planning treatment. First-line treatment of most of these B-cell lymphoproliferative disorders consists of chemoimmunotherapy. In relapsed and refractory disease, there is a growing role for therapies targeting the B-cell receptor signaling pathway.

Multiple myeloma (MM) and monoclonal gammopathy of undetermined significance (MGUS) are plasma cell disorders of aging. The landscape of the diagnosis and management of MM and MGUS is rapidly changing. This article provides an updated understanding of the clinical presentation, evaluation, diagnosis, and management of older adults with MM and

MGUS. Because most oncology providers are not formally trained in geriatric medicine, geriatricians play a key role in providing oncologists with a broader understanding of patient health status in the hope of improving outcomes for older adults with MM.

CLINICS IN GERIATRIC MEDICINE

ISSUE OF RELATED INTEREST

Hematology/Oncology Clinics of North America, February 2015 (Vol. 29, No. 1)
Colorectal Cancer
Leonard B. Saltz, *Editor*
http://www.hemonc.theclinics.com/

THE CLINICS ARE AVAILABLE ONLINE!
Access your subscription at:
www.theclinics.com

Preface

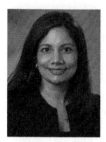 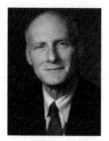

Arati V. Rao, MD   Harvey Jay Cohen, MD
Editors

Cancer is the second leading cause of death after heart disease in the United States. Age is the single most important risk factor for developing cancer with ~60% of all newly diagnosed malignant tumors and 70% of all cancer deaths occurring in persons 65 years or older. It has been estimated that by the year 2030, 20% of the US population (70 million people) will be older than age 65 years. The median age range for diagnosis for most major tumors is 68 to 74 years, and the median age range at death is 70 to 79 years.

One concerning issue is that the death rate is disproportionately higher for the elderly population. There are several reasons for this, including more aggressive biology, competing comorbid medical conditions, decreased physiologic reserve compromising the ability to tolerate therapy, physicians' reluctance to provide aggressive therapy, and barriers in the elderly person's access to care. Communication between health care providers and elderly patients may be hampered by deficits in hearing, vision, and cognition. The elderly patient with cancer often has an elderly caregiver, and the diagnosis of cancer often affects the health-related quality of life of both individuals. All of these challenges contribute to defining "geriatric-oncology" as a true subspecialty, and this issue of the *Clinics in Geriatric Medicine* aims to address some specific and special scenarios with respect to our senior patients with cancer.

The past two decades have led to significant discoveries in cancer therapeutics, and the advent of monoclonal antibodies, tyrosine kinase inhibitors, and other targeted agents has led to increased numbers of elderly patients receiving therapy. Sixty-one percent of cancer survivors are senior adults, and a large number of these patients may follow-up with their geriatricians and oncologists. Geriatric cancer research is much needed, and better clinical trial data are needed to guide the care of this patient population. Historically, older patients with cancer were excluded from or underrepresented in clinical trials. More recent estimates suggest that approximately 30% of accruals to all phase II and III cancer cooperative group trials are patients 65 years or older. Oncologists are less likely to offer trial participation to older patients—yet when offered, older patients are as likely to participate as younger patients.

We have gathered a number of well-recognized specialists within the geriatric-oncology community to educate the reader about the various challenges that they

Clin Geriatr Med 32 (2016) xiii–xiv
http://dx.doi.org/10.1016/j.cger.2015.09.001
0749-0690/16/$ – see front matter © 2016 Published by Elsevier Inc.

may face in clinic while caring for this unique patient population. Why are older patients more prone to developing cancer; how and when to screen these patients is important, and when to stop screening is perhaps even more important. How to optimize therapy in older patients with cancer by identifying geriatric syndromes and risk factors for toxicity by utilizing comprehensive geriatric assessment is a well-studied area in the field. We have attempted to cover the most common tumor types in both men and women, prostate and breast cancers, respectively. In addition, several acute and chronic hematologic malignancies, and the long-term toxicities and sequelae from cancer therapy, are covered. We discuss the importance of supportive and palliative care during the entire trajectory of care for the elderly patient with cancer. Finally, the elephant in the room: "the cost of cancer care" and several ideas on models of care for this patient population are also covered. We hope that the readers will be empowered with a better understanding of the care of this special patient population, be able to identify geriatric syndromes in patients and survivors, and work as a team with oncology professionals to ultimately improve the survival and enrich the quality of life of our senior adult patients with cancer.

Arati V. Rao, MD
Division of Hematologic Malignancies and Cell Therapy
Division of Geriatrics
Duke University Medical Center
Box 3961 DUMC
Durham, NC 27710, USA

Harvey Jay Cohen, MD
Center for the Study of Aging
Duke University Medical Center
Durham, NC 27710, USA

E-mail addresses:
arati.rao@dm.duke.edu (A.V. Rao)
harvey.cohen@duke.edu (H.J. Cohen)

Erratum

In the November 2015 issue of *Clinics in Geriatric Medicine* (Volume 31, Number 4), the author disclosures were inadvertently omitted from the article, "Late-Onset Hypogonadism and Testosterone Replacement in Older Men." Dr. Rajib K. Bhattacharya, corresponding author, is a speaker for AbbVie Pharmaceuticals and Endo Pharmaceuticals.

Clin Geriatr Med 32 (2016) xv
http://dx.doi.org/10.1016/j.cger.2015.10.001
0749-0690/16/$ – see front matter © 2016 Elsevier Inc. All rights reserved.

geriatric.theclinics.com

Erratum

In the Discussion in Chapter 2 (Cortical Bone Metabolism (Volume 22, Number 4), the author was inadvertently omitted from the article "Labral Dysplasia: The Radiographic Presentation and Treatment" (Odem-Mari, Dr. Ralph R. Prokopenko, corresponding author). is a Surgeon for Adult Reconstruction and Hip Preservation Care.

http://dx.doi.org/10.1016/j.cger.2015.10.001
generic.theclinics.com
0749-0690/16/$ – see front matter © 2016 Elsevier Inc. All rights reserved.

Cancer and Aging

General Principles, Biology, and Geriatric Assessment

Daneng Li, MD[a], Nienke A. de Glas, MD, PhD[b], Arti Hurria, MD[a],*

KEYWORDS

• Cancer • Aging • Biology • Biomarker • Geriatric assessment

KEY POINTS

- The biology of cancer and aging remains complex and is likely intertwined through multiple molecular, cellular, and physiologic interactions.
- Geriatric assessment can identify areas of vulnerability in older adults and be used to predict potential treatment toxicity and overall survival among elderly patients with cancer.
- Biomarkers of functional aging along with geriatric assessment may help facilitate personalized treatment decisions among older adults with cancer, through weighing the risks and benefits of cancer treatment in the setting of overall life expectancy and health status.

INTRODUCTION

Cancer is a disease of aging as older adults are much more likely to develop cancer compared with their younger counterparts. In the United States, approximately 60% of all cancer diagnoses and 70% of cancer-related mortalities occur in patients 65 years or older.[1] As the population continues to age, an estimated 70% of all cancer diagnoses will occur in patients over the age of 65 by the year 2030.[2] Understanding the biology of cancer and aging remains complex, and numerous theories regarding the relationship between the 2 have been proposed. Furthermore, treatment decisions regarding older adults with cancer are often difficult due to limited evidence on which to base treatment decisions given the poor representation of this patient population in cancer clinical trials.[3] In this article, the topic of cancer and aging in terms of general principles, biology, and the role of geriatric assessment in older adults with cancer is discussed.

[a] Department of Medical Oncology, City of Hope Comprehensive Cancer Center, 1500 East Duarte Road, Duarte, CA 91010, USA; [b] Department of Internal Medicine, Tergooi Hospitals, Van Riebeeckweg 212, Hilversum 1213XZ, The Netherlands
* Corresponding author.
E-mail address: Ahurria@coh.org

Clin Geriatr Med 32 (2016) 1–15
http://dx.doi.org/10.1016/j.cger.2015.08.003
0749-0690/16/$ – see front matter © 2016 Elsevier Inc. All rights reserved.

GENERAL PRINCIPLES

Chronologic age has been identified as a risk factor for numerous malignancies.[4] However, chronologic age alone is not reliable in predicting overall life expectancy, physical function, or the ability to tolerate treatment in older adults with cancer.[5] Rather, aging is a heterogeneous process in regards to individual changes in physiologic status, comorbidities, and cancer biology. In fact, for certain malignancies, the tumor biology and its response to treatment are integrally related to age.[6]

In treating older adults with cancer, chronologic age alone should not exclude patients from the use of therapies that could prolong survival.[7,8] However, the benefit of treatment in terms of prolonging survival must be weighed against potential treatment toxicities and the overall impact on quality of life. Although large randomized clinical trial data for the treatment of older adults with various malignancies are limited, some studies have shown that older patients with good performance status are often able to tolerate and benefit from the same therapies compared with younger patients.[9–11] Nevertheless, individualization of treatments for older adults with cancer requires more data beyond just chronologic age.[12] Use of tools to predict life expectancy,[13,14] establishment of objective biomarkers to predict functional age,[12] and incorporation of geriatric assessment to identify older adults at risk for adverse outcomes and pinpoint interventions to decrease this risk are needed.[15] These tools may ultimately help guide physicians in the shared decision-making process with older adults contemplating cancer treatment, thus facilitating and personalizing care for the older adult.

BIOLOGY OF CANCER AND AGING

A better understanding of the biology of aging may provide valuable clues to understanding cancer development. The term senescence is often synonymous with biologic aging and is characterized by a decrease in stress response, disruptions in homeostatic balance, and an increased risk of chronic illnesses such as cancer. At the cellular level, senescence is characterized by the cessation of replicative division within normal cells of the human body. The relationship between aging, cellular senescence, and cancer is complex, and numerous theories have been proposed to elucidate the relationship (**Table 1**).

Theories on Aging and Potential Impact on Cancer

Mutation accumulation
One of the early theories of aging focused on the accumulation of mutations throughout a lifetime. In this theory, mutations that are not affected by natural selection early in life tend to accumulate and ultimately result in aging.[16] Building on this concept, Denham Harman[17] proposed the free radical theory initially in 1954. Through various oxidative stress reactions occurring within organisms, free radicals are generated that lead to damaging effects in DNA and proteins, thereby contributing to aging and potential carcinogenesis. Furthermore, scientists have also reported that changes in the composition of chromatin such as general hypomethylation,[18] hypermethylation of CpG islands, and accumulation of heterochromatin are associated with an aging phenotype as well. The DNA damage response is essential to the maintenance of the human genome and epigenome. For severe damage, programmed cell death or cell-cycle arrest occurs, allowing for potential anti-cancer protection. However, the cost of this response could be a further depletion of stem-cell reserves, which may promote an aging phenotype. Furthermore, DNA and chromatin repair in itself can be error prone, leading to the accumulation of additional mutations. Interestingly,

Table 1 Theories on aging and potential impact on cancer			
Theories on Aging	**Description**	**Aging Impact**	**Cancer Impact**
Mutation accumulation	Oxidative stress → free radicals → DNA and protein damage or alterations	Increase	Increase
Antagonist pleiotropy	Genes that promote reproduction and anti-cancer protection (ie, tumor suppressors) early in life result in aging later in life	Increase	Decrease
Disposable soma (includes cellular senescence and role of telomeres)	Maintenance of somatic cells become less important beyond reproductive years → accumulation of cellular damage	Increase	Increase
Role of stem cells	Stem cells decline in ability to proliferate and differentiate → DNA damage → activation of senescence or apoptosis	Likely increase	Likely increase
Hyperfunction and role of metabolic pathways	Overactivity of biosynthetic and metabolic pathways → hypertrophy and inflammation in tissue systems → cell failure and loss of homeostasis	Increase	Increase

many syndromes that have defective DNA damage response are associated with premature aging and an increased risk of cancer.[19] Overall, the theories of mutation accumulation suggest that aging and cancer are driven by the same increased burden of mutations resulting in cellular degeneration.

The antagonist pleiotropy

In addition to mutation accumulation, the antagonist pleiotropy theory by George Williams[20] was also initially developed in the 1950s. In relation to aging, antagonist pleiotropy refers to the concept that a gene may cause both increased reproduction early in life followed by aging later in life. For instance, tumor suppressors such as p16 regulate apoptosis and cellular senescence leading to potential cancer protection. Although mutations of p16 have been found to promote carcinogenesis,[21] upregulated expression of p16 has also been reported to be associated with age in many tissues.[22–24] Interestingly, data on patients with breast cancer who received adjuvant chemotherapy showed a near doubling of p16 expression in peripheral T cells consistent with a comparable increase of 14.7 years of chronologic aging.[25] Overall, tumor suppressors such as p16 support the theory of antagonist pleiotropy by providing an example of reproductive advantage through initial cancer protection at the overall cost of potential tissue aging.

Disposable soma theory

The third major historic theory on aging involves the concept of disposable soma. In 1977, Thomas Kirkwood proposed this theory wherein a finite amount of energy exists that must be divided between reproduction (germ cells) and maintenance (somatic cells) of an organism.[26] This theory is fundamentally based on time because the greatest amount of energy is dedicated to reproduction during the early reproductive years in order to maximize an evolutionary selective advantage. Aging was therefore thought to be the result of accumulation of damage over time as maintenance of somatic cells became less important beyond the initial reproductive years.

Both replicative and cellular senescence further support the theory of disposable soma with regards to aging. Replicative senescence specifically refers to the systemic arrest of human primary cell lines after several specific cell divisions.[27] However, replicative senescence is only a part of the component for overall cellular senescence because pathways involved with tumor suppressors, lysosomal activity, and chromatin remodeling have been described as well.[26] Furthermore, as cells enter senescence, the secretion of numerous proinflammatory cytokines, growth factors, and proteases through the process of senescence-associated secretory phenotype (SASP) have been described.[28] The release of cytokines, such as interleukin (IL) -6, IL-8, and additional proteins responsible for inflammation by senescent cells and the SASP, has been hypothesized to contribute to both aging and many age-related diseases, including cancer. For example, age-related breast changes, pulmonary artery hypertrophy, and premature skin aging have all been described as a potential consequence of senescent cell accumulation and the release of multiple factors during the SASP process to the surrounding tissues.[28] In addition, many SASP released factors, such as stromelysin, vascular endothelial growth factor, and amphiregulin, appear to have the ability to stimulate tumor growth in mouse xenograft studies.[29,30] Furthermore, the secretion of IL-6 and IL-8 by senescent fibroblasts in culture has been specifically shown to induce epithelial-to-mesenchymal transition, which is a crucial step in the development of metastatic cancer.[31] Overall, as senescent cells accumulate with age, the SASP could be creating a potential tissue microenvironment suitable for the development or progression of many chronic diseases such as cancer.

The discovery of telomeres and telomerase also provides additional molecular support for the disposable soma theory. Telomeres are repetitive nucleotide sequences located at the ends of linear chromosomes. Normal telomere length and function have been found to be crucial for many cell processes, such as stem-cell renewal and tissue development. However, with each cell replication and division process, there is incomplete replication of the ends of chromosomes at the location of telomeres. This incomplete replication results in telomere shortening over time, and once a critical threshold telomere length is reached, replicative senescence or apoptotic events are triggered.[32,33] Telomere shortening can be compensated for by telomerase, a reverse transcriptase enzyme responsible for synthesis of telomeres. However, for most cells in the human body, telomerase expression is halted beginning in embryogenesis, thereby creating a molecular clock whereby each additional replication leads ultimately to senescence and aging.

Although telomere erosion appears to play a crucial role in replicative senescence leading to aging, it may also contribute to both cancer development and prevention. In mice, eroded telomeres have been shown to limit cancer formation by triggering senescence.[34,35] However, other studies suggest that telomere shortening may lead to genomic instability and chromosome loss, leading to the process of tumor development.[36] For example, shortened telomeres have been seen in a variety of cancers, including pancreatic, prostate, bladder, kidney, lung, and bone tumors. Patients with the shortest versus longest telomeres have been shown to have an increased risk of cancer development.[37,38] Furthermore, telomerase, the enzyme that promotes telomere repair, has been reported to be activated in up to 80% of tumors.[39] Therefore, the relationship of telomeres to cancer development and prevention is complex and is likely dependent on both the specific cell types involved and the overall genomic context.[40,41]

Stem cells, aging, and cancer

In addition to somatic cells, stem cells are also likely to have a significant impact on both aging and cancer. Stem cells are characterized by their capability of self-renewal. With aging, stem cells decline in their ability to proliferate and differentiate.[26] Intrinsically, DNA damage tends to accumulate in an age-dependent manner in stem cells of different organs.[42–44] However, the overall effect of accumulated DNA damage in stem cells on tissue aging and cancer is not fully understood. DNA damage in stem cells has been shown to trigger pathways leading to the activation of tumor suppressors such as p16 or p53,[45–47] resulting in senescence or apoptosis; this suggests that the functional decline in stem cells could be due to the result of cancer suppression and supports the antagonist pleiotropy theory as described above. However, studies in mice have also demonstrated the opposite, whereby increases in the gene dose of numerous tumor suppressors resulted in both improved cancer suppression and overall longevity.[48] In addition, extrinsic mechanisms may also contribute to cancer development during the aging process of stem cells. As DNA damage accumulates with aging, there is a loss of proliferative competition[49] from the decrease of undamaged stem cells. Therefore, overall selection of potential premalignant clones is increased.[50] Furthermore, impaired immune clearance of senescent cells may also result in decreased tissue integrity and possibly contribute to cancer development.[51,52]

Hyperfunction theory and role of metabolic pathways

In the hyperfunction theory,[53,54] aging is the result of overactivity through biosynthetic processes during adulthood, leading to hypertrophy and inflammation in multiple tissue systems and ultimately resulting in cell failure and loss of homeostasis. Furthermore, hyperfunction has been shown to increase the activity of DNA damage repair pathways despite a lack of accumulation of actual DNA damage.[54] Metabolic pathways associated with hyperfunction are additional areas of research in the field of aging and its relationship to cancer development. For example, excess caloric intake is associated with the activation of insulin, insulin growth factor 1 (IGF-1), and a target of rapamycin pathways. Interestingly, controlled caloric restriction and suppression of overactivity in insulin and IGF-1 pathways in mice have been shown to be associated with a decrease in the rate of aging and delay of many chronic illnesses such as cancer.[55,56] Therefore, reduction of the overactivity of certain metabolic pathways such as IGF-1 may ultimately result in protection against aging and development of cancer. Further research of metabolic pathways associated with longevity and identification of potential molecular targets[57] is needed in order to provide better understanding of aging pathways and their roles in cancer development.

THE ROLE OF AGE-RELATED BIOMARKERS IN CANCER

As the understanding for the biology of aging continues to grow, identification of potential aging biomarkers represents the next step in the development of personalized cancer care among older adults by more accurately characterizing a patient's functional age. Several potential age-related biomarkers have been previously described in the literature[12] and are highlighted in this section for their potential use during the treatment of older adults with cancer (**Table 2**).

Markers of chronic inflammation such as C-reactive protein (CRP) and IL-6 and markers of coagulation such as D-dimer have been found to be associated with physical function or frailty.[12] Even after controlling for age, comorbidities, and physical function, these markers have the ability to predict functional decline and overall mortality.[58–60] The potential advantage for the use of chronic inflammatory markers or

Table 2
Potential aging biomarkers for use in cancer

Markers	Advantages	Challenges
Chronic inflammation (CRP, IL-6, TNFα, IL-1RA)	1. Correlation with physical function and mortality 2. Ease of measurement from ELISA of serum or plasma	Possible production by cancer itself resulting in interpretation difficulties
Coagulation (D-dimer, sVCAM)	1. Correlation with physical function and mortality 2. Ease of measurement from ELISA of serum or plasma	Possible production by cancer itself resulting in interpretation difficulties
Telomere length	1. Correlation with physical function and mortality 2. Association with poor prognosis of various malignancies	1. Expertise laboratory equipment required for analysis 2. Genetic and environmental confounders influence length
p16^{INK4a}	Strong association with aging from breast cancer studies	Special expertise required for processing of T-lymphocyte RNA samples

Abbreviations: ELISA, enzyme-linked immunosorbent assay; IL-1RA, interleukin-1 receptor antagonist; sVCAM, soluble vascular cell adhesion molecule; TNFα, tumor necrosis factor α.

markers of coagulation is the overall ease of measurement through enzyme-linked immunosorbent assays, which are widely commercially available. However, a direct mechanistic link between these inflammatory and coagulation markers and functional decline has not been clearly established. Furthermore, in patients with cancer, when the tumor has not been removed, these markers are often produced by the actual cancer itself, resulting in difficulties for accurate interpretation of correlation with overall functional age.[61] Therefore, chronic inflammatory markers or markers of coagulation may have potentially better utility in the setting of early stage cancer when the tumors have been completely removed.

Cellular senescence appears to be associated with aging as previously described in the section on Theories on Aging. Therefore, markers associated with cellular senescence such as p16 and telomeres have also been explored as potential biomarkers for aging. Studies have shown that p16^{INK4a} levels increase with age and also correlate with high expressions of IL-6.[22,62,63] Although p16^{INK4a} levels require special expertise to process due to the requirement of performing quantitative real-time polymerase chain reaction on T-lymphocyte RNA,[64] it does have tremendous promise as a biomarker for aging in patients with cancer because its expression has been reported to increase in women undergoing chemotherapy for breast cancer.[65] The role of p16 levels is currently being evaluated in the geriatric oncology population as part of an ongoing clinical trial (NCT00849758).

Similar to p16, telomere length has been shown to correlate with age, functional status, and mortality.[66,67] In addition, shorter telomere length is associated with poorer prognosis in patients with soft tissue sarcomas, or colorectal, breast, or lung cancers.[64] Telomere length can be measured with routine blood draws but requires sophisticated laboratory methods for analysis.[68,69] Furthermore, several caveats need to be considered. First, the assumption is that the telomere length found in peripheral blood leukocytes is equivalent to telomere length in other tissues; however, this may not be the case. In addition, several processes can impact telomere length, including genetic processes, environmental exposure, and dietary intake.[69] However, similar to markers of inflammation such as CRP and IL-6, establishing a correlation between telomere length and functional status alone may be enough to provide insights to help treatment decisions in older adults with cancer. Interestingly, dysfunctional telomeres could also be a potential aging biomarker as early laboratory studies have shown its ability to not only distinguish between old and young adults but also differentiate healthy older adults from those with multiple chronic illnesses.[70]

In addition to markers of chronic inflammation, coagulation, and cellular senescence, less well-defined age-related biomarkers with associations with physical function such as oxidative stress, lymphopenia, genes associated with longevity, and single nucleotide polymorphisms may prove to be predictors of oncology outcomes in an aging population.[12] Ultimately, a collection of potential aging biomarkers as part of ongoing clinical trials in older adults with cancer will be needed in order to elucidate their potential utility in predicting endpoints, such as treatment tolerance, quality of life, and survival of older adults with cancer.

GERIATRIC ASSESSMENT IN OLDER PATIENTS WITH CANCER

Cancer in older patients occurs in the background of physiologic decline. The geriatric assessment is a tool that can be used to assess the whole spectrum of health issues and functional status in older adults with cancer. It consists of validated measurements of functional status, comorbidity (including medications taken), nutrition, cognition, social support, and psychological state.[15] Currently, the International Society for Geriatric Oncology as well as the National Comprehensive Cancer Network guidelines recommend performing a geriatric assessment in all older patients with cancer.[15,71] Previous studies have shown that performing a geriatric assessment is feasible in daily clinical practice and in the research setting.[72–74] The main applications of geriatric assessment are summarized in **Table 3**.

Applications of Geriatric Assessment in Older Patients with Cancer

Predict treatment toxicity
A geriatric assessment can identify older adults at risk for chemotherapy toxicity. Currently, there are 2 tools available that predict chemotherapy toxicity in older adults with cancer. The CRASH score (Chemotherapy Risk Assessment Scale for High-Age Patients) was developed in a prospective cohort of adults age 70 and older who were starting chemotherapy.[75] It consists of 2 parts: first, a hematologic score, which included diastolic blood pressure, activities of daily living (ADL), lactate dehydrogenase level, and the toxicity of the chemotherapy regimen; and second, the nonhematologic score, which includes the Eastern Cooperative Oncology Group (ECOG) performance status, Mini Mental Status score, Mini Nutritional Assessment score, and the toxicity of the chemotherapy regimen.

In addition, the chemotherapy prediction tool of the Cancer and Aging Research Group (CARG) was developed in a prospective cohort of adults aged 65 years and older. This tool uses tumor and treatment variables (age, cancer type, chemotherapy dosing, number of chemotherapy drugs), laboratory values (hemoglobin level, creatinine clearance), as well as geriatric assessment variables (hearing, number of falls in previous 6 months, the need for assistance with taking medications, the ability to walk 1 block, and social activity). This score was compared with the ability of the Karnofsky Performance Status (KPS) to predict chemotherapy toxicity. It was shown that KPS is not predictive of toxicity of chemotherapy in older adults with cancer, whereas the prediction tool can discriminate the risk of chemotherapy toxicity in older adults with cancer.[76]

Table 3	
Applications of the geriatric assessment in older adults with cancer	
Application	**Examples**
Predict treatment toxicity	• CRASH score: developed in a prospective cohort of older adults with cancer starting chemotherapy. The score predicts hematological and nonhematological toxicity in older adults with cancer • Chemotherapy prediction tool of CARG: developed in a cohort of older adults with cancer starting chemotherapy. The tool predicts severe (grade III and above) chemotherapy toxicity in older adults with cancer • PACE Study: showed that a summary deficit score based on Geriatric Assessment variables can predict 30-day morbidity in older adults with cancer who were undergoing cancer surgery[77]
Predict survival	Geriatric assessment can predict survival in older adults with cancer and may aid in treatment decisions by weighing the risk of dying from cancer vs the risk of dying from other comorbid conditions[78–81]
Identify areas of vulnerability	Geriatric assessment can identify geriatric problems that are not picked up by routine history and physical examination, such as functional impairment, poor nutritional status, depression, cognitive impairment, and risk of falls[74,83]
Assist in clinical decision-making	20%–50% of treatment decisions are changed when a Geriatric Assessment is used[73]
Inclusion in clinical trials	• Geriatric assessment can be used in clinical research because it can provide a more accurate descriptor of the study population[86] • Geriatric assessment can be used in research as a predictor of toxicity to treatment • Geriatric assessment can be used as a predictor of ability to complete treatment, and as a stratification factor that defines subgroups

Data from Refs.[73,74,77–81,83,86]

Furthermore, the Preoperative Assessment of Cancer in the Elderly (PACE) Study showed that a summary deficit score that was based on geriatric assessment was predictive of 30-day postoperative morbidity.[77] Hence, the geriatric assessment may not only be useful in the chemotherapy setting but also in surgical decision-making.

Predict survival of older adults with cancer

A geriatric assessment can also be used to predict survival of older adults with cancer. A recent systematic review that included 51 publications from 37 studies showed that data gathered in a geriatric assessment can predict mortality in older patients with cancer.[78] For example, a retrospective study that included patients with cancer aged 70 years and older showed that several domains of a comprehensive geriatric assessment are independent predictors of mortality (including ECOG performance status, geriatric depression scale, and the DETERMINE nutritional index).[79] In addition, a study by Klepin and colleagues[80] showed that geriatric assessment is predictive of overall survival in older patients with hematologic malignancies, specifically in patients with acute myelogenous leukemia.

A key part of cancer treatment decisions is to weigh the risk of dying from cancer versus another comorbid condition. For example, in cancer types that are not very aggressive (eg, prostate or hormone receptor positive breast cancer), the risk of dying from other comorbid conditions may exceed the risk of dying from cancer. On the other hand, in aggressive cancer types, such as acute myelogenous leukemia or diffuse large cell lymphoma, the cancer is likely going to be the disease that limits life expectancy, and the decisions will focus on the preferences for treatment and the specific treatments considered in light of the patient's health status and other co-morbid illnesses. Hence, it is important to consider the risk of competing mortality when deciding on whether to treat the cancer. There are several prediction tools that are currently used to estimate the risk of cancer mortality, of which Adjuvant! Online is the most well-known and widely used.[81] However, Adjuvant! Online does not incorporate geriatric assessment measures and only a brief assessment of comorbidity is included. It was recently shown that Adjuvant! Online may not accurately predict breast cancer outcome in older patients because it overestimated 10-year overall survival by 10% in a large cohort of unselected older patients with breast cancer. In addition, 10-year cumulative recurrence was overestimated by 9%.[82] Hence, new prediction tools that can predict cancer outcomes in older patients are needed that include geriatric assessment parameters in order to weigh the risk of cancer recurrence and mortality against the risk of other competing health conditions.

Identify areas of vulnerability
A geriatric assessment can identify areas of vulnerability beyond that commonly identified by routine history and physical examination. Furthermore, it adds substantial information even in patients with a good performance status (defined as an ECOG score <2).[83] For example, among patients with an ECOG score of less than 2, it was shown that the geriatric assessment detected the need for functional assistance, as measured by ADL and IADL score, in 9% and 38% of patients, respectively.[83] In addition, a large cohort study including 1967 older patients with cancer identified unknown geriatric problems that were not identified in routine history and physical examination in 51.2% of all patients (such as poor physical functioning [40.1%], poor nutritional status [37.6%], falls [30.5%], depression [27.2%], and cognitive impairment [19.0%]).[74]

Assist in clinical decision-making
A geriatric assessment could also be used to facilitate decisions in older patients with cancer. It has been reported that 20% to 50% of treatment decisions are influenced by geriatric assessment when it is performed.[72–74] For example, the French ELPACA Study showed that the initial treatment plan was modified based on findings of a geriatric assessment in 20.8% of all patients.[84]

Inclusion in clinical trials to provide a more accurate descriptor of the study population
A geriatric assessment can be used in clinical research, because it provides a more extensive description of baseline characteristics of older patients included in clinical trials. It has been widely acknowledged that older patients are underrepresented in randomized clinical trials.[85–87] In addition, it has been shown that older patients who are included in clinical trials are not representative of the general older population, because they tend to have better functional status, less comorbidity, and a higher socioeconomic status.[88] Several research collaborative groups, such as the Alliance for Clinical Trials in Oncology and European Organisation for Research and Treatment of Cancer, advocate that studies in older patients with cancer should incorporate some

form of geriatric assessment in their trial design.[86] In addition, the geriatric assessment can be used in clinical research as a predictor of ability to complete treatment and as a stratification factor that defines subgroups.

Future Research Directions

The ultimate goal of a geriatric assessment is to guide rational interventions and facilitate treatment decision-making. For example, a geriatric assessment could be used to initiate interventions to improve general health status before cancer treatment commences. Studies are underway to identify how geriatric assessment–guided interventions can potentially improve treatment tolerance. For example, an ongoing randomized clinical trial by Mohile and colleagues assesses a geriatric assessment intervention for reducing chemotherapy toxicity in older patients with cancer (NCT02054741, NCT01915056). Furthermore, another recently published study compared 2 cohorts of older patients with cancer undergoing chemotherapy. The intervention group used a geriatric assessment to identify high-risk patients, who received geriatric interventions based on issues identified by geriatric assessment. It was shown that patients undergoing a geriatric assessment were more likely to complete cancer treatment and required less treatment modifications, although the overall toxicity rate was not significantly different.[89]

Last, a geriatric assessment could be used to guide cancer treatment based on the risk for treatment toxicity. For example, patients with a lower than average risk for treatment toxicity could receive a standard dose and schedule, whereas patients at higher risk for treatment toxicity could receive modified treatment, such as dose reducing the first cycle and subsequently increasing to the standard dosing if it well tolerated. Alternatively, novel treatments could be studied in those at high risk of treatment toxicity. Finally, studies should focus on the development of cutoff points that can be used to aid clinical decision-making.

SUMMARY

As the US population continues to age, an increasing proportion of patients diagnosed with cancer will be over the age of 65. A better understanding of the aging process and its relationship to cancer is needed. Biomarker development to better assess the functional age of older patients with cancer is an active area of research. In addition, geriatric assessment plays an important role in determining physiologic reserves and capacity to tolerate treatment. Further research is needed to determine specific interventions that can decrease treatment toxicity as well as improve cancer and noncancer outcomes and quality of life after treatment.

REFERENCES

1. Howlader N, Noone AM, Krapcho M, et al. SEER cancer statistics review, 1975-2012. Bethesda (MD): National Cancer Institute; 2015. based on November 2014 SEER data submission, posted to the SEER web site Available at: http://seer.cancer.gov/csr/1975_2012/.
2. Smith BD, Smith GL, Hurria A, et al. Future of cancer incidence in the United States: burdens upon an aging, changing nation. J Clin Oncol 2009;27:2758–65.
3. Crome P, Lally F, Cherubini A, et al. Exclusion of older people from clinical trials: professional views from nine European countries participating in the PREDICT study. Drugs Aging 2011;28:667–77.
4. Hansen J. Common cancers in the elderly. Drugs Aging 1998;13:467–78.

5. Wedding U, Honecker F, Bokemeyer C, et al. Tolerance to chemotherapy in elderly patients with cancer. Cancer Control 2007;14:44–56.
6. Balducci L. Management of cancer in the elderly. Oncology (Williston Park) 2006; 20:135–43.
7. Saltzstein SL, Behling CA. 5- and 10-year survival in cancer patients 90 and older. A study of 37,218 patients from SEER. J Surg Oncol 2002;81:113–6.
8. Extermann M. Management issues for elderly patients with breast cancer. Curr Treat Options Oncol 2004;5:161–9.
9. Chen H, Cantor A, Meyer J, et al. Can older cancer patients tolerate chemotherapy? A prospective pilot study. Cancer 2003;97:1107–14.
10. Christman K, Muss HB, Case LD, et al. Chemotherapy of metastatic breast cancer in the elderly. The Pidemont Oncology Association experience. JAMA 1992; 268:57–62.
11. Sargent DJ, Goldberg RM, Jacobson SD, et al. A pooled analysis of adjuvant chemotherapy for resected colon cancer in elderly patients. N Engl J Med 2001;345:1091–7.
12. Hubbard JM, Cohen HJ, Muss HB. Incorporating biomarkers into cancer and aging research. J Clin Oncol 2014;32:2611–6.
13. Walter LC, Covinsky KE. Cancer screening in elderly patients: a framework for individualized decision making. JAMA 2001;285:2750–6.
14. Lee SJ, Lindquist K, Segal MR, et al. Development and validation of a prognostic index for 4-year mortality in older adults. JAMA 2006;295:801–8.
15. Wildiers H, Heeren P, Puts M. International Society of Geriatric Oncology consensus on geriatric assessment in older patients with cancer. J Clin Oncol 2014;32:2595–603.
16. Medawar PB. Unsolved problems of biology. London: H.K. Lewis; 1952.
17. Harman D. Extending functional life span. Exp Gerontol 1998;33:95–112.
18. Slagboom PE, Vijg J. The dynamics of genome organization and expression during the aging process. Ann N Y Acad Sci 1992;673:58–69.
19. Cheng WH, Muftic D, Muftuoglu M, et al. WRN is required for ATM activation and the S-phase checkpoint in response to interstrand cross-link-induced DNA double-strand breaks. Mol Biol Cell 2008;19:3923–33.
20. Williams GC. Pleiotropy, natural selection, and the evolution of senescence. Evolution 1957;11:398–411.
21. Holst CR, Nuovo GJ, Esteller M, et al. Methylation of p16(INK4a) promoters occurs in vivo in histologically normal human mammary epithelia. Cancer Res 2003;63:1596–601.
22. Krishnamurthy J, Torrice C, Ramsey MR, et al. Ink4a/Arf expression is a biomarker of aging. J Clin Invest 2004;114:1299–307.
23. Munro J, Barr NI, Ireland H, et al. Histone deacetylase inhibitors induce a senescence-like state in human cells by a p16-dependent mechanism that is independent of a mitotic clock. Exp Cell Res 2004;295:525–38.
24. Liu Y, Johnson SM, Fedoriw Y, et al. Expression of a p16(INK4a) prevents cancer and promotes aging in lymphocytes. Blood 2011;117:3257–67.
25. Sanoff HK, Deal AM, Krishnamurthy J, et al. Effect of cytotoxic chemotherapy on markers of molecular age in patients with breast cancer. J Natl Cancer Inst 2014; 106:dju057.
26. Falandry C, Bonnefoy M, Freyer G, et al. Biology of cancer and aging: a complex association with cellular senescence. J Clin Oncol 2014;32:2604–10.
27. Hayflick L, Moorhead PS. The serial cultivation of human diploid cell strains. Exp Cell Res 1961;25:585–621.

28. Campisi J. Aging, cellular senescence, and cancer. Annu Rev Physiol 2013;75: 685–705.
29. Coppe JP, Kauser K, Campisi J, et al. Secretion of vascular endothelial growth factor by primary human fibroblasts at senescence. J Biol Chem 2006;281: 29568–74.
30. Liu D, Hornsby PJ. Senescent human fibroblasts increase the early growth of xeno-graft tumors via matrix metalloproteinase secretion. Cancer Res 2007;67:3117–26.
31. Laberge RM, Awad P, Campisi J, et al. Epithelial-mesenchymal transition induced by senescent fibroblasts. Cancer Microenviron 2012;5:39–44.
32. D'Adda di Fagagna F, Reaper PM, Clay-Farrace L, et al. A DNA damage check-point response in telomere-initiated senescence. Nature 2003;426:194–8.
33. Gilson E, Geli V. How telomeres are replicated. Nat Rev Mol Cell Biol 2007;8: 825–38.
34. Feldser DM, Greider CW. Short telomeres limit tumor progression in vivo by inducing senescence. Cancer Cell 2007;11:461–9.
35. Cosme-Bianco W, Shen MF, Lazar AJ, et al. Telomere dysfunction suppresses spontaneous tumorigenesis in vivo by initiating p53-dependent cellular senes-cence. EMBO Rep 2007;8:497–503.
36. Raynaud CM, Sabatier L, Philipot O, et al. Telomere length, telomeric proteins and genomic instability during the multistep carcinogenic process. Crit Rev Oncol Hematol 2008;66:99–117.
37. Ma H, Zhou Z, Wei S, et al. Shortened telomere length is associated with increased risk of cancer: a meta-analysis. PLoS One 2011;6:e20466.
38. Wentzensen IM, Mirabello L, Pfeiffer RM, et al. The association of telomere length and cancer: a meta-analysis. Cancer Epidemiol Biomarkers Prev 2011;20: 1238–50.
39. Aschacher T, Wolf B, Enzmann F, et al. LINE-1 induces hTERT and ensures telo-mere maintenance in tumour cell lines. Oncogene 2015;1–11. [Epub ahead of print].
40. Chin L, Artandi SE, Shen Q, et al. P53 deficiency rescues the adverse effects of telomere loss and cooperates with telomere dysfunction to accelerate carcino-genesis. Cell 1999;97:527–38.
41. Greenberg RA, Chin L, Femino A, et al. Short dysfunctional telomeres impair tumorigenesis in the INK4a(delta2/3) cancer-prone mouse. Cell 1999;97:515–25.
42. Vaziri H, Dragowska W, Alllsopp RC, et al. Evidence for a mitotic clock in human hematopoietic stem cells: loss of telomeric DNA with age. Proc Natl Acad Sci U S A 1994;91:9857–60.
43. Rossi DJ, Seita J, Czechowicz A, et al. Hematopoietic stem cell quiescence at-tenuates DNA damage response and permits DNA damage accumulation during aging. Cell Cycle 2007;6:2371–6.
44. Rube CE, Fricke A, Widmann TA, et al. Accumulation of DNA damage in hemato-poietic stem and progenitor cells during human aging. PLoS One 2011;6: e17487.
45. TelKippe M, Harrison DE, Chen J. Expansion of hematopoietic stem cell pheno-type and activity in Trp53-null mice. Exp Hematol 2003;31(6):521–7.
46. Berfield AK, Andress DL, Abrass CK. IGFBP-5(201-208) stimulates Cdc42GAP aggregation and filopodia formation in migrating mesangial cells. Kidney Int 2000;57:1991–2003.
47. Chen J, Ellison FM, Keyvanfar K, et al. Enrichment of hematopoietic stem cells with SLAM and LSK markers for the detection of hematopoietic stem cell function in normal and Trp53 null mice. Exp Hematol 2008;36:1236–43.

48. Matheu A, Maraver A, Klatt P, et al. Delayed aging through damage protection by the Arf/p53 pathway. Nature 2007;448:375–9.
49. Bondar T, Medzhitov R. p53-mediated hematopoietic stem and progenitor cell competition. Cell Stem Cell 2010;6:309–22.
50. Porter CC, Baturin D, Choudhary R, et al. Relative fitness of hematopoietic progenitors influences leukemia progression. Leukemia 2011;25:891–5.
51. Xue W, Zender L, Miething C, et al. Senescence and tumour clearance is triggered by p53 restoration in murine liver carcinomas. Nature 2007;445:656–60.
52. Kang TW, Yevsa T, Woller N, et al. Senescence surveillance of pre-malignant hepatocytes limits liver cancer development. Nature 2011;479:547–51.
53. Blagosklonny MV. Revisiting the antagonistic pleiotropy theory of aging: TOR-driven program and quasi-program. Cell Cycle 2010;9:3151–6.
54. Blagosklonny MV. Answering the ultimate question "what is the proximal cause of aging?". Aging 2012;4:861–77.
55. Gems D, Doonan R. Antioxidant defense and aging in C. elegans: is the oxidative damage theory of aging wrong? Cell Cycle 2009;8:1681–7.
56. Gems D, de la Guardia Y. Alternative perspectives on aging in Caenorhabditis elegans: reactive oxygen species or hyperfunction? Antioxid Redox Signal 2013; 19:321–9.
57. Berman AE, Leontieva OV, Natarajan V, et al. Recent progress in genetics of aging, senescence and longevity: focusing on cancer-related genes. Oncotarget 2012;3:1522–32.
58. Cohen HJ, Harris T, Pieper CF. Coagulation and activation of inflammatory pathways in the development of functional decline and mortality in the elderly. Am J Med 2003;114:180–7.
59. Reuben DB, Chen AI, Harris TB, et al. Peripheral blood markers of inflammation predict mortality and functional decline in high-functioning community-dwelling older persons. J Am Geriatr Soc 2002;50:638–44.
60. Pieper CF, Rao KM, Currie MS, et al. Age, functional status, and racial differences in plasma D-dimer levels in community-dwelling elderly persons. J Gerontol A Biol Sci Med Sci 2000;55:M649–57.
61. Flandry C, Gilson E, Rudolph KL. Are aging biomarkers clinically relevant in oncogeriatrics? Crit Rev Oncol Hematol 2013;85:257–65.
62. Liu Y, Sanoff HK, Cho H, et al. Expression of p16(INK4a) in peripheral blood T-cells is a biomarker of human aging. Aging Cell 2009;8:439–48.
63. Song Z, von Figura G, Liu Y, et al. Lifestyle impacts on the aging-associated expression of biomarkers of DNA damage and telomere dysfunction in human blood. Aging Cell 2010;9:607–15.
64. Pallis AG, Hatse S, Brouwers B, et al. Evaluating the physiological reserves of older patients with cancer: the value of potential biomarkers of aging? J Geriatr Oncol 2014;5:204–18.
65. Muss HB, Krishnamurthy J, Alston SM, et al. P16INK4a expression after chemotherapy in older women with early-stage breast cancer. J Clin Oncol 2011;29: 550s (suppl; abstract: 9002).
66. Cawthon RM, Smith KR, O'Brien E, et al. Association between telomere length in blood and mortality in people aged 60 years or older. Lancet 2003;361:393–5.
67. Risques RA, Arbeev KG, Yashin AL, et al. Leukocyte telomere length is associated with disability in older US population. J Am Geriatr Soc 2010;58: 1289–98.
68. Harley CB, Futcher AB, Greider CW. Telomeres shorten during aging of human fibroblasts. Nature 1990;345:458–60.

69. Mather KA, Jorm AF, Parslow RA, et al. Is telomere length a biomarker of aging? A review. J Gerontol A Biol Sci Med Sci 2011;66:202–13.

70. Jiang H, Schiffer E, Song Z, et al. Proteins induced by telomere dysfunction and DNA damage represent biomarkers of human aging and disease. Proc Natl Acad Sci U S A 2008;105:11299–304.

71. National Comprehensive Cancer Network (NCCN). Older Adult Oncology (Version 2.2015). Available at: http://www.nccn.org/professionals/physician_gls/pdf/senior. pdf. Accessed June 20, 2015.

72. Puts M, Hardt J, Monette J, et al. Use of geriatric assessment for older adults in the oncology setting: a systematic review. J Natl Cancer Inst 2012;104:1133–63.

73. Hamaker ME, Schiphorst AH, ten Bokkel Huinink D, et al. The effect of a geriatric evaluation on treatment decisions for older cancer patients—a systematic review. Acta Oncol 2014;53:289–96.

74. Kenis C, Bron D, Libert Y, et al. Relevance of a systematic geriatric screening and assessment in older patients with cancer: results of a prospective multicentric study. Ann Oncol 2013;24:1306–12.

75. Extermann M, Boler I, Reich R, et al. Predicting the risk of chemotherapy toxicity in older patients: the Chemotherapy Risk Assessment Scale for High-Age Patients (CRASH) score. Cancer 2012;118:3377–86.

76. Hurria A, Togawa K, Mohile S, et al. Predicting chemotherapy toxicity in older adults with cancer: a prospective multicenter study. J Clin Oncol 2011;29: 2457–65.

77. Kenig J, Olszewska U, Zychiewicz B, et al. Cumulative deficit model of geriatric assessment to predict the postoperative outcomes of older patient with solid abdominal cancer. J Geriatr Oncol 2015. [Epub ahead of print].

78. Hamaker ME, Vos AG, Smorenburg CH, et al. The value of geriatric assessments in predicting treatment tolerance and all-cause mortality in older patients with cancer. Oncologist 2012;17:1439–49.

79. Kanesvaran R, Li H, Koo KN, et al. Analysis of prognostic factors of comprehensive geriatric assessment and development of a clinical scoring system in elderly Asian patients with cancer. J Clin Oncol 2011;29:3620–7.

80. Klepin HD, Geiger AM, Tooze JA, et al. Geriatric assessment predicts survival for older adults receiving induction chemotherapy for acute myelogenous leukemia. Blood 2013;121:4287–94.

81. Ravdin PM, Siminoff LA, Davis GJ, et al. Computer program to assist in making decisions about adjuvant therapy for women with early breast cancer. J Clin Oncol 2001;19:980–91.

82. de Glas NA, van de Water W, Engelhardt EG, et al. Validity of Adjuvant! Online program in older patients with breast cancer: a population-based study. Lancet Oncol 2014;15:722–9.

83. Repetto L, Fratino L. Geriatric assessment adds information to Eastern Cooperative Oncology Group performance status in elderly cancer patients: an Italian Group for Geriatric Oncology study. J Clin Oncol 2002;20:494–502.

84. Caillet P, Canoui-Poitrine F, Vouriot J, et al. Comprehensive geriatric assessment in the decision-making process in elderly patients with cancer: ELCAPA study. J Clin Oncol 2011;29:3636–42.

85. Pallis AG, Ring A, Fortpied C, et al. EORTC workshop on clinical trial methodology in older individuals with a diagnosis of solid tumors. Ann Oncol 2011;22: 1922–6.

86. Wildiers H, Mauer M, Pallis A, et al. End points and trial design in geriatric oncology research: a joint European organisation for research and treatment of

cancer—Alliance for Clinical Trials in Oncology-International Society of Geriatric Oncology position article. J Clin Oncol 2013;31:3711–8.

87. Hurria A, Dale W, Mooney M, et al. Designing therapeutic clinical trials for older and frail adults with cancer: U13 conference recommendations. J Clin Oncol 2014;32:2587–94.

88. van de Water W, Kiderlen M, Bastiaannet E, et al. External validity of a trial comprised of elderly patients with hormone receptor-positive breast cancer. J Natl Cancer Inst 2014;106:dju051.

89. Kalsi T, Babic-Illman G, Ross PJ, et al. The impact of comprehensive geriatric assessment interventions on tolerance to chemotherapy in older people. Br J Cancer 2015;112:1435–44.

Cancer Screening in Older Adults

Sarah A. Wingfield, MD[a], Mitchell T. Heflin, MD, MHS[b],*

KEYWORDS

- Cancer screening • Shared decision making • Older adults • Guidelines
- Risk versus benefit

KEY POINTS

- Screening is an important tool for reducing cancer-related morbidity and mortality in the elderly.
- Little direct evidence exists to inform decisions regarding cancer screening in older adults.
- The decision to screen for cancer in an elderly patient should take into account the patient's functional status, personal preferences/goals, medical comorbidities, and life expectancy.

INTRODUCTION

Cancer is a devastating disease that exerts a significant impact on the public health of the United States. In 2015, an estimated 1,658,370 new cases of cancer will be diagnosed and approximately 589,430 people will die of the disease.[1] Moreover, cancer disproportionately affects older adults, with a combined median age at diagnosis of 65 years for malignancies of all types. When stratified by age, the greatest percentage of cancer deaths occurs in people aged 75 to 84 years (27.4% of deaths caused by cancer of all sites combined). Although other articles in this issue focus on the evolving options for diagnosing and treating cancer in the elderly, early detection through screening remains a critical tool for reducing cancer-related morbidity and mortality in the elderly.

A brief review of the key characteristics of screening tests is worthwhile. Most fundamentally, the cancer or precancerous lesion that tests are designed to detect should have an asymptomatic preclinical phase in which intervention improves patient

Disclosure: Dr M.T. Heflin writes questions for the American Board of Internal Medicine self-evaluation process modules for geriatrics.
[a] Geriatric Medicine, Duke University Medical Center, Box 3003, Durham, NC 27710, USA;
[b] Department of Medicine, Division of Geriatrics, Center for the Study of Aging and Human Development, Duke University Medical Center, Duke University, Box 3003, Durham, NC 27710, USA
* Corresponding author.
E-mail address: mitchell.heflin@duke.edu

outcomes. Like any diagnostic test, the screening test should be highly sensitive (meaning that it is able to detect the disease when it is present with few false-negatives) and specific (meaning that there are few false-positives). However, unlike other diagnostic tests, screening tests are intended for performance on large numbers of otherwise asymptomatic, average-risk individuals with an ultimate goal of further risk stratification, not final diagnosis. As a result, identifying a small number of cases of cancer in a large population may, by necessity, expose those being screened to large numbers of false-positives. As a result, any screening test should have limited or acceptable side effects and costs.

In addition to considering the factors discussed earlier, specific issues arise in cancer screening in the elderly population. Significant heterogeneity in baseline health and functional status exists among older adults. Life expectancy varies based on level of frailty and number of medical comorbidities. **Fig. 1** shows the upper, middle, and lower quartiles for life expectancy of US men and women based on age.[2] Those in the upper quartile have fewer comorbid illnesses and higher functional status, whereas those in the lowest quartile have multiple medical comorbidities and functional impairment, which limits their life expectancy and makes it more likely that they would be harmed rather than helped by cancer screening. This idea is illustrated by the concept of time lag to benefit.[3] The harms of a particular screening test may be immediate (eg, anxiety caused by a false-positive mammogram), whereas the benefits are not seen until years later. Benefits of screening come from identifying a cancer in an early, asymptomatic stage that can be treated before it causes symptoms and death years in the future. As an illustrative example, it takes an average of 4.8 years before 1 death from colorectal cancer is prevented per 5000 patients screened with fecal occult blood testing (FOBT) and 10.3 years before 1 death from colon cancer is prevented for every 1000 patients screened with FOBT. About 1 in 10 patients screened with FOBT has a false-positive result leading to anxiety and colonoscopy. Day and colleagues[4] estimated that the composite adverse event rate for colonoscopy, including perforation, bleeding, or cardiopulmonary events, is 25.9 per 1000 patients screened after the age of 65 years. Therefore, the benefit of colorectal cancer screening does not outweigh the risk unless the patient has a life expectancy of greater than 10 years.

This article describes the evidence (or lack thereof) for use of common cancer screening tests in older adults, including those for colorectal, prostate, lung, breast, and cervical cancers. Decisions regarding cancer screening in this population are complex and require shared decision making between patients and their health care providers. In short, any decision to screen or not to screen should take into account the individual patient's preferences, medical comorbidities, life expectancy, and functional status.

COLORECTAL CANCER SCREENING

Colon cancer is the third most common cancer in both men and women in the United States and it is the second leading cause of cancer-related death.[5] In 2015, an estimated 132,700 people in the United States will be diagnosed with colorectal cancer and 49,700 will die of the disease.[1] About 4.5% of US men and women are diagnosed with the disease at some point during their lifetimes. As with other cancers that are discussed in this article, localized disease is associated with a higher 5-year relative survival at 90.1% compared with 13.1% for metastatic disease. As such, screening plays an important role in minimizing the morbidity and mortality associated with this malignancy.

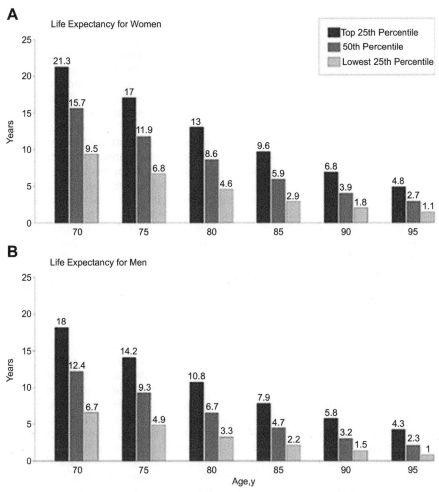

Fig. 1. Upper, middle, and lower quartiles for life expectancy for older women (A) and men (B). For example, 25% of women aged 85 years will live about 10 years, 50% will live 5 years, and 25% will live 3 years. Those in the upper quartile have few comorbid conditions and good functional status, whereas those in the lowest quartile have a high burden of comorbid disease and functional impairment. Those in the lowest quartile are generally not likely to benefit from cancer screening. (*Data from* Walter LC, Lewis CL, Barton MB. Screening for colorectal, breast, and cervical cancer in the elderly: a review of the evidence. Am J Med 2005;118(10):1079.)

There are several modalities used to screen for colorectal cancer. These modalities include FOBT with 3 stool samples, sigmoidoscopy, and colonoscopy. Computed tomography (CT) colonography and stool DNA have been suggested for screening but they are not currently recommended by the US Preventive Services Task Force (USPSTF) because of insufficient evidence of their associated benefits and harms, and therefore they are not discussed further here. FOBT testing can be performed with standard guaiac, sensitive guaiac (Hemoccult SENSA, Beckman Coulter), and immunochemical methods. These different methods are associated with sensitivities of 33% to 50%, 50% to 75%, and 60% to 85% for cancer, respectively.[6] Sigmoidoscopy is associated with a sensitivity of greater than 95% for cancers in the distal colon, whereas colonoscopy is associated with a sensitivity of greater than 95% for cancers throughout the colon.

Incidence of colon cancer and incidence of adenomatous polyps increase with age.[7] In a cross-sectional study by Lin and colleagues,[8] 1244 asymptomatic individuals in 3 age groups (50–54 years, 75–79 years, and ≥80 years) who underwent colonoscopy at a US teaching hospital and clinic were examined to determine the prevalence of colon neoplasia and estimated gain in life expectancy. The prevalence of neoplasia was 13.8% in the 50 to 54 years age group, 26.5% in the 75 to 79 years age group, and 28.6% in those more than the age of 80 years. Despite the increased prevalence of colonic neoplasia in the more elderly patients, mean extension in life expectancy was significantly less in the patients more than the age of 80 years compared with those in the 50 to 54 years age group (0.13 vs 0.85 years). Day and colleagues[7] postulated that this decrease in net benefit observed with age is potentially related to mortality because of competing comorbidities in elderly patients and increased risks associated with screening in this population. One modeling study estimating the risks and benefits of screening colonoscopy in elderly patients found that the number needed to screen to prevent 1 death from colorectal cancer is 227 for male patients aged 80 to 84 years, 140 for female patients aged 80 to 84 years, and 61 to 63 in 50-year-old to 54-year-old controls.[9] For FOBT, the number needed to screen is higher at 945 for male patients aged 80 to 84 years, 581 for female patients aged 80 to 84 years, and 255 to 263 in 50-year-old to 54-year-old controls.

As noted earlier, there are increased risks associated with colonoscopy in elderly patients. In a systematic review by Day and colleagues,[4] which examined data regarding the elderly and colonoscopy complications, a composite adverse event rate (defined as perforation, bleeding, and cardiovascular/pulmonary events) was 25.9 per 1000 colonoscopies for patients more than the age of 65 years and 34.8 per 1000 colonoscopies for patients more than the age of 80 years. Risk of perforation in particular has been found to be associated with age, with individuals more than the age of 65 years having a 30% higher risk of developing perforation compared with younger patients and a 13-fold higher risk compared with age-matched controls who have not had a colonoscopy. Patients more than the age of 80 years are also at greater risk of having an inadequate prep and therefore compromising the ability to complete the procedure successfully in these patients.

The recommendations of the USPSTF are to screen for colorectal cancer using FOBT, sigmoidoscopy, or colonoscopy in adults beginning at age 50 years and continuing to age 75 years (grade A).[10] **Table 1** provides grade definitions. **Table 2** provides USPSTF guidelines for screening by cancer type. The USPSTF recommends against routine screening in patients aged 76 to 85 years (grade C) and recommends against screening in adults more than 85 years old (grade D). In elderly adults, it is important to consider the individual patient's preferences, comorbid conditions, life expectancy, and functional status when considering colorectal cancer screening. The physician should have a discussion with the patient regarding risks and benefits of screening versus not screening and elicit the patient's thoughts and opinions. A study by Lewis and colleagues[11] in which physicians were given 3 clinical vignettes involving 80-year-old patients in good, fair, and poor health examined this issue. The physicians were then surveyed about whether they would initiate a discussion about colorectal cancer screening and whether they would seek patient input for their screening recommendation. Ninety-one percent of the physicians stated that they would discuss colorectal cancer screening with the patient in good health compared with 66% and 44% for the patients in fair and poor health. A greater proportion of

Table 1		
USPSTF grade definitions		
Grade	**Definition**	**Recommendations for Practice**
A	The USPSTF recommends the service. There is high certainty that the net benefit is substantial	Offer or provide this service
B	The USPSTF recommends this service. There is high certainty that the net benefit is moderate or there is moderate certainty that the net benefit is moderate to substantial	Offer or provide this service
C	The USPSTF recommends selectively offering or providing this service to individual patients based on professional judgment and patient preferences. There is at least moderate certainty that the net benefit is small	Offer or provide this service for selected patients depending on individual circumstances
D	The USPSTF recommends against the service. There is moderate or high certainty that the service has no net benefit or that the harms outweigh the benefits	Discourage the use of this service
I	The USPSTF concludes that the current evidence is insufficient to assess the balance of benefits and harms of the service. Evidence is lacking, of poor quality, or conflicting, and the balance of benefits and harms cannot be determined	Read the clinical considerations sections of the USPSTF Recommendation Statement. If the service is offered, patients should understand the uncertainty about the balance of benefits and harms

From Grade Definitions. U.S. Preventive Services Task Force. October 2014. Available at: http://www.uspreventiveservicestaskforce.org/Page/Name/grade-definitions. Accessed September 21, 2015.

physicians would seek patient input for their screening recommendation for the patients in good or fair health compared with the patient in poor health (45% and 49% vs 26% respectively). This finding suggests that physicians are appropriately weighing potential benefits versus harms and considering elderly patients' health status when offering colorectal cancer screening.

LUNG CANCER SCREENING

Lung cancer is the second most frequently diagnosed type of cancer in the United States and the leading cause of cancer death in both men and women.[5] Risk factors for developing lung cancer include increasing age and smoking history. Based on data from 2009 to 2011, 3 to 4 out of 100 US men who are 70 years old will develop lung cancer over the next 10 years.

Despite advances in lung cancer treatment, 5-year relative survival of those diagnosed with lung cancer is a mere 18.4%.[1] Five-year relative survival decreases with age, with a rate of 18.4% in patients between 65 and 74 years old and 12.8% in those 75 years and older compared with a rate of 20.4% in those less than the age of 65 years. The 5-year survival rate is significantly higher at 54.8% for those patients with localized disease at the time of diagnosis compared with a rate of 4.2% in patients with distant metastases. Given the high prevalence of the disease and that advanced disease is more deadly, there has been interest in developing a screening

Table 2
USPSTF guidelines for screening by cancer type

Type of Cancer	Recommendations
Colorectal	• Screen for colorectal cancer using FOBT, sigmoidoscopy, or colonoscopy in adults beginning at age 50 y and continuing until age 75 y (grade A) • Recommend against routine screening for colorectal cancer in adults aged 76–85 y. There may be considerations that support colorectal cancer screening in individual patients (grade C) • Recommend against screening for colorectal cancer in adults more than the age of 85 y (grade D) • Evidence is insufficient to assess the benefits and harms of CT colonography and fecal DNA testing as screening modalities for colorectal cancer (I)
Lung	Recommend annual screening for lung cancer with low-dose LDCT in adults aged 55–80 y who have at least a 30-pack-year smoking history and currently smoke or have quit within the past 15 y. Screening should be discontinued once a person has not smoked for 15 y or develops a health problem that substantially limits life expectancy or willingness to have curative lung surgery (grade B)
Prostate	Recommend against PSA-based screening for prostate cancer (grade D)
Breast	• Recommend biennial screening mammography for women 50–74 y (grade B) • Decision to start regular biennial screening mammography before the age of 50 y should be an individual one and take patient context into account, including patient's values regarding specific benefits and harms (grade C) • Current evidence is insufficient to assess the benefits and harms of screening mammography in women aged 75 y and older (I) • Recommend against teaching BSE (grade D) • Current evidence is insufficient to assess the additional benefits and harms of CBE beyond screening mammography in women aged 40 y or older (I) • Current evidence is insufficient to assess additional benefits and harms of either digital mammography or MRI instead of film mammography as screening modalities for breast cancer (I)
Cervical	• Recommend screening for cervical cancer in women aged 21–65 y with cytology (Pap smear) every 3 y or, for women aged 30–65 y who want to lengthen the screening interval, screening with a combination of cytology and HPV testing every 5 y (grade A) • Recommend against screening for cervical cancer with HPV testing, alone or in combination with cytology, in women younger than 30 y (grade D) • Recommend against screening for cervical cancer in women less than 21 y old (grade D) • Recommend against screening for cervical cancer in women more than 65 y old who have had adequate prior screening and are not otherwise at high risk for cervical cancer (grade D) • Recommend against screening for cervical cancer in women who have had a hysterectomy with removal of the cervix and who do not have a history of a high-grade precancerous lesion (CIN grade 2 or 3) or cervical cancer (grade D)

Abbreviations: BSE, breast self-examination; CBE, clinical breast examination; CIN, cervical intrae-pithelial neoplasia; I, insufficient evidence; LDCT, low-dose CT; HPV, human papillomavirus; PSA, prostate-specific antigen.

test for lung cancer since the 1970s. Several screening tests have been examined, including sputum cytology; chest radiography; and, most recently, low-dose CT (LDCT).

Randomized controlled trials examining sputum cytology and chest radiography for screening found that although these methods do detect more lung cancers at earlier stages, they do not seem to have an impact on the number of advanced cancers detected or lung cancer–related mortality.[11] The Prostate, Lung, Colorectal, and Ovarian (PLCO) randomized trial examined the effect on mortality of screening for lung cancer using chest radiography.[12] The study included 154,901 patients aged 55 to 74 years who were randomized to screening with annual posteroanterior chest radiograph for 4 years or usual care. Patients were followed for 13 years with the primary outcome measure of mortality caused by lung cancer. Over the 13 year follow-up period, there were 1213 lung cancer deaths in the intervention group and 1230 lung cancer deaths in the group that received usual care (mortality relative risk [RR], 0.99; 95% confidence interval [CI], 0.87–1.22). The study concluded that annual chest radiography does not decrease lung cancer–related mortality compared with usual care.

The National Lung Screening Trial (NLST) randomized more than 50,000 patients aged 55 to 74 years with at least 30 pack years of smoking history who were current smokers or who had quit no earlier than 15 years before either screening with 3 rounds of annual LDCT or chest radiography.[13] There was a 20% decrease in lung cancer mortality in the group that received screening with LDCT compared with the group screened with annual chest radiographs (274 vs 309 lung cancer–related deaths per 100,000 patient years of follow-up). This finding corresponds with 310 people who need to be screened to prevent 1 lung cancer–related death.[14] According to a review by Gould,[15] this magnitude of benefit is at least as great as that conferred by annual mammographic screening for women between the ages of 50 and 59 years. Two smaller randomized controlled trials examining the effects of LDCT screening on lung cancer–related mortality failed to show beneficial effects of screening.[15]

Based on the results of the NLST, LDCT has a 93.8% sensitivity for the detection of lung cancer and a specificity of 73.4%. Chest radiograph has a 73.5% sensitivity and a 91.3% specificity. No studies have been performed on the test characteristics of sputum cytology for the detection of lung cancer.

Although data collected in the NLST seem to support using annual LDCT for lung cancer screening, there are several issues to consider in an elderly population. First, the NLST only included patients up to the age of 74 years. The oldest patient screened during the study was 76 years old. Fewer than 10% of the study participants were more than 70 years of age.[13] The study excluded patients with significant comorbid conditions and patients who were unlikely to undergo surgery for early-stage disease. These exclusions make it difficult to generalize the results of the study to a geriatric population.

Pinsky and colleagues[16] performed a secondary analysis of the NLST data examining the findings of the study in Medicare-eligible adults compared with those less than 65 years of age. The false-positive rate was higher in adults more than 65 years of age (27.7% vs 22.0%; P<.001) and older adults were more likely to undergo invasive diagnostic procedures following a false-positive result (3.3% vs 2.7%; P = .039). Prevalence and positive predictive value were higher in the cohort more than 65 years of age (positive predictive value, 4.9% vs 3.0%). Resection rates of cancers detected based on screening were the same in both groups.

A study performed by Varlotto and colleagues[17] examined whether women aged 75 to 84 years who underwent aggressive treatment of early-stage cancer experienced similar survival benefits to their younger counterparts. Survival benefits for those in the 75 to 84 years age group were similar to those in the 55 to 74 years age group, suggesting that the older age group may benefit from lung cancer screening, assuming that they are able to undergo aggressive management of any early-stage cancer that is detected.

Although screening with LDCT has the potential benefit of decreasing lung cancer–related mortality, there are also potential harms that must be kept in mind. In the NLST, about 20% of patients in each annual round of screening had positive test results, whereas only 1% of those screened were found to have lung cancer.[14] Restated, this means that more than 90% of the nodules discovered on screening were benign. Although follow-up imaging studies were most frequently performed for further evaluation of nodules discovered on screening, invasive diagnostic tests were performed in some cases. About 1.2% of patients with benign lesions underwent needle biopsy or bronchoscopy, whereas 0.7% of those ultimately discovered to be free of malignancy underwent thoracoscopy, mediastinoscopy, or thoracotomy. Summarized by Gould,[15] per 1000 patients screened in the NLST, 375 had a false-positive result, 41 had a biopsy performed for a benign nodule, 10 had a surgical procedure for a benign nodule, and about 3 had a complication from an invasive procedure performed for a benign nodule.[15] See **Table 3** for a summary of the benefits and harms of various cancer screening tests. Other potential harms of screening that have not been clearly characterized include the potential for development of radiation-induced cancers (less likely from LDCT directly but potentially from increased radiation exposure caused by follow-up imaging required for incidentally discovered nodules) and the potential for decreased smoking cessation rates if patients are falsely reassured by a negative screening test.

The USPSTF released a recommendation in 2014 supporting annual screening for lung cancer with LDCT for all adults aged 55 to 80 years with at least a 30-pack-year smoking history who are current smokers or who quit within the last 15 years (see **Table 2**).[18] Screening should be discontinued after a person has not smoked for more than 15 years or after they develop a health problem that significantly limits their life expectancy. This recommendation is a B grade recommendation. The American College of Chest Physicians, American Society of Clinical Oncology, and the American Thoracic Society all recommend offering screening to patients who meet NLST eligibility criteria and suggest that screening should be conducted in centers similar to those included in the NLST (grade 2B recommendation). They place an emphasis on the importance of shared decision making. The American Geriatrics Society has not released a recommendation regarding lung cancer screening.

As in all areas of geriatric practice, it is important for the clinician to consider many different factors when deciding whether lung cancer screening with LDCT is appropriate for an individual older adult. Functional status, comorbid conditions, and patient values are all essential pieces of information to take into account. If the patient meets eligibility criteria for the NLST (age 65–74 years, 30-pack-year smoking history, current smoker or quit within the last 15 years) and is willing and able to undergo surgical resection should an early-stage cancer be discovered, screening should be offered along with a frank discussion of potential benefits/harms of screening and gaps in current knowledge related to screening with LDCT. Although there is no current evidence for offering screening outside of this population, it may be reasonable to offer screening to patients more than 75 years of age with high risk of lung cancer if they are able to undergo surgical resection of a cancer discovered through screening and if they have no other significantly life-limiting conditions. Shared decision making between patient and physician should be used to determine whether screening will

Table 3
Screening outcomes per 1000 persons tested

Screening Test	Population	Cancer-specific Deaths Prevented per 1000 Patients Screened	Harms per 1000 Patients Screened
FOBT for colorectal cancer[6]	Men aged 80–84 y	1	—
	Men aged 50–54 y	5	
	Women aged 80–84 y	2	
	Women aged 50–54 y	5	
Colonoscopy for colorectal cancer[6,7]	Men aged 80–84 y	5	25.9 composite adverse event rate (perforation, bleeding, and cardiovascular/pulmonary events) in patients more than 65 y old
	Men aged 50–54 y	15–20	
	Women aged 80–84 y	10–15	34.8 composite adverse event rate (perforation, bleeding, and cardiovascular/pulmonary events) in patients more than 80 y old
	Women aged 50–54 y	15–20	
LDCT for lung cancer[14,15]	Patients aged 55–74 y with at least a 30-pack-year smoking history who quit within the previous 15 y	3–4	375 false-positives 41 biopsies for benign nodules 10 surgical procedures for benign nodules 3 complications from invasive procedures for benign nodules
Mammography for breast cancer[31]	Women more than 75 y old who continue screening for 10 y	1	200 false-positives 15 new diagnoses of DCIS
Prostate cancer with PSA test[20]	Men aged 50–69 y screened for 10 y	0–1	100–120 false-positives 110 new diagnoses of prostate cancer 29 with erectile dysfunction 18 with urinary incontinence

Abbreviations: DCIS, ductal carcinoma in situ; FOBT, fecal occult blood test; LDCT, low dose computed tomography; PSA, prostate specific antigen.
Data from Refs.[6,7,10,12,20,31]

be pursued. Medicare covers annual screening with LDCT for patients aged 55 to 77 years with a 30-pack-year smoking history who are currently smoking or quit within the last 15 years. Note that no screening program for lung cancer supersedes or surpasses the importance of smoking cessation.

PROSTATE CANCER SCREENING

Prostate cancer, like most other malignancies, is a disease of late life. The annual incidence rate of adenocarcinoma of the prostate is 137.9 per 100,000 men in the US population.[1] The median age at diagnosis is 66 years, with nearly 20% of new cases occurring in men more than 75 years of age. Prostate cancer kills men at a rate of 21.4 per 100,000 per year in the United States with most (69.1%) of those aged more than 75 years. However, it is not a so-called equal opportunity disease. Black men have higher rates of prostate cancer and die at a rate twice that of white men. Although it is a disease of aging, its impact on overall morbidity and mortality is variable, partly because older men with prostate cancer are more likely to die of other causes regardless of cancer treatment. In addition, older men may be more prone to have adverse effects from both the search for the cancer and the subsequent treatment if it is found.

Measurement of serum prostate-specific antigen (PSA) level has served as the foundation of screening for prostate cancer since its initial widespread adoption in clinical practice in the early 1990s. Complementary testing with digital rectal examination (DRE) or ultrasonography has been proposed but lacks specific evidence. The PSA test has long been a source of controversy, partly because of the inherent inaccuracy of the test (similar to other screening tests), the long intervals required to discern benefit of treatment, and the short-term harms that can result. The evidence concerning the effectiveness of PSA testing was augmented in 2012 with the publication of 2 long-awaited randomized controlled trials of screening. The PLCO screening trial randomized 76,685 men aged 55 to 74 years to annual testing with PSA for 6 years. After 13 years of follow-up, prostate cancer–specific mortality was nearly equal in the two groups (0.37 vs 0.34 per 1000 person-years in screened vs nonscreened, RR of prostate cancer death = 1.09; CI, 0.87–1.36).[19] The study had significant contamination between the two arms, with nearly 50% of the men randomized to no screening receiving at least 1 PSA test during the trial. The European Randomized Study of Screening for Prostate Cancer randomized 182,160 men aged 55 to 69 years to PSA screening without DRE. Prostate cancer–specific mortality was significantly lower in the screened group (0.39 vs 0.50 per 1000 person-years) after 11 years of follow-up.[20] Contamination in this study was low, with only 20% of the men randomized to no screening having a PSA. However, concerns were raised about equitable treatment in light of lower rates of aggressive forms of treatment in men diagnosed with cancer in the unscreened arm. After much anticipation, the conflicting results of the two trials left older men and their providers without the definitive answer they expected. Despite their shortcomings, the studies did confirm 2 issues useful for those caring for older men: (1) the range of benefit for prostate cancer–specific mortality is somewhere between no benefit and 1 prostate cancer death prevented for 1000 men screened, and (2) a man has to have a life expectancy of at least 10 years (if not more) to garner any possible benefit.

The evidence for benefit must be balanced with an understanding of the potential problems, both immediate and lasting, for older men from PSA screening. The test, like other cancer screening measures, is nonspecific. After 4 annual PSA tests, 12.9% of those tested have a false-positive result (PSA>4 µg/L) and 5.5% have a biopsy with no cancer found.[21] The psychological stress and physical harms associated with the uncertainty of a positive test and biopsy are well documented. Further, most men diagnosed with prostate cancer via screening do not experience a survival benefit. The recent Prostate Cancer Intervention Versus Observation Trial (PIVOT) compared watchful waiting and radical prostatectomy in men with early-stage disease. No difference in prostate cancer mortality was found, although a difference was found in a subgroup analysis of men with a higher PSA levels ($\geq$10 µg/L) at baseline (RR, 0.79; 95% CI, 0.63–0.99), indicating that there may be utility in increasing the cutoff value for screening.[22] Besides the immediate risks of postoperative complications, such as cardiovascular events and venous thromboembolism, substantial numbers of men have longer term complications that may primarily affect function and quality of life, including erectile dysfunction and incontinence (29 and 18 in 1000 respectively).

Guidelines, predictably, differ substantially on their recommendations for prostate cancer screening. The USPSTF in 2012, invoking recent evidence, changed its overall recommendation from C (no evidence to support screening) to D (do not screen using PSA because of evidence to support more harm than benefit), and as a result asserted that screening with PSA should not be offered (see **Table 2**).[23] Other groups, including the American Urological Association and American Society of Clinical Oncology, continue to support offers of screening with PSA with or without DRE beginning at age 50 to 55 years and continuing as long as life expectancy is greater than 10 to 15 years.[24,25] The American College of Physicians (ACP) in 2013 updated its recommendations with more cautionary language about the limited benefit in men aged 50 to 69 years and real and substantial harms in men of all ages.[26] All organizations supporting screening emphasize the importance of shared decision making with prior discussions of the associated risks. Most also identify the substantially higher risk of diagnosis and death in African American men and those with a positive family history and an earlier age at initiation of screening. Although a man more than 75 years of age in vigorously good health and at average risk of prostate cancer might live long enough to garner benefit from screening, most face only the potential harm of either complications and stress from the diagnostic process or, more importantly, the risk of more substantial, life-altering injury from treatment of a cancer that would not otherwise have affected their health and well-being.

BREAST CANCER SCREENING

Breast cancer is the leading cause of cancer and the third leading cause of cancer-related deaths among women in the United States. In 2015, an estimated 231,840 women will be diagnosed with breast cancer and 40,000 women will die of the disease. Older women continue to experience most of the morbidity and mortality from breast cancer. The median age at diagnosis is 61 years and the median age of breast cancer-related death is 68 years, with 58% of all breast cancer deaths occurring in those more than 65 years old.[1]

Breast cancer has a more favorable prognosis with early detection. For localized disease, 5-year survival rates in patients more than 50 years old are 98.6%. With spread to regional lymph nodes at diagnosis, the 5-year survival in this group decreases to 84.9%, and, with distant metastases, to 25.9%.[1] These rates do not seem to change with advancing age, particularly for early-stage disease. Among women with higher levels of comorbidity diagnosed with early-stage cancer, survival seems to be primarily limited by preexisting conditions.[27] In addition, evidence exists that tumors diagnosed in the elderly seem to be more slow growing and therefore more amenable to screening detection and eradication with treatment, particularly hormonal agents.[28,29]

Mammography is the mainstay of breast cancer screening in that it detects smaller, deeper breast masses, and, thereby, allows the discovery of cancer earlier than physical examination alone. Overall, the sensitivity of mammography has been estimated at approximately 75% to 90%, varying with age, breast density, and screening interval. Specificity ranges from 83% to 98.5%.[30] Evidence shows that mammography has improved test performance in older patients, possibly because of a decrease in overall breast density and increased fat content. Clinical breast examination (CBE) may augment screening with mammography. A cohort study of the accuracy of mammography and CBE among postmenopausal women revealed that CBE has a lower false-positive rate, albeit at the expense of a lower sensitivity.[31] Fewer false-positives may mean fewer extended work-ups for women without cancer or with in-situ lesions with a low likelihood of progression. However, no evidence supports the use of CBE alone as an independent screening test.

Results of experimental trials of mammography have been mixed. The Health Insurance Plan of Greater New York study, an early trial, showed a 23% reduction in mortality at 18 years of follow-up. Survival analysis in this trial and others revealed that significant benefits did not appear in the screened group until 5 years or more after initial screening. However, almost all trials excluded older women. Only the Swedish Two County Trial and the Malmö Trial included women more than 65 years of age at the time of randomization. The Two County Trial reported an RR reduction of death from breast cancer of between 25% and 44% for patients aged 50 to 74 years. However, a subgroup analysis of patients aged 70 to 74 years among all the Swedish trials revealed no significant reduction in breast cancer mortality (RR = 0.94; 95% CI, 0.63–1.53) at 12 years of follow-up.[32] This analysis cast further doubt on the extension of the mortality benefit from breast cancer screening in the elderly population. A Cochrane Collaboration review of evidence from prospective trials indicates a discrepancy in findings between high-quality studies focused on breast cancer mortality that show no advantage for screening and other studies more prone to bias that show modest mortality benefit. The review also emphasizes the magnitude of potential overdiagnosis and overtreatment.[33] These assertions continue to fuel debate within the medical community and the lay press about the quality of evidence supporting breast cancer screening with mammography. The fact remains that mammography, although widely accepted, remains largely untested in elderly women.

Given the paucity of evidence examining mammography in older women, researchers have turned to creating models to support decision making. In a recent review, Walter and Schonberg[34] summarized evidence from prior studies, including observational studies and decision models. Overall, these studies support a small sustained benefit of screening mammography in women more than 69 years old as long as their remaining life expectancy is at least 10 years. The investigators estimate that about 50% of 80-year-olds and 25% of 85-year-olds in the United States would satisfy this survival criteria based on current health status (see **Fig. 1**). This finding is consistent with the results of a meta-analysis of screening trials examining time lag to benefit, which found that, after approximately 10 years of biennial screening, 1 additional breast cancer death was prevented among 1000 women screened.[3]

High rates of false positivity also translate into substantial stress and real harm to thousands of women undergoing regular screening. Recall that for each woman diagnosed with breast cancer via screening mammography, approximately 8 to 10 women experience a work-up for a false-positive study. Studies of women undergoing extended evaluations for suspicious lesions reveal significant levels of anxiety that persist even after they have learned that they did not have cancer.[35] In addition, among older women with cognitive or physical disabilities, the test itself can present significant discomfort and distress.

Even among patients diagnosed with breast cancer through mammography, the potential for harm exists. Screening mammograms can detect both invasive disease and ductal carcinoma in situ (DCIS). Approximately 0.1% to 0.5% of older women undergoing mammography have DCIS identified. Although the minority of these cases progress to cancer (7%–25% over 5–10 years), DCIS is usually considered a preinvasive form of malignancy and is treated by surgical resection and, in some cases, with adjuvant hormonal or radiation therapy. Many older women with DCIS would have never discovered their cancer without screening and would likely have lived to die of other causes. For those diagnosed with invasive disease, the possibility of having a clinically insignificant cancer still exists.

Published guidelines reflect a diversity of interpretations of the existing evidence for mammography. The American Cancer Society cautions against setting an upper age limit for screening and recommends that any decision to stop mammography "should be individualized based on the potential benefits and risks of screening in the context of overall health and estimated longevity."[36] In contrast, the USPSTF simply states that there is insufficient evidence to support screening in women more than 75 years of age, mainly because of the lack of trial data.[37] The Canadian Task Force for Preventive Health Care offers a compromise, suggesting a tailored approach in women more than 70 years of age with a life expectancy of at least 5 to 10 years.[38] Most recently, as part of their Choosing Wisely campaign, the American Geriatrics Society and American Board of Internal Medicine included mammography among the tests and treatments that older patients and their providers should question.[39] The investigators agree with the general consensus of continuing to offer biennial screening mammography to women more than 70 years of age if they have sufficient life expectancy. In our estimation, an expected survival of 10 or more years with reasonable quality of life warrants an offer of screening.

CERVICAL CANCER SCREENING

Cervical cancer is a significant cause of morbidity and mortality among women. In 2011, more than 12,000 women were diagnosed with cervical cancer and 4092 women died of the disease.[5] The widespread implementation of screening with the Pap smear has decreased the number of cases diagnosed and the number of deaths from cervical cancer over the last 40 years. Five-year survival is 48.5% for women more than 65 years of age.[1]

There is often confusion among clinicians about when to stop cervical cancer screening in elderly women. Observational studies indicate that women who have never been screened have a higher risk of developing cervical cancer.[40] In a retrospective chart review of all women diagnosed with cervical cancer at Kaiser Permanente Medical Center from 1988 to 1994, older women were less likely than younger women to have been screened within the 3 years before diagnosis and older women were more likely to be found to have an advanced stage at the time of diagnosis. They were also more likely to die of their disease in the 3 years following their diagnosis, likely because of more advanced-stage disease. A study examining the association between midlife screening and late-life incidence of cervical cancer found that women with adequate negative screening (defined as 3 Pap tests between 50–64 years of age with the most recent test being negative and no tests with high-grade squamous epithelial lesions or higher grade cytology) at age 50 to 64 years had one-sixth of the risk of developing cervical cancer at age 65 to 83 years compared with those who were not screened (8 cancers per 10,000 women in the adequate negative screening group vs 49 cancers per 10,000 women in the never-screened group).[41] Regular screening between the ages of 50 and 64 years was associated with a low risk of cervical cancer until age 75 years, and then the benefit of screening waned. By the age of 80 years, the risk of cervical cancer in adequately screened women was only half that of unscreened women.

In a systematic review by Nanda and colleagues,[42] the accuracy of the Papanicolaou test was examined. The ThinPrep Pap smear had a sensitivity of 94.2% and a specificity of 57.7%, and conventionally prepared Pap smears had a sensitivity of 84.6% and a specificity of 37.0%. It is possible that these test characteristics may be altered in elderly women. Sawaya and colleagues[43] found that the positive predictive value of cervical smears in postmenopausal women who had a negative smear within the previous 2 years was very low. The investigators found that 231 additional interventions were performed as a result of a positive smear in order to find 1 potentially significant cervical lesion.

The ACP recommends that physicians stop screening after age 65 years for average-risk women (no history of high-grade, precancerous cervical lesions or cervical cancer; not immunocompromised; and no in utero exposure to diethylstilbestrol), assuming that the patient has had 3 consecutive negative results on cytology or 2 consecutive negative results on cytology plus human papillomavirus testing within the previous 10 years and the most recent test performed within 5 years. The investigators also recommend no further screening after the patient has had a hysterectomy with removal of the cervix.[44] These recommendations are in line with those issued by the USPSTF and the American College of Obstetricians and Gynecologists. These authors agree with these recommendations but add that a clinician should consider screening in women more than 65 years of age if they have never been screened before, because never-screened women are at particularly high risk of cervical cancer, and that a clinician should perform an initial pelvic examination on a patient with a history of hysterectomy to clarify the anatomy if it is not clear whether or not the patient has a cervix.

SUMMARY

There has been increasing awareness that cancer screening tests are procedures that are associated with both benefits and harms. The ACP recently released 2 articles discussing the need for high-value cancer screening.[45,46] They emphasize the importance of viewing a cancer screening as a cascade of events rather than a single test. One positive screening test can have a series of downstream events, each with its own potential for harm. The investigators emphasize that the number of people harmed in some way by screening is always larger than the number of cancer deaths prevented. It is important for patients to be informed of the risks and benefits of cancer screening. Screening for cancer should involve shared decision making and should take into account patient preferences, medical comorbidities, life expectancy, and functional status.

REFERENCES

1. Howlader N, Noone AM, Krapcho M, et al, editors. SEER cancer statistics review, 1975-2012. Bethesda (MD): National Cancer Institute; 2014. based on November 2014 SEER data submission, posted to the SEER Web site, April 2015. Available at: http://seer.cancer.gov/csr/1975_2012/.
2. Walter LC, Lewis CL, Barton MB. Screening for colorectal, breast, and cervical cancer in the elderly: a review of the evidence. Am J Med 2005;118(10):1079.

3. Lee SJ, Boscardin WJ, Stijacic-Cenzer I, et al. Time lag to benefit after screening for breast and colorectal cancer: meta-analysis of survival data from the United States, Sweden, United Kingdom, and Denmark. BMJ 2013;346:e8441.
4. Day LW, Somsouk M, Inadomi JM. Adverse events in older patients undergoing colonoscopy: a meta-analysis [abstract]. Gastroenterology 2010;138(5 Suppl): S-126.
5. US Cancer Statistics Working Group. United States cancer statistics: 1999–2011 incidence and mortality web-based report. Atlanta (GA): Department of Health and Human Services, Centers for Disease Control and Prevention, and National Cancer Institute; 2014.
6. Lieberman DA. Screening for colorectal cancer. N Engl J Med 2009;361:1179–87.
7. Day LW, Walter LC, Velayos F. Colorectal cancer screening and surveillance in the elderly patient. Gastroenterology 2011;106:1197–206.
8. Lin OS, Kozarek RA, Schembre DB, et al. Screening colonoscopy in very elderly patients: prevalence of neoplasia and estimated impact on life expectancy. JAMA 2006;295:2357–65.
9. Ko CW, Sonnenberg A. Comparing risks and benefits of colorectal cancer screening in elderly patients. Gastroenterology 2005;129:1163–70.
10. US Preventative Services Task Force. Screening for colorectal cancer: U.S. Preventative Services Task Force recommendation statement. Ann Intern Med 2008; 149:627–37.
11. Lewis CL, Esserman D, DeLeon C, et al. Physician decision making for colorectal cancer screening in the elderly. J Gen Intern Med 2013;28:1202–7.
12. Oken MM, Hocking WG, Kvale PA. Screening by chest radiograph and lung cancer mortality: the Prostate, Lung, Colorectal and Ovarian (PLCO) randomized trial. JAMA 2011;306:1865–73.
13. The National Lung Screening Trial Research Team. Reduced lung-cancer mortality with low-dose computed tomographic screening. N Engl J Med 2011;36: 395–409.
14. Bach PB, Mirkin JN, Oliver TK, et al. Benefits and harms of CT screening for lung cancer: a systematic review. JAMA 2012;307:2418–29.
15. Gould MK. Lung-cancer screening with low-dose computed tomography. N Engl J Med 2014;371:1813–20.
16. Pinsky PF, Gierada DS, Hocking W, et al. National Lung Screening Trial findings by age: Medicare-eligible versus under-65 population. Ann Intern Med 2014;161: 627–34.
17. Varlotto JM, DeCamp MM, Flickinger JC, et al. Would screening for lung cancer benefit 75- to 84-year-old residents of the United States? Front Oncol 2014;4:1–9.
18. Moyer VA. Screening for lung cancer: U.S. Preventative Services Task Force recommendation statement. Ann Intern Med 2014;160:330–8.
19. Andriole GL, Crawford ED, Grubb RL III, et al, PLCO Project Team. Prostate cancer screening in the randomized Prostate, Lung, Colorectal, and Ovarian cancer screening trial: mortality results after 13 years of follow-up. J Natl Cancer Inst 2012;104(2):125–32.
20. Schröder FH, Hugosson J, Roobol MJ, et al, ERSPC Investigators. Prostate-cancer mortality at 11 years of follow-up. N Engl J Med 2012;366(11):981–90.
21. Hayes JH, Barry MJ. Screening for prostate cancer with the prostate-specific antigen test: a review of current evidence. JAMA 2014;311(11):1143–9.
22. Wilt TJ, Brawer MK, Jones KM, et al, Prostate Cancer Intervention versus Observation Trial (PIVOT) Study Group. Radical prostatectomy versus observation for localized prostate cancer. N Engl J Med 2012;367(3):203–13.

23. Moyer VA, US Preventive Services Task Force. Screening for prostate cancer: US Preventive Services Task Force recommendation statement. Ann Intern Med 2012;157(2):120–34.
24. Carter HB, Albertsen PC, Barry MJ, et al. Early detection of prostate cancer: AUA guideline. J Urol 2013;190(2):419–26.
25. Basch E, Oliver TK, Vickers A, et al. Screening for prostate cancer with prostate-specific antigen testing: American Society of Clinical Oncology provisional clinical opinion. J Clin Oncol 2012;30(24):3020–5.
26. Qaseem A, Barry MJ, Denberg TD, et al. Screening for prostate cancer: a guidance statement from the Clinical Guidelines Committee of the American College of Physicians. Ann Intern Med 2013;158(10):761–9.
27. McPherson CP, Swenson KK, Lee MW. The effects of mammographic detection and comorbidity on the survival of older women with breast cancer. J Am Geriatr Soc 2002;50:1061–8.
28. Balducci L, Extermann M, Carreca I. Management of breast cancer in the older woman. Cancer Control 2001;8:431–41.
29. Clark GM. The biology of breast cancer in older women. J Gerontol 1992;47: 19–23.
30. Kerlikowske K, Grady D, Barclay J, et al. Effect of age, breast density and family history on the sensitivity of first screening mammography. JAMA 1996; 276:33–8.
31. Elmore JG, Barton MB, Moceri VM, et al. Ten-year risk of false positive screening mammograms and clinical breast examinations. N Engl J Med 1998;338: 1089–96.
32. Nystrom L, Rutqvist LE, Wall S, et al. Breast cancer screening with mammography: overview of the Swedish randomised trials. Lancet 1993;341:973–8.
33. Gøtzsche PC, Jørgensen K. Screening for breast cancer with mammography. Cochrane Database Syst Rev 2013;(6):CD001877.
34. Walter LC, Schonberg MA. Screening mammography in older women: a review. JAMA 2014;311(13):1336–47.
35. Lerman C, Trock B, Rimer B, et al. Psychological and behavioral implications of abnormal mammograms. Ann Intern Med 1991;114:657–61.
36. Smith RA, Cokkinides V, Brooks D, et al. Cancer screening in the United States, 2010: a review of current American Cancer Society guidelines and issues in cancer screening. CA Cancer J Clin 2010;60(2):99–119.
37. U.S. Preventative Services Task Force. Screening for breast cancer: U.S. Preventative Services Task Force recommendation statement. Ann Intern Med 2009;151: 716–26.
38. Warner E, Heisey R, Carroll JC. Applying the 2011 Canadian guidelines for breast cancer screening in practice. CMAJ 2012;184(16):1803–7.
39. American Geriatric Society Choosing Wisely Workgroup. New York: AGS Choosing Wisely Workgroup; 2013–2014. Available at: www.americangeriatrics. org/choosingwisely. Accessed July 2, 2015.
40. Sawaya GF, Sung H, Kearney KA, et al. Advancing age and cervical cancer screening and prognosis. J Am Geriatr Soc 2001;49:1499–504.
41. Castanon A, Landy R, Cuzick J, et al. Cervical screening at age 50-64 year and the risk of cervical cancer at age 65 years and older: population based case control study. PLoS Med 2014;11:1–13.
42. Nanda K, McCrory DC, Myers ER, et al. Accuracy of the Papanicolaou test in screening for and follow-up of cervical cytologic abnormalities: a systematic review. Ann Intern Med 2000;132:810–9.

43. Sawaya GF, Grady D, Kerlikowske K, et al. The positive predictive value of cervical smears in previously screened postmenopausal women: the heart and estrogen/progestin replacement study (HERS). Ann Intern Med 2000;133: 942–50.
44. Sawaya GF, Kulasingam S, Denberg T, et al. Cervical cancer screening in average-risk women: best practice advice from the Clinical Guidelines Committee of the American College of Physicians. Ann Intern Med 2015;162(12):851–9.
45. Harris RP, Wilt TJ, Qaseem A. A value framework for cancer screening: advice for high-value care from the American College of Physicians. Ann Intern Med 2015; 162:712–8.
46. Wilt TJ, Harris RP, Qaseem A. Screening for cancer: advice for high-value care from the American College of Physicians. Ann Intern Med 2015;162:718–26.

Socioeconomic Considerations and Shared-Care Models of Cancer Care for Older Adults

 CrossMark

William Dale, MD, PhD[a,b,]*, Selina Chow, MD[a,b], Saleha Sajid, MD[a,b]

KEYWORDS

- Models of care • Geriatrics • Oncology • Geriatric oncology • Aging • Cancer

KEY POINTS

- Older patients are the largest and fastest-growing group of patients with cancer.
- Older adults currently account for the most expensive segment of the population in overall costs of cancer care, which is growing with the advent of costly new therapies.
- Principles of care and assessment tools from geriatrics can be used to assessment life expectancy, identify age-associated deficits, and target therapies to optimize care for older patients with cancer.
- Specific models of care exist to implement a geriatric oncology approach into clinical practice that can optimize and improve quality, reduce costs, and optimize care for older adults with cancer.

GERIATRICS APPROACH TO CANCER CARE CAN IMPROVE THE DELIVERED VALUE

The geriatrics approach to the care of older adults is centered on decision-making for complex patients in the face of uncertainty, based on 2 fundamental principles:

1. Using the highest-quality evidence available appropriately applied to clinical circumstances
2. Incorporating patients' goals to maximize quality of life.

By matching the available evidence to those goals, then communicating clearly with the patient, an informed and shared decision guides all management. These principles must be kept clearly in mind when treating older patients with cancer.

[a] Section of Geriatrics and Palliative Medicine, Department of Medicine, University of Chicago, 5841 South Maryland Avenue, Chicago, IL 60637, USA; [b] Section of Hematology/Oncology, Department of Medicine, University of Chicago, 5841 South Maryland Avenue, Chicago, IL 60637, USA
* Corresponding author. Section of Geriatrics and Palliative Medicine, Department of Medicine, University of Chicago, MC6098, 5841 South Maryland Avenue, Chicago, IL 60643.
E-mail address: wdale@medicine.bsd.uchicago.edu

Clin Geriatr Med 32 (2016) 35–44
http://dx.doi.org/10.1016/j.cger.2015.08.007
0749-0690/16/$ – see front matter © 2016 Elsevier Inc. All rights reserved.

What challenges currently prevent an evidence-based care for older adults with cancer? First, there is a dearth of sufficient high-quality evidence on which to base management decisions. Too often, older patients are excluded from clinical trials. Even when included, those older adults are typically not representative, being sicker and frailer, and therefore not generalizable, to older adults most commonly being treated. Management decisions are typically made in a busy clinical setting with little time to weigh treatment alternatives, making subtle decisions even more difficult.

Although better evidence is awaited, a practical approach to cancer care for older adults with cancer is necessary. Such an approach will bring the "art" of geriatrics to the oncology clinic, providing an approach for providers to use based on current evidence. Broadly speaking, there are 2 common errors made in treating older patients: undertreatment and overtreatment. Undertreatment results from ageism— making management choices based on chronologic age rather than physiologic age. Medical decisions for fit older adults should be indistinguishable from any other patient with cancer—they should be treated with the most appropriate treatment compatible with their care goals. Conversely, overtreatment results from inappropriately aggressive cancer-directed therapy while ignoring patient vulnerability, remaining life expectancy (RLE), and treatment toxicities. Treating older adults with cancer requires navigating between undertreatment due to ageism—denying life-enhancing treatment to fit older patients with cancer—and overtreatment—giving toxic therapy to vulnerable older patients and lowering the quality of their survival. Delivering high-value care requires avoiding both errors.

With this is mind, the authors recommend the following a 3-step approach to deliver such high-value care and guide care models. First, a clinician should use geriatric assessment (GA) to estimate remaining life-expectancy for an older adult with cancer. Estimating remaining life-expectancy is done through the application of the validated tools from GA to older patients, allowing the assignment of patients into 3 categories: fit, vulnerable, or frail. This categorization avoids undertreating the fit elderly, avoids overtreating the frail elderly, and targets further assessment for the vulnerable. Second, it is important to both stage the cancer and "stage the aging" to predict the likelihood of complication and toxicities from possible treatment. Finally, one must match the available care options with the preferences and goals of patients, communicating carefully to reach an informed, shared decision. In taking such an approach, one can be sail safely through the troubled waters of caring for older adults with cancer.

SOCIOECONOMIC CONSIDERATIONS OF PROVIDING HIGH-VALUE CANCER CARE

It has long been recognized that age is associated with increased costs of care. According to the 1992 to 1998 Medicare Current Beneficiary survey data, older adults in better health had a longer RLE than those in poorer health, but had similar cumulative health care expenditures until death.[1] A person with no functional limitations at 70 had an RLE of 14.3 years and expected cumulative health care expenditures of $136,000, whereas a person with a limitation in at least one activity of daily living had a life expectancy of 11.6 years and expected cumulative expenditures of $145,000. Expenditures varied little according to self-reported health at the age of 70. Persons who were institutionalized at the age of 70 had cumulative expenditures that were much higher than those for persons who were not institutionalized. Age is clearly an important contributor to the costs of care.

Medicare's expenditures on cancer care are substantial and vary by phase of care, tumor site, stage at diagnosis, and survival. A SEER (Surveillance, Epidemiology, and End Results) database review (2008) found the mean net costs of cancer care were highest in the initial and last year-of-life phases of care and lowest in the continuing phase.[2,3] Mean 5-year net costs varied significantly by tumor type, from less than $20,000 for patients with breast cancer or melanoma to more than $40,000 for patients with cancers of the brain, esophageal, gastric, ovarian cancers, or lymphoma. In patients with acute myeloid leukemia, 80% of costs are related to inpatient hospitalization. In 2004, the 5-year net costs of cancer care to Medicare for older patients were approximately $21.1 billion. In short, cancer costs have long been substantial.

With the creation of several new agents in the last decade, the per month costs of anticancer agents has more than doubled, from $4500 to more than $10,000. Of the 12 anticancer drugs approved by the US Food and Drug Administration in 2012, only 3 prolonged survival (2 of them by <2 months): 9 were priced at more than $10,000 per month.[4] Many so-called targeted agents have been priced between $6000 to 12,000 per month or approximately $70,000 to 115,000 per patient annually.[5] The high cost may prevent many older patients from being able to obtain such medications, leading to nonadherence. This nonadherence, in turn, results in costs exceeding $100 billion annually, due to increased health services utilization, higher hospital admission rates, and adverse drug events associated with nonadherence.[6] The economic impact of cancer survivorship is considerable, remains high years after a cancer diagnosis, and is approximately the same in younger and older cancer survivors.

Given the high and rising costs of cancer care for older adults, combined with the rapidly rising numbers of older adults with cancer as the baby boomers age, it is more important than ever to use resources wisely and is best accomplished through a geriatrics approach to cancer for older patients. Creating care models based on a geriatrics approach and using geriatrics tools are the most economical way to deliver such care.

GERIATRIC ASSESSMENT AND TARGETED INTERVENTIONS ACROSS THE CANCER CARE CONTINUUM

Coordination and collaboration across the cancer care continuum are emerging ideals. A geriatric oncology model of care consists of constructing a multilevel clinical and organizational system that:

1. Provides cancer-specific, fitness-appropriate, and individualized geriatric care;
2. Provides strong integration between medical care, supportive care, and social services;
3. Can design and implement age-appropriate health care policies and practices.

Older patients with cancer are a heterogeneous group with a high prevalence of comorbid conditions and vulnerabilities to cancer treatment.[7] Identifying first those at highest risk of chemotherapy or surgical morbidity during subsequent therapy may improve treatment and prognosis in these patients and generally requires a 3-step approach. First, they should be assessed using validated tools such as the comprehensive geriatric assessment (CGA) before treatment.[8] Second, the risk of therapy-related toxicity during treatment should be completed using validated tools such as Cancer and Aging Research Group and the Chemotherapy Risk-Assessment Scale for High-Age Patients.[9,10] Third, those at highest risk for toxicity should receive appropriate interventions to mitigate against these risks.

CGA helps determine a patient's level of frailty, thereby guiding treatment choices.[11] However, institutions often have organizational constraints limiting providers' ability to administer CGA.[12] For this reason, attention to using prescreening tests such as the Vulnerable Elders Survey-13.[13–17] Using screening tools decreases resources needed for assessments of older adults. The CGA is best administered at times of clinical decision-making to identify vulnerable patients such as during initial treatment consultations or during changes in clinical condition, including new or worsening pain, fatigue, hospitalizations, or disease progression requiring a change in therapy.[9] The impact of CGA for informing treatment decisions was of greatest value when unidentified medical problems were found, which occurred in 70% of patients.[18] Screening during the course of chemotherapy found that the CGA directly influenced oncologic treatment in 40% of patients; it ensured continuity/coordination of care in 70%, and the success rate in addressing problems was 87%, in which Functional Assessment of Cancer Treatment–Breast scores improved and function and independence were maintained during therapy.[19,20] Sequential CGA assessment is appropriate as patients progress through the continuum of cancer experience. Consideration must be given to the phase of disease where disability or death from the cancer will outpace treatment-related toxicities. Several studies have showed that frail patients identified using CGA had poorer outcomes compared with fit patients, and specifically shortened overall survival.[21,22] CGA can help to frame discussions with patients and families, during the course of cancer therapy, allowing for realistic expectations from offered treatments. Studies have shown that the use of chemotherapy in frail patients is associated with increased risk of cardiopulmonary resuscitation, mechanical ventilation, or both, and dying in an intensive care unit.[23–30] Thus, treatment-related decisions, before, during, and after chemotherapy, are complex and should be individualized.

Geriatric assessments can predict treatment-related toxicities and adverse geriatrics outcomes, which are independent from oncologic, tumor-based predictors. Appropriate geriatrics parameters to predict adverse outcomes to guide treatment modifications have not yet been established for different cancer types or treatments.[31] Nevertheless, results from this assessment can be effectively used to guide various treatment options across tumor types (**Fig. 1**).

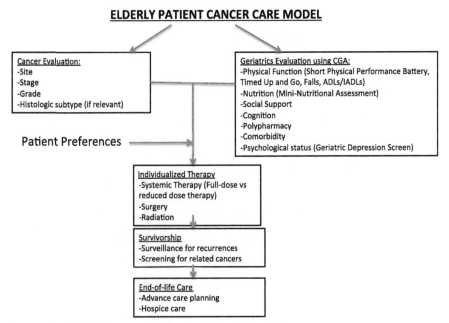

Fig. 1. Individualized treatment plan in older adults with cancer.

The International Society of Geriatric Oncology has created a task force to address tumor-specific therapies in the elderly, including for screening, surgery, radiation, (neo)adjuvant therapies, chemotherapies, and metastatic diseases on several tumor types in the elderly.[32–34] The CGA can help identify deficits within geriatrics domains to guide targeted interventions. The CGA has been used in patient selection for multi-modality treatment in cancers, such as head and neck, breast, and colorectal cancers, which has improved geriatrics outcomes.[35,36] In patients with head and neck cancer where prevalence of malnutrition is high, the CGA identifies nutritional deficiencies early and allows timely interventions, thus improving quality of life.[37] In leukemia patients undergoing bone marrow transplant, the CGA identifies fit older patients who have an overall survival benefit from reduced-intensity conditioning hematopoietic stem cell transplantation.[38] Regardless of the tumor type, the approach remains the same: use the CGA to predict competing causes of morbidity and mortality before cancer therapy (surgery, radiation, chemotherapy, or multimodality therapy), use it as a tool to define patient fitness, use it to longitudinally assess patient frailty during therapy, and potentially to decide when to discontinue therapy (see **Fig. 1**).

ORGANIZATIONAL MODELS OF CANCER CARE

Geriatric oncology has evolved over the past 2 decades, combining these 2 disciplines to develop the optimal approach to care for older patients with cancer. Bringing the principles of care from geriatrics, applying them to older adults with cancer, and coordinating that care to deliver high-value, cost-effective care is more important than ever. Cancer centers in the United States have taken several approaches to develop different models of geriatric oncology care that may be specific to their treatment populations, to availability of specialty-trained providers, and that operates within their local institutional infrastructure and constraints. Although there is not a universal model of geriatric oncology care, the rationale for developing a geriatric oncology clinic includes[39]:

- Identifying patients potentially at risk for cancer treatment toxicity;
- Reducing the time required by the medical oncologist to manage the complexity of older patients;
- Crafting treatment plans after CGA or by managing the nononcologic issues of older patients with cancer in separate clinics;
- Providing patient-centered care with an assessment that takes into account a patient's values and social support network;
- Being a research hub to further the understanding of treating older patients with cancer;
- Providing fellow, resident, and medical student education in geriatric oncology.

The first geriatric oncology clinic that opened in the United States was at the H. Lee Moffitt Comprehensive Cancer Center in Tampa, Florida in 1993 under the leadership of Lodovico Balducci, MD. Since then, a small number of such clinics have evolved. Over these past 2 decades, 4 distinct geriatric oncology clinical models have been described:

1. Screen-and-referral model
2. Primary-provider model
3. Multidisciplinary consultative model
4. Embedded, geriatrics-driven, comprehensive care model.

Of course, some of these models can overlap, and blended care models are possible. However, for reasons of conceptual clarity, each is considered separately in later discussion.

Primary Provider Model

This care model incorporates a formally trained geriatric oncologist, geriatrician, and palliative medicine provider as the primary medical care provider for older patients with cancer. In cancer centers such as H. Lee Moffitt Comprehensive Cancer Center, John Theurer Cancer Center at Hackensack University Medical Center in New Jersey, UNC Lineberger Comprehensive Cancer Center, and the Specialized Oncology Care and Research in the Elderly (SOCARE) clinic at the University of Chicago and University of Rochester, these programs have the ability to perform the initial comprehensive assessment, devise the overall treatment plan, and manage a patient's care from the time of diagnosis to the end of life.[40–42] The advantages of this primary provider model include care continuity for this vulnerable patient population, a medical home for patients with complex care needs, and a concentration of resources on the most vulnerable patients with cancer. The disadvantages to this care model are the limits of expertise due to the small number of dually trained geriatric oncologists that could carry out this role, the limits on numbers of patients as panel sizes grow, and the need for specialized resources (eg, space, equipment, time, training) to be invested. Such care models are difficult to develop outside of large organizations with the ability to invest in these resources; however, they typically deliver the highest value care for frail older adults with cancer.

Multidisciplinary Consultative Model

In this care model, used by centers such as the SOCARE Clinics at the University of Rochester and University of Chicago, Thomas Jefferson University, and the Cleveland Clinic, the use of a cancer-specific GA is the basis for these clinics with self-reported assessments and in-clinic evaluations.[39,43,44] These consultative clinics typically evaluate older, frailer patients with cancer with solid tumor malignancies, typically at the request of other oncologists. At the University of Chicago, with the Transplant in Older Patients program, and the Dana-Farber/Brigham and Women's Cancer Center with their Older Adult Hematology Malignancy Program, some centers have developed disease-specific multidisciplinary consultative clinics for older patients with leukemia and related blood disorders.[45,46] As described above, GA is used to develop appropriate treatment plans adapted for older adults with cancer.[13,47] Typically, GA is performed in the outpatient setting by a multidisciplinary team led by a geriatrician or geriatric oncologist. Other key members of this multidisciplinary team may include advanced practice nurses or physician assistants, pharmacists, social workers, nutritionists, physical therapists, occupational therapists, and patient navigators. The availability of these providers varies depending on local resources, but the goal is to provide a comprehensive evaluation that leads to a personalized treatment plan for patients and their treating oncologists. A significant advantage of this care model is that a larger number of patients can be evaluated, receive advice, and derive benefit to their cancer care while maintaining continuity with their primary oncologist. However, the ability to provide continued guidance from experts in the care of aging patients during a patient's treatment course is more limited with this clinical model.

Geriatrics-Driven and Embedded Consultative Model

At centers such as Memorial Sloan-Kettering Cancer Center, MD Anderson Cancer Center, and the University of California, Los Angeles, geriatricians have been either embedded within the oncology clinics or perform the GA assessments within their own, separate location.[48,49] This model has emerged within larger cancer centers, but where geriatrics' expertise has a notable, but geographically separate existence. This care model is similar to the multidisciplinary consultative model, in which geriatrics expertise is infused into an on-going oncology care plan. This model works best where geriatrics has a strong institutional presence, but where dually trained geriatric oncologists are not readily available to provide comprehensive assessments and the ability to assume care for patients. In some institutions, a geriatrician-led team may be available to assist with non-oncologic-related issues as they arise during a patient's treatment course. This care model is a partnership, with the infusion of aging expertise into ongoing cancer care.

Screen and Refer Clinic Model

This care model typically takes place at a university setting, with assessments that can take several hours to complete, and is resource-intensive due to coordination of a multidisciplinary team of health care providers. With most cancer care taking place in a community practice setting, geriatric oncology providers have developed ways to conduct GA evaluations that could be feasible in the busy community clinical practices. In a study conducted by Williams and colleagues[50] from the UNC Lineberger Comprehensive Cancer Center, a validated GA tool consisting of a self-reported questionnaire with a brief in-clinic assessment by a health professional is used to determine the feasibility of performing this assessment in a community setting. The median time to completing the entire assessment was comparable to the academic setting (30 minutes vs 22 minutes, respectively) with a modest commitment of professional time. The authors are now examining the feasibility of providing timely GA-based recommendations for referrals and services similar to that practiced at the academic institution level. In a study performed at the Joan Karnell Cancer Center at Pennsylvania Hospital, a community affiliate of the University of Pennsylvania Health System, a brief screening tool was administered by the geriatric social worker evaluating for nursing, social work, psychological, nutrition, prescription, and caregiver needs.[51] If older patients were identified as having needs beyond that which could be provided through social work intervention, referrals were made to appropriate clinicians and outside community resources. In both of these cases, it was shown that significant elements of GA can be implemented in busy community settings with relatively limited resources. Whether this care model will prove cost-effective is not known.

REFERENCES

1. Lubitz J, Cai L, Kramarow E, et al. Health, life expectancy, and health care spending among the elderly. N Engl J Med 2003;349(11):1048–55.
2. Yabroff KR, Lamont EB, Mariotto A, et al. Cost of care for elderly cancer patients in the United States. J Natl Cancer Inst 2008;100(9):630–41.
3. Kantarjian HM, Fojo T, Mathisen M, et al. Cancer drugs in the United States: Justum Pretium–the just price. J Clin Oncol 2013;31(28):3600–4.
4. Dusetzina SB, Winn AN, Abel GA, et al. Cost sharing and adherence to tyrosine kinase inhibitors for patients with chronic myeloid leukemia. J Clin Oncol 2014; 32(4):306–11.
5. IMS Institute for Healthcare Informatics Avoidable costs in U.S. healthcare: The $200 billion opportunity from using medicines more responsibly. Available at: http://www.imshealth.com/deployedfiles/imshealth/Global/Content/Corporate/IMS%20Institute/RUOM-2013/IHII_Responsible_Use_Medicines_2013.pdf. Accessed August 15, 2015.

6. Guy GP Jr, Ekwueme DU, Yabroff KR, et al. Economic burden of cancer survivorship among adults in the United States. J Clin Oncol 2013;31(30):3749–57.

7. Stafford RS, Cyr PL. The impact of cancer on the physical function of the elderly and their utilization of health care. Cancer 1997;80:1973–80.

8. Rubenstein LZ, Wieland D. Comprehensive geriatric assessment. Annu Rev Gerontol Geriatr 1989;9:145–92.

9. Hurria A, Togawa K, Mohile SG, et al. Predicting chemotherapy toxicity in older adults with cancer: a prospective multicenter study. J Clin Oncol 2011;29(25): 3457–65.

10. Extermann M, Boler I, Reich RR, et al. Predicting the risk of chemotherapy toxicity in older patients: the Chemotherapy Risk Assessment Scale for High-Age Patients (CRASH) score. Cancer 2012;118(13):3377–86.

11. Hurria A, Gupta S, Zauderer M, et al. Developing a cancer-specific geriatric assessment. Cancer 2005;104(9):1998–2005.

12. McCarthy AL, Cook PS, Yates P. Engineering the fitness of older patients for chemotherapy: an exploration of Comprehensive Geriatric Assessment in practice. Health (London) 2014;18(2):196–212.

13. Ingram SS, Seo PH, Martell RE, et al. Comprehensive assessment of the elderly cancer patient: the feasibility of self-report methodology. J Clin Oncol 2002;20(3): 770–5.

14. Saliba D, Elliott M, Rubenstein LZ, et al. The Vulnerable Elders Survey: a tool for identifying vulnerable older people in the community. J Am Geriatr Soc 2001; 49(12):1691–9.

15. Mohile SG, Bylow K, Dale W, et al. A pilot study of the Vulnerable Elders Survey-13 compared with the comprehensive geriatric assessment for identifying disability in older patients with prostate cancer who receive androgen ablation. Cancer 2007;109(4):802–10.

16. Kim J, Hurria A. Determining chemotherapy tolerance in older patients with cancer. J Natl Compr Canc Netw 2013;11(12):1494–502.

17. Luciani A, Ascione G, Bertuzzi C, et al. Detecting disabilities in older patients with cancer: comparison between comprehensive geriatric assessment and vulnerable elders survey-13. J Clin Oncol 2010;28(12):2046–50.

18. Horgan AM, Leighl NB, Coate L, et al. Impact and feasibility of a comprehensive geriatric assessment in the oncology setting: a pilot study. Am J Clin Oncol 2012; 35(4):322–8.

19. Extermann M, Meyer J, McGinnis M, et al. A comprehensive geriatric intervention detects multiple problems in older breast cancer patients. Crit Rev Oncol Hematol 2004;49(1):69–75.

20. Extermann M, Bonetti M, Sledge GW, et al. MAX2—a convenient index to estimate the average per patient risk for chemotherapy toxicity: validation in ECOG trials. Eur J Cancer 2004;40(8):1193–8.

21. Merli F, Luminari S, Rossi G, et al. Outcome of frail elderly patients with diffuse large B-cell lymphoma prospectively identified by Comprehensive Geriatric Assessment: results from a study of the Fondazione Italiana Linfomi. Leuk Lymphoma 2014;55(1):38–43.

22. Aaldriks AA, Maartense E, le Cessie S, et al. Predictive value of geriatric assessment for patients older than 70 years, treated with chemotherapy. Crit Rev Oncol Hematol 2011;79(2):205–12.

23. Wright AA, Zhang B, Keating NL, et al. Associations between palliative chemotherapy and adult cancer patients' end of life care and place of death: prospective cohort study. BMJ 2014;348:g1219.

24. Goldstein NE, Morrison RS. The intersection between geriatrics and palliative care: a call for a new research agenda. J Am Geriatr Soc 2005;53(9): 1593–8.
25. AGS Panel on Persistent Pain in Older Persons. The management of persistent pain in older adults. J Am Geriatr Soc 2002;50(6 Suppl):S205–24.
26. Coleman EA, Boult C. Improving the quality of transitional care for persons with complex care needs. J Am Geriatr Soc 2003;51(4):556–7.
27. Schulz R, Beach SR. Caregiving as a risk factor for mortality: the Caregiver Health Effects Study. JAMA 1999;282(23):2215–9.
28. Waltson J, Fried L. Frailty and its implications for care. In: Meier DE, Morrison RS, editors. Geriatric palliative care. New York: Oxford University Press; 2003. p. 93–109.
29. Penrod JD, Morrison RS. Challenges for palliative care research. J Palliat Med 2004;7(3):398–402.
30. Casarett DJ. The future of the palliative medicine fellowship. J Palliat Med 2000; 3(2):151–5.
31. Wildiers H, Heeren P, Puts M, et al. International Society of Geriatric Oncology consensus on geriatric assessment in older patients with cancer. J Clin Oncol 2014;32(24):2595–603.
32. Wildiers H, Kunkler I, Biganzoli L, et al. Management of breast cancer in elderly individuals: recommendations of the International Society of Geriatric Oncology. Lancet Oncol 2007;8(12):1101–15.
33. Pallis AG, Gridelli C, van Meerbeeck JP, et al. EORTC Elderly Task Force and Lung Cancer Group and International Society for Geriatric Oncology (SIOG) experts' opinion for the treatment of non-small-cell lung cancer in an elderly population. Ann Oncol 2010;21(4):692–706.
34. Droz JP, Balducci L, Bolla M, et al. Management of prostate cancer in older men: recommendations of a working group of the International Society of Geriatric Oncology. BJU Int 2010;106(4):462–9.
35. Bernardi D, Barzan L, Franchin G, et al. Treatment of head and neck cancer in elderly patients: state of the art and guidelines. Crit Rev Oncol Hematol 2005; 53(1):71–80.
36. Kristjansson SR, Nesbakken A, Jordhøy MS, et al. Comprehensive geriatric assessment can predict complications in elderly patients after elective surgery for colorectal cancer: a prospective observational cohort study. Crit Rev Oncol Hematol 2010;76(3):208–17.
37. Ortholan C, Benezery K, Dassonville O, et al. A specific approach for elderly patients with head and neck cancer. Anticancer Drugs 2011;22(7):647–55.
38. Koreth J, Pidala J, Perez WS, et al. Role of reduced-intensity conditioning allogeneic hematopoietic stem-cell transplantation in older patients with de novo myelodysplastic syndromes: an international collaborative decision analysis. J Clin Oncol 2013;31(21):2662–70.
39. Magnuson A, Dale W, Mohile S, et al. Models of care in geriatric oncology. Curr Geriatr Rep 2014;3(3):182–9.
40. McNeil C. Geriatric oncology clinics on the rise. J Natl Cancer Inst 2013;105(9): 585–6.
41. Geriatric Oncology Program. UNC Linberger Comprehensive Cancer Center. Available at: https://unclineberger.org/patientcare/programs/geriatric. Accessed August 15, 2015.
42. Geriatric Oncology. SOCARE Clinic. Available at: http://www.uchospitals.edu/specialties/cancer/geriatric-oncology/. Accessed August 15, 2015.

43. Chapman AE, Swartz K, Schoppe J, et al. Development of a comprehensive multidisciplinary geriatric oncology center, the Thomas Jefferson University Experience. J Gen Orthod 2014;5:164–70.
44. Taussig Oncology Program for Seniors (TOPS). Cleveland Clinic. Available at: http://my.clevelandclinic.org/services/cancer/treatments-procedures/taussig-oncology-program-for-seniors. Accessed August 15, 2015.
45. Blood and Bone Marrow Stem Cell Transplantation for Older Adults. Older Adults: Blood and Bone Marrow Stem Cell Transplantation. Available at: http://www.uchospitals.edu/specialties/cancer/stem-cell-transplant/older-adults.html. Accessed August 15, 2015.
46. Older Adult Hematologic Malignancy (OHM) Program - Dana-Farber Cancer Institute | Boston, MA. Older Adult Hematologic Malignancy (OHM) Program - Dana-Farber Cancer Institute|Boston, MA. Available at: http://www.dana-farber.org/Adult-Care/Treatment-and-Support/Treatment-Centers-and-Clinical-Services/Hematologic-Oncology-Treatment-Center/Older-Adult-Hematologic-Malignancy-(OHM)-Program.aspx. Accessed August 15, 2015.
47. Hurria A, Wildes T, Blair SL, et al. Senior adult oncology, version 2.2014: clinical practice guidelines in oncology. J Natl Compr Canc Netw 2014;12(1):82–126.
48. Help for Older Patients. Counseling & Support. Available at: https://www.mskcc.org/cancer-care/treatments/symptom-management/help-older-patients. Accessed August 15, 2015.
49. Geriatric Oncology | David Geffen School of Medicine at UCLA. Geriatric Oncology David Geffen School of Medicine at UCLA. Available at: http://people.healthsciences.ucla.edu/education/institution/groups-detail?group_id=13268. Accessed August 15, 2015.
50. Williams GR, Deal AM, Jolly TA, et al. Feasibility of geriatric assessment in community oncology clinics. J Gen Orthod 2014;5:245–51.
51. Lynch MP, Marcone D, Kagan SH, et al. Developing a multidisciplinary geriatric oncology program in a community cancer center. Clin J Oncol Nurs 2007;11(6):929–33.

Palliative Care and Symptom Management in Older Patients with Cancer

Koshy Alexander, MD[a,b,*], Jessica Goldberg, MSN, AGPCNP-BC[c],
Beatriz Korc-Grodzicki, MD, PhD[a,b]

KEYWORDS

- Geriatrics • Cancer • Symptom management • Palliative care

KEY POINTS

- Palliative care (PC) should be part of the care of older patients with cancer throughout the trajectory of the disease.
- Its focus on symptom management and maximization of function is essential in maintaining quality of life.
- Pain, a frequent symptom in all patients with cancer, presents specific barriers for evaluation and treatment in older patients with cancer.
- Nonpain symptoms are multiple, frequent, and debilitating. They need to be addressed comprehensively.
- Nonpharmacologic interventions should be considered first in the treatment of older adults in order to minimize drug-drug interactions and serious side effects.
- Timely referral to PC could decrease patient and caregiver distress.

PALLIATIVE CARE IN GERIATRIC ONCOLOGY

Medical care for older patients with cancer is complicated by many factors, including the heterogeneity of their health status, polypharmacy, frailty, dementia, delirium, and functional impairment. They are best served by a multidisciplinary approach with palliative care (PC) playing an integral role, primarily focusing on symptom control and quality of life. Older patients with cancer benefit from a palliative approach that prioritizes the patient's individual goals, and strives to maintain the patient's independence

Disclosure: The authors have nothing to disclose.
[a] Geriatrics, Memorial Sloan Kettering Cancer Center, 1275 York Avenue, Box 205, New York, NY 10065, USA; [b] Department of Medicine, Weill Cornell Medical College, 425 East 61st Street, New York, NY 10065, USA; [c] Palliative Medicine, Memorial Sloan Kettering Cancer Center, 1275 York Avenue, New York, NY 10065, USA
* Corresponding author. Memorial Sloan Kettering Cancer Center, 1275 York Avenue, Box 205, New York, NY 10065.
E-mail address: alexandk@mskcc.org

Clin Geriatr Med 32 (2016) 45–62
http://dx.doi.org/10.1016/j.cger.2015.08.004
0749-0690/16/$ – see front matter © 2016 Elsevier Inc. All rights reserved.

and physical, emotional, and spiritual health. For most older patients living with cancer, both life-prolonging and palliative treatments can be necessary and appropriate. PC should not be associated only with terminal care, and should be part of older patients' cancer care throughout the trajectory of their disease with various levels of involvement as the disease progresses. In some cases, introduction of PC may have an even greater impact at earlier time points when the focus is on cure. Closer to, during, and after death, attention to the caregivers may increase in importance. National organizations' guidelines recommend that PC be routinely integrated into comprehensive cancer care.[1,2]

SYMPTOM MANAGEMENT

Symptom management, whether related to the disease or to the treatment, influences the quality of life of patients with cancer. For older adults, serious illness is frequently characterized by a high prevalence of untreated symptoms that result in progressive functional dependence. The focus on symptom management and maximization of function provide the patients and their caregivers with relief from one of the largest sources of stress. Advanced age is also associated with physiologic changes that affect the pharmacokinetics and pharmacodynamics of medications, further complicating the treatment of cancer-related symptoms. Age-related physiologic changes must be considered when making treatment decisions in older adults.[3] In addition, cognitive impairment, functional difficulties, and caregiver issues play a role in errors and compliance. To prescribe appropriately for symptom management, clinicians must consider not only the pharmacologic properties of the drugs but also clinical, epidemiologic, social, cultural, and economic factors.[3]

ASSESSMENT AND MANAGEMENT OF PAIN

Pain is difficult to evaluate and manage. Many barriers exist to the optimal evaluation and adequate treatment of pain in older patients with cancer. These barriers include cognitive and functional impairments, underreporting, bias in prescribing, comorbid conditions, and polypharmacy, as well as drug administration in institutional living settings.[4] The consequences of poorly managed pain extend to behavioral domains (ie, depression, anxiety, and substance abuse), cardiovascular domains (ie, hypertension, increased incidence of deep vein thrombosis caused by impaired mobility), delirium, insomnia, functional impairment, and increased health care use.

Pain is one of the most common symptoms experienced by patients with cancer. Up to two-thirds of all older patients develop pain as a result of the cancer or as a consequence of its treatment.[5] Treatment-related pain, such as chemotherapy-induced peripheral neuropathy, is most likely to affect the elderly. Pain may also be caused by non–cancer-related painful comorbidities, which are more frequent in the elderly patients, such as degenerative disk disease or osteoporosis-related fractures. The assessment of pain in patients with cancer should involve a comprehensive evaluation with a thorough physical examination and pain review (**Box 1**). In addition, clinicians need to be familiar with common cancer pain syndromes (eg, plexopathies, peripheral neuropathy) in order to identify the correct cause.[6]

There are several assessment tools for the evaluation of pain in the elderly (**Box 2**). Pain scales should be used even if the patient has mild or moderate cognitive impairment. As dementia progresses, the ability to self-report pain decreases. For these patients clinicians should anticipate the kinds of conditions that may cause pain and patient behaviors that may indicate pain (eg, agitation, restlessness, irritability, facial expressions, labored breathing, or withdrawal), and possibly use surrogate reports

---

Box 1
Assessment of pain

1. Questions about the onset, location, duration, quality, and any aggravating and alleviating factors of the pain.
2. Questions to determine the tolerable level of pain.
3. Questions about prior experiences with pain medications, their side effects, and barriers to use.
4. Assessment for medical comorbidities that may affect the perception and experience of pain.
5. Assessment of the patient's cognitive status and functional ability.

---

of pain from caregivers and nurses. If a patient shows behaviors that could be caused by pain, it should be assumed that the patient is experiencing pain and a trial of analgesics is appropriate. A decrease in those behaviors can be considered a positive response to the analgesics.

Management of Pain

The standard pain management algorithm is based on the World Health Organization (WHO) analgesic ladder (**Table 1**).[20] The cause of pain should be identified and addressed properly in order to correct the underlying disease process causing the pain. Ideally the treatment of the cancer eliminates the cause of pain. If this approach is not possible, is only partially successful, or while the patient is awaiting treatment, nonpharmacologic and/or pharmacologic interventions are warranted.

Box 2
Summary of validated pain assessment tools in the elderly population

Pain Assessment Checklist for Seniors with Limited Ability to Communicate (PACSLAC)[7]

Pain Assessment in Advanced Dementia (PAINAD)[8]

Doloplus-2 Scale[9]

Abbey Pain Scale[10]

Rotterdam Elderly Pain Observation Scale (REPOS)[11]

Pain Assessment Tool in Confused Older Adults (PATCOA)[12]

Pain Assessment in Noncommunicative Elderly Persons (PAINE)[13]

Pain Assessment for the Demented Elderly (PADE)[14]

Mahoney Pain Scale[15]

Elderly Pain Caring Assessment-2 (EPCA-2)[16]

Discomfort Scale-Dementia Alzheimer Type (DS-DAT)[17]

Certified Nurse Assistant Pain Assessment Tool (CPAT)[18]

Checklist of Nonverbal Pain Indicators (CNPI)[19]

Data from Refs.[7–19]

Table 1
WHO analgesic ladder and recommendations for elderly patients

Step	Recommendations	Suggested Medications
Step 1: mild pain	Nonopioid	NSAIDs, acetaminophen
	± Adjuvant	Neurontin, pregabalin
Step 2: moderate pain	Weak opioid	Codeine
	± Nonopioid	NSAIDs, acetaminophen
	± Adjuvant	Neurontin, pregabalin
Step 3: severe pain	Strong opioid	Morphine, oxycodone, hydromorphone, fentanyl, methadone
	± Nonopioid	NSAIDs, acetaminophen
	± Adjuvant	Neurontin, pregabalin

Abbreviation: NSAIDs, nonsteroidal antiinflammatory drugs.

Nonpharmacologic interventions

All treatment plans for older patients with cancer should incorporate nonpharmacologic interventions such as massage, relaxation techniques, exercise, and rehabilitation.[6] Cognitive behavior therapy may be helpful in patients who are cognitively intact. It is also important to ensure the involvement of a multidisciplinary team that includes a geriatrician, PC specialist, social worker, and chaplain.

Pharmacologic interventions

Nonopioid therapy

Acetaminophen Acetaminophen is used for the relief of mild to moderate pain and is the first line for pain control in older patients with cancer. However, because of potential liver toxicity, patients should be counseled not to consume more than 3000 mg of acetaminophen per day. It is also important to educate patients and their caregivers that many other medications, including over-the-counter medications, contain acetaminophen and require caution when used in combination.[21]

Nonsteroidal antiinflammatory drugs Nonsteroidal antiinflammatory drugs (NSAIDs) are also effective for the treatment of mild to moderate pain, especially bone pain. However, NSAIDs are associated with increased risks in older patients, and have been linked to gastrointestinal bleeds, renal toxicity, myocardial infarction, and stroke. Patients taking concomitant nephrotoxic agents and those with compromised renal function caused by aging or other comorbidities are at higher risk of NSAID-related renal toxicity. NSAID-associated side effects are dose and time dependent and therefore, in this population, NSAIDs should be used only for short intervals.[22] If NSAIDs are used, they should be prescribed in conjunction with a gastroprotective medication such as a proton pump inhibitor.[23] Absolute contraindications for the use of NSAIDs include chronic kidney disease, active peptic ulcer disease, and heart failure.

Opioid therapy Opioids are used in the treatment of moderate to severe cancer-related pain. These medications can be administered in many preparations (eg, oral, intravenous, and transdermal) and, compared with nonopioids, have no analgesic ceiling dose (**Table 2**). Before initiating treatment it is important to evaluate the hepatic and renal function, cognitive ability, level of social support, and potential drug-drug interactions with other active medications (**Box 3**). In older patients with cancer, oral administration is preferred because of ease of use and affordability.[22] Weak opioids (codeine, hydrocodone, tramadol, tapentadol, and buprenorphine) are the second

Table 2
Opioid medications in older patients

Drug	Equianalgesic PO Dose (mg)	PO Starting Dose in Elderly[a] (mg)	Equianalgesic IV Dose	IV Starting Dose in Elderly[a]	Half-life (h)	Duration of Action (h)	Cautions
Morphine	30	2.5–7.5	10 mg	1.25–2.5 mg	1.5–3	3–7	Renal failure
Oxycodone	20	2.5	—	—	2–4	3–6	Patients with abuse potential
Hydromorphone	7.5	0.5–1	1.5 mg	0.2 mg	2–3	2–5	Renal failure
Methadone[b]	2	1.25–2.5	1 mg	1.25 mg	12–190	4–12	—
Fentanyl[c]	—	—	250 µg	12.5–25 µg	3–4	4–6	—

Abbreviations: IV, intravenous; PO, by mouth.
[a] Opioid-naive patients.
[b] Use restricted to experienced practitioners.
[c] Not for use in opioid-naive patients.

Box 3
Important considerations in the treatment of cancer pain with opioids

- Strong opioids are the mainstay of the management of moderate to severe cancer pain.
- Most patients tolerate morphine well, including the elderly.
- Occasional cancer-related pain can be managed with PRN opioid medications, but patients who require more than 4 PRN doses per day should be started on a long-acting scheduled medication.
- It is helpful to use the same drug for short-acting and long-acting doses (eg, morphine immediate and extended release). Rescue doses should be calculated at 10% to 15% of the total daily dose and should be scheduled based on the half-life of the medication.[6]
- In older patients with cancer an ideal starting dose is 30% to 50% lower than the standard for younger patients and it is important to adhere to the adage start low and go slow.[22]
- Reduce dose of morphine in patients with renal failure to avoid accumulation of the active metabolite morphine-6-glucuronide.
- Dose titration in this population must be done carefully to balance any side effects with the level of analgesia.
- It is appropriate to increase the daily opioid dose by 25% to 50% every 24 hours until pain relief is achieved.[4]
- Close follow-up is important in order to evaluate for safe opioid storage, adherence, and frequency of use.[6]
- Opioid rotation is required in approximately 25% of patients started on morphine who develop dose-limiting side effects.
- All patients prescribed opioids should be started on a prophylactic bowel regimen that includes a stimulant laxative to prevent opioid-induced constipation.

Abbreviation: PRN, as needed.
Data from Refs.[4,6,22]

---

step in the WHO analgesic ladder and are recommended for mild to moderate pain. However, lower doses of stronger opioids have been shown to be more effective than weak opioids and many experts skip the second step of the ladder and use a strong opioid instead to treat cancer-related pain.[24] At the same time consider starting stool softeners and laxatives to avoid opioid-induced constipation (see **Box 3**).

Opioid adverse effects The side effect profile of opioid pain medications is no different based on age, although older patients with cancer are more likely to show symptoms.[22] The most common opioid-related adverse effects include constipation, sedation, confusion, and hallucinations. Constipation in older adults is multifactorial; opioid-induced constipation is likely caused by a combination of mu-receptor binding within the gastrointestinal tract, delayed motility, and increased water resorption. All patients prescribed opioids should be started on a prophylactic bowel regimen that includes a stimulant laxative.[25] The development of sedation, confusion, or hallucinations is usually managed with dose reduction or opioid rotation. The use of benzodiazepines should be avoided in this population if possible.[26] Other less common opioid-associated adverse effects seen in older patients with cancer include nausea, dry mouth, pruritus, myoclonus, and urinary retention.

Adjuvant medications Adjuvant medications are given to enhance the pain relief provided by an opioid. Some of them are used primarily for other indications (eg, antidepressants, muscle relaxers, anticonvulsants, corticosteroids). Neuropathic cancer-related pain (eg, chemotherapy-related pain) is best treated with adjuvant medications, including tricyclic antidepressants and antiepileptics. However, tricyclic antidepressants are rarely indicated in older patients with cancer because of their association with significant anticholinergic side effects and subsequent cognitive changes. The most commonly prescribed antiepileptics are gabapentin and pregabalin. In older patients with cancer, these medications should be renally dosed and escalated slowly. Serotonin-norepinephrine reuptake inhibitors (venlafaxine, duloxetine) have been shown to be effective and well tolerated.

ASSESSMENT AND MANAGEMENT OF NONPAIN SYMPTOMS
Fatigue

Fatigue is one of the most common and debilitating symptoms experienced by patients with cancer. Cancer-related fatigue (CRF) is characterized by feelings of tiredness, weakness, and lack of energy, and is distinct from that experienced by healthy individuals in that it is not relieved by rest or sleep.[27] The prevalence of fatigue in patients receiving anticancer treatment has been estimated to be more than 80%.[28] Fatigue has been found to be associated with distress, depression, anxiety, and low performance status, as well as other symptoms such as nausea, vomiting, lack of appetite, sleep disturbance, dyspnea, dry mouth, restlessness, and problems with concentration.[29]

Management of fatigue
Nonpharmacologic interventions
1. Aerobic exercise: is considered beneficial for individuals with CRF, specifically those with solid tumors during and after cancer therapy.[30,31] Combined aerobic and resistance exercise regimens with or without stretching should be included as part of rehabilitation programs for people who have been diagnosed with cancer.
2. Psychological interventions: fatigue in terminally ill patients with cancer is determined by both physical and psychological factors and it may be important to include psychological interventions.[32] Individual sessions during which participants were educated on fatigue and learned activity management have been found to be effective.[33]
3. Complementary therapies: a wide range of practical interventions and complementary therapies are likely to be helpful. These therapies include acupressure and acupuncture, stress management and relaxation, energy conservation measures, anticipatory guidance and preparatory information, and attention-restoring activities.[34]

Pharmacologic interventions
1. Modafinil: recent studies and reviews show that modafinil has no effect on CRF and should not be prescribed outside a clinical trial setting.[35]
2. Corticosteroids have been shown to improve fatigue in various studies.[36,37]
3. Methylphenidate: existing trials of methylphenidate on CRF provide limited evidence for its use.[38]
4. Antidepressants: paroxetine shows benefit in the treatment of fatigue, primarily when it is a symptom of clinical depression. Bupropion sustained release may have psychostimulantlike effects and, therefore, may be beneficial in treating fatigue.[39]
5. Cholinesterase inhibitors: donepezil has been studied. However, there is no evidence of a significant improvement in CRF.[40]

6. Other: traditional Chinese medicine (TCM) is widely used in the treatment of CRF in China. TCM seems to be effective in alleviating the fatigue in people with CRF. However, because of the high risk of bias in the literature, larger, well-designed studies are needed to confirm the potential benefit.[41]

Delirium

Delirium is a fluctuating disturbance in attention and awareness that represents a decline from baseline status, accompanied by cognitive dysfunction. It is the most common serious neuropsychiatric complication in patients with cancer. It is associated with increased morbidity and mortality, increased length of hospitalizations, higher health care cost, and significant distress for patients, family members, and health professionals. The prevalence of delirium in cancer ranges from 20% to 40% in hospitalized patients and can be as high as 88% in terminally ill patients with cancer.[42] The development of delirium may be an indicator of impending death in patients who are terminally ill.

The cause of delirium is usually multifactorial, involving multiple medical conditions, such as infections, organ failure, or adverse reactions to medications (**Box 4**). In patients with cancer, its complexity is enhanced by the direct effects of cancer on the central nervous system (CNS) (ie, brain metastatic disease) and the indirect CNS effects of the disease or its treatment.[43] Delirium may interfere with the recognition of other symptoms such as pain. At times, agitation may be misinterpreted as uncontrolled pain and patients may be given increasing doses of opioids, which, in turn, can exacerbate the delirium state.

The work-up of delirium should always include a history and physical examination assessing for potentially reversible causes, with a thorough review of medications and doses. Laboratory tests may be necessary for the assessment of metabolic abnormalities, hypoxia, or other medical problems. Brain imaging to evaluate for brain metastasis, ischemia, or bleed as well as electroencephalography and/or lumbar puncture to rule out leptomeningeal carcinomatosis may be indicated. The diagnosis of delirium can be made using specific instruments such as the Confusion Assessment Method (CAM)[44] (**Box 5**) or the CAM-ICU (CAM for the Intensive Care Unit) for intubated patients.[45]

Box 4
Causes of delirium frequently seen in the patients with cancer

Multiple medical causes (ie, infections, organ failure, malignant hypercalcemia)

Uncontrolled pain

Metastatic brain lesions

CNS effects of chemotherapeutic/immunotherapeutic agents (eg, vincristine, interferon)

Medications used for supportive care (eg, steroids, opioids, antiemetics, benzodiazepines)

Paraneoplastic syndromes

Constipation

Withdrawal from alcohol, illicit drugs, benzodiazepines

Sleep deprivation caused by environmental factors

Strange/new environment

Abbreviation: CNS, central nervous system.

Box 5
CAM criteria for a positive diagnosis of delirium

1. Acute onset and fluctuating course of the mental status

2. Inattention: difficulty focusing and easily distracted

3. Disorganized thinking: disorganized or incoherent speech, and/or illogical flow of ideas

4. Altered level of consciousness, vigilant, hyperalert, lethargic, or stuporous.

1 and 2 plus 3 or 4 should be present for a positive diagnosis of delirium.
Adapted from Inouye SK, Westendorp RG, Saczynski JS. Delirium in elderly people. Lancet 2014;383:911–22 [supplementary appendix.]

Management of delirium

Nonpharmacologic interventions The incidence of delirium can be reduced by minimizing exposure to known risk factors. Interventions are multifactorial and should include a thorough search for the underlying cause.[46]

Pharmacologic interventions When nonpharmacologic interventions are not sufficient, treatment with psychotropic medications is necessary. To date, no medication has been approved by the US Food and Drug Administration for the treatment of delirium. The main classes of medications studied in the treatment and prevention of delirium are antipsychotics, cholinesterase inhibitors, and alpha-2 agonists.[43]

Anxiety and Depression

Anxiety and depression are the most common manifestations of psychological distress in patients with cancer, and the prevalence varies considerably depending on many factors, such as the type and stage of the disease, the patients' coping abilities, and psychosocial support. Among patients with cancer, 47% have a formal psychiatric disorder. Approximately 85% of these patients have a disorder with depression or anxiety as the central symptom.[47] These symptoms tend to increase as death approaches.

Anxiety frequently invokes hopelessness and often causes patients to reject advice given by clinicians.[48] Goals of care conversations are central components of cancer care. However, anxiety about death contributes to decreased communication between patients and family members regarding the patient's end-of-life care wishes.[49] Untreated anxiety is frequently detrimental to patients' quality of life.

Terminally ill patients with cancer experience progressive functional decline, accelerating symptom severity, and deteriorating social support, and perceive themselves to be a burden to others, predisposing them to depressive symptoms.[50] Fatigue and confusion are associated with mild to moderate depressive symptoms and anxiety is frequently associated with severe depressive symptoms.[51]

Management of Anxiety and Depression

A careful history and physical are important for determining effective interventions. Emphasis should be placed on identifying treatable conditions causing anxiety or depression, including pain and dyspnea, and managing them appropriately.

Nonpharmacologic interventions

Nonpharmacologic approaches for the treatment of anxiety should be tried first. Multidisciplinary assessments and short-term psychotherapy can be used in managing symptoms. Providing updated information on the prognosis, establishing short-term goals and expectations, identifying strengths and coping techniques, as well as the use of relaxation techniques can be helpful. In patients with depression and serious illness, pharmacologic and nonpharmacologic interventions should be used concurrently.

Pharmacologic interventions

Short-acting or long-acting oral benzodiazepines are the mainstay in treating anxiety symptoms in patients with serious illness. If the anxiety is severe and associated with paranoia or hallucinations, antipsychotics such as haloperidol may be needed (**Table 3**).

For the treatment of depression in older adults with terminal cancer, initial dosing of antidepressants should be reduced because of decreased drug clearance and potential side effects. Selective serotonin reuptake inhibitors (SSRIs) cause less sedation and fewer autonomic side effects than other antidepressant medications but may not show efficacy for 4 to 6 weeks. The tricyclics are the best studied and can be given as a single dose at bedtime. In some cases psychostimulants may be needed because of their rapid effect, but they may exacerbate anxiety and restlessness (**Table 4**). Patients should be referred to psychiatry when there is poor response to initial treatment and when there is a complex presentation with psychosis or suicidal ideation.

Cachexia and Anorexia

Cachexia is a complex metabolic syndrome associated with underlying illness and is characterized by loss of muscle with or without loss of fat mass.[52] Anorexia is loss of appetite. Although anorexia with weight loss is common among patients with cancer, the profound weight loss in patients with cachexia cannot be entirely attributed to poor caloric intake. The overall prevalence of cancer anorexia-cachexia syndrome ranges from 40% at cancer diagnosis to 70% to 80% in advanced phases of the disease.[53] Anorexia and cachexia may be more distressing to the families than to the patients, and treatment should include education of caregivers regarding the underlying disease.

Management of cachexia and anorexia

The best approach to the treatment of the cachectic syndrome is multifactorial. An improvement of cachexia may not be possible in all patients, but a reasonable goal could be to delay or prevent further decline.

Table 3
Pharmacologic management of anxiety in patients with terminal cancer

Medication	Dosage	Route	Comments
Short-acting Benzodiazepines			
Lorazepam	0.5–2 mg 2–4 times a day	PO	Available as PO, sublingual, rectal, and IV preparations
Alprazolam	0.25–2 mg 3–4 times a day	PO	Peaks in 30 min. Useful for quick relief of acute anxiety
Long-acting Benzodiazepines			
Clonazepam	0.25–0.5 mg 2–3 times a day	PO	—
Diazepam	2–20 mg once to 3 times a day	PO	Parenteral form available
Others			
Haloperidol	0.5–4 mg q4 h PRN	PO	Parenteral forms available. Use in severe cases with psychotic features

Abbreviations: PRN, as needed; q, every.

Table 4
Pharmacologic management of depression

Medication	Maximum Dosage (mg)	Route	Comments
SSRIs			
Citalopram	20–40 daily	PO	Taper when discontinuing. Dose adjustment in patient with severe renal impairment
Escitalopram	10–20 daily	PO	Taper when discontinuing
Fluoxetine	10–60 daily	PO	—
Tricyclic Antidepressants			
Amitriptyline	10–75 (150)	PO HS	Sedating. Analgesic effects. Anticholinergic side effects
Nortriptyline	10–25 (75)	PO HS	Less side effects than amitriptyline
Psychostimulants			
Methylphenidate	2.5 once to twice a day (60 daily)	PO	Adjuvant in patients with prognosis of days to weeks. Administer in morning and at noon
Modafinil	100–400 daily	—	Adjuvant in patients with prognosis of days to weeks
Miscellaneous			
Bupropion	100 bid (450)	PO	Contraindicated with seizures
Mirtazapine	15 (45)	PO HS	Possible sedation, may improve oral intake
Venlafaxine	37.5 bid (375)	PO	Available as extended release

Abbreviations: bid, 2 times a day; HS, at bedtime.

Nonpharmacologic interventions
1. Patients should be assessed and treated for causes interfering with appetite, such as a dry mouth, uncontrolled pain, nausea, and constipation.
2. Encourage small, frequent meals and assist with feeding if needed.
3. Oral nutritional supplementation may be beneficial.

Pharmacologic interventions Many drugs, including appetite stimulants, thalidomide, cytokine inhibitors, steroids, NSAIDs, branched-chain amino acids, eicosapentaenoic acid, and antiserotoninergic drugs have been proposed and used in clinical trials, whereas others are still under investigation in experimental animal models.[54] Appetite stimulants are not always successful; however, some patients benefit from them. When appetite stimulants are indicated, megestrol, prednisone, or dronabinol[55] may be considered, but they have not been proved to extend life.

Artificial nutrition and hydration During the curative phase of cancer, optimal enteral or parenteral nutrition intake can reduce morbidity and mortality, and improve quality of life, but when the main goal of treatment becomes palliative, introduction of artificial nutrition is controversial.[56] In patients at the end of life, artificial hydration and nutrition pose clinical, ethical, and logistical dilemmas. No strong evidence exists supporting the use of parenteral hydration or nutrition for most terminally ill patients.[57] For patients with refractory cachexia, it is important to discuss the risks and benefits of parenteral nutrition and hydration with the patient, family members and health care team to set up realistic nutritional care goals. Previous studies on artificial hydration found no beneficial effects on terminal delirium, thirst, chronic nausea, and fluid overload, but identified negative effects such as increased incidence of ascites and intestinal drainage.[58]

Nausea and Vomiting

Nausea and vomiting are common in patients with advanced cancer.[59] The prevalence in patients with cancer is estimated at between 30% and 70% and the most common causes are chemotherapy, radiation, opioids, bowel obstruction, and constipation. Because many factors can contribute to these symptoms, a history and physical focused on identification of specific causes is extremely important.

Management of nausea and vomiting

Nonpharmacologic interventions Small, frequent meals of the patient's own choosing, providing adequate liquids, relaxation techniques, companionship, and a pleasant atmosphere during meals can be of help. Acupuncture in patients with cancer can be associated with a significantly reduced intensity of nausea during chemotherapy and in the final phase of life.[60]

Pharmacologic interventions Drugs used to control nausea and vomiting include prokinetics, antihistamines, neuroleptics, serotonin receptor antagonists, benzodiazepines, corticosteroids, cannabinoids, and others such as scopolamine (**Table 5**).

Dyspnea

Dyspnea is defined as an uncomfortable awareness of breathing and is a common symptom in patients receiving PC. Acute dyspnea is the most frequent reason for an emergency admission in PC and severely affects the quality of life.[61] In the terminally ill, dyspnea can have multiple causes. Common causes include effusions,

Table 5
Pharmacologic management of nausea and vomiting in elderly patients with cancer

Medication	Dose (Oral)	Route	Comments
Metoclopramide	5–15 mg before meals	PO, SC, or IV	May cause dystonia
Domperidone	Divided doses before meals to maximum of 80 mg/d	PO	May cause dystonia
Diphenhydramine	1 mg/kg/dose q4 h	PO, SC, or IV	May cause drowsiness
Haloperidol	0.01–0.05 mg/kg/dose q8 h	PO, SC, or IV	May prolong QT interval. Can cause EPS
Prochlorperazine	0.15 mg/kg/dose q4 h	PO, PR, or IV	May cause EPS and dystonias
Ondansetron	0.15 mg/kg/dose q6 h	PO or IV	Used particularly in chemotherapy-induced nausea
Diazepam	0.05–0.2 mg/kg/dose q6 h	PO or IV	Helpful in anticipatory nausea
Dexamethasone	2–4 mg bid to qid	PO, SC, or IV	Use for nausea with increased intracranial pressure
Dronabinol	2.5 mg bid	PO	May cause dysphoria, drowsiness, hallucinations
Scopolamine	0.5 mg transdermal q72 h	Transdermal	May cause dry mouth, blurred vision, confusion

Abbreviations: EPS, extrapyramidal symptoms; PR, by rectum; qid, 4 times a day; SC, subcutaneous.

bronchospasm, thick airway secretions and airway obstructions, anemia, anxiety, and even unresolved emotional issues.

Management of dyspnea

Evaluation of patients complaining of dyspnea should include a thorough history and physical as well as imaging and/or other tests to rule out reversible causes.

Nonpharmacologic interventions

1. Repositioning the patient, usually to a more upright position
2. Improving air circulation by opening windows or using fans
3. Relaxation techniques and breathing retraining
4. Addressing anxiety issues and providing reassurance may be beneficial

Supplementary oxygen is often unnecessary in the PC setting. Oxygen delivered by a nasal cannula provides no additional symptomatic benefit for relief of refractory dyspnea in patients with life-limiting illness compared with room air.[62]

Pharmacologic interventions

1. Patients with specific diagnoses may benefit from treatments with diuretics, bronchodilators, or corticosteroids.
2. Opioids are recommended for emergency medical therapy for dyspnea in patients receiving PC.[63] Opioids are the first-choice treatment of most nonspecific dyspnea because they suppress respiratory awareness effectively. Patients may report substantial relief of dyspnea with opiates without a change in respiratory rate. One of the most serious but infrequent side effects is respiratory depression. Studies have shown that opioids are both safe and effective in the treatment of dyspnea in terminal cancer[64] (**Table 6**). Oxycodone 5 to 10 mg every 4 hours as needed or morphine syrup 5 to 15 mg every 4 hours as needed may be considered. In patients already on opioids and for those with high levels of anxiety, these doses may be increased by 50% every 4 to 12 hours until the patient experiences relief.
3. Benzodiazepines may also be helpful to relieve anxiety, which worsens dyspnea.

END-OF-LIFE CARE

Most referrals to PC and hospice occur late in the trajectory of the disease despite the fact that an earlier intervention could decrease patients' symptoms of distress.[65] Benefits are seen to extend to the caregivers as well; caregivers of patients referred early to PC had lower depression scores at 3 months and lower depression and stress burden in the terminal period.[66] Many patients with end-stage cancer are offered chemotherapy in an attempt to improve quality of life. Chemotherapy at the end of life has been shown not

Table 6
Pharmacologic management of dyspnea in the patients with end-stage cancer

Medication	Oral Dose	Comments
Mild Dyspnea		
Hydrocodone	5 mg q4 h	Additional 5 mg q2 h PRN
Acetaminophen codeine	1 tab (30 mg) q4 h	Additional tab q2 h PRN
Severe Dyspnea		
Oxycodone	3–10 mg q4 h	Additional PRN doses
Morphine syrup	5–15 mg q4 h	
Hydromorphone	1–3 mg q4 h	

Abbreviation: tab, tablet.

> **Box 6**
> **Four essential drugs needed for quality care of patients dying of cancer**
>
> 1. Morphine (ie, an opioid)
>
> 2. Midazolam (a benzodiazepine)
>
> 3. Haloperidol (a neuroleptic)
>
> 4. Anticholinergic (ie, glycopyrrolate)
>
> *Data from* Lindqvist O, Lundquist G, Dickman A, et al. Four essential drugs needed for quality care of the dying: a Delphi-study based international expert consensus opinion. J Palliat Med 2013;16:38–43.

only to be futile in that it is not associated with improved patient survival but also to be harmful by impairing the quality of life near death of these patients.[67] Terminally ill patients experience a variety of symptoms in the last hours and days of life, including delirium, agitation, anxiety, restlessness, dyspnea, pain, vomiting, and psychological distress. Patients and families are usually unaware of the typical changes that occur in the last hours of life and at the moment of death, which can lead to last-minute confusion and panic. The purposeless movements and facial expressions that occur at this time can be misinterpreted as physical discomfort or emotional distress. The gurgling sounds of air passing over accumulated oropharyngeal secretions may be interpreted as choking. Caregiver education regarding what to expect in the final hours can help alleviate stress and prevent panic. This education is particularly helpful for families planning a home death.

Management of Refractory Terminal Symptoms and Agitation

In the terminal phase of life, symptoms may become refractory and poorly controlled by supportive and palliative therapies that specifically target these symptoms. Palliative sedation can be used to provide relief from these refractory symptoms that are not controlled by other methods. It is designed to induce a state of decreased awareness or in some cases, if necessary, unconsciousness. Sedative drugs, typically short-acting benzodiazepines, are administered in a monitored setting and titrated to achieve the desired level of sedation (**Box 6**). The level of sedation can be easily maintained and the effect is reversible. A systematic review found that palliative sedation did not hasten death, which has been a concern of physicians and families in prescribing this treatment.[68]

SUMMARY

Patients with cancer can develop several symptoms that impair comfort and quality of life. They should be managed by a combination of nonpharmacologic and pharmacologic interventions. After initiation of treatment, patients should be reassessed frequently until the distressing symptoms are controlled while looking out for medication side effects. Caregiver education regarding what to expect in the final hours significantly alleviates stress.

REFERENCES

1. Levy MH, Back A, Benedetti C, et al. NCCN clinical practice guidelines in oncology: palliative care. J Natl Compr Cancer Netw JNCCN 2009;7:436–73.
2. Fogel JF, Hyman RB, Rock B, et al. Predictors of hospital length of stay and nursing home placement in an elderly medical population. J Am Med Dir Assoc 2000;1:202–10.

3. Korc-Grodzicki B, Boparai MK, Lichtman SM. Prescribing for older patients with cancer. Clin Adv Hematol Oncol 2014;12:309–18.
4. Tracy B, Sean Morrison R. Pain management in older adults. Clin Ther 2013;35: 1659–68.
5. Rao A, Cohen HJ. Symptom management in the elderly cancer patient: fatigue, pain, and depression. J Natl Cancer Inst Monogr 2004;(32):150–7.
6. Makris UE, Abrams RC, Gurland B, et al. Management of persistent pain in the older patient: a clinical review. JAMA 2014;312:825–36.
7. Fuchs-Lacelle S, Hadjistavropoulos T. Development and preliminary validation of the Pain Assessment Checklist for Seniors with Limited Ability to Communicate (PACSLAC). Pain Manag Nurs 2004;5:37–49.
8. Warden V, Hurley AC, Volicer L. Development and psychometric evaluation of the Pain Assessment in Advanced Dementia (PAINAD) scale. J Am Med Directors Assoc 2003;4:9–15.
9. Lefebvre-Chapiro S. The DOLOPLUS 2 scale - evaluating pain in the elderly. Eur J Palliat Care 2001;8:191–4.
10. Abbey J, Piller N, De Bellis A, et al. The Abbey Pain Scale: a 1-minute numerical indicator for people with end-stage dementia. Int J Palliat Nurs 2004;10:6–13.
11. van Herk R, et al. The Rotterdam Elderly Pain Observation Scale (REPOS): a new behavioral pain scale for non-communicative adults and cognitively impaired elderly persons. J Pain Management 2009;1:367–78.
12. Decker SA, Perry AG. The development and testing of the PATCOA to assess pain in confused older adults. Pain Manag Nurs 2003;4:77–86.
13. Cohen-Mansfield J. Pain Assessment in Noncommunicative Elderly Persons—PAINE. Clin J Pain 2006;22:569–75.
14. Villanueva MR, Smith TL, Erickson JS, et al. Pain Assessment for the Dementing Elderly (PADE): reliability and validity of a new measure. J Am Med Directors Assoc 2003;4:1–8.
15. Mahoney AE, Peters L. The Mahoney Pain Scale: examining pain and agitation in advanced dementia. Am J Alzheimers Dis Other Demen 2008;23:250–61.
16. Morello R, Jean A, Alix M, et al. A scale to measure pain in non-verbally communicating older patients: the EPCA-2 Study of its psychometric properties. Pain 2007;133:87–98.
17. Hurley AC, Volicer BJ, Hanrahan PA, et al. Assessment of discomfort in advanced Alzheimer patients. Res Nurs Health 1992;15:369–77.
18. Cervo FA, Raggi RP, Bright-Long LE, et al. Use of the Certified Nursing Assistant Pain Assessment Tool (CPAT) in nursing home residents with dementia. Am J Alzheimers Dis Other Demen 2007;22:112–9.
19. Feldt KS. The cheCklist of Nonverbal Pain Indicators (CNPI). Pain Manag Nurs 2000;1:13–21.
20. Zech DF, Grond S, Lynch J, et al. Validation of World Health Organization guidelines for cancer pain relief: a 10-year prospective study. Pain 1995;63: 65–76.
21. Taylor R Jr, Lemtouni S, Weiss K, et al. Pain management in the elderly: an FDA safe use initiative expert panel's view on preventable harm associated with NSAID therapy. Curr Gerontol Geriatr Res 2012;2012:196159.
22. American Geriatrics Society Panel on Pharmacological Management of Persistent Pain in Older Persons. Pharmacological management of persistent pain in older persons. J Am Geriatr Soc 2009;57:1331–46.
23. Medlock S, Eslami S, Askari M, et al. Co-prescription of gastroprotective agents and their efficacy in elderly patients taking nonsteroidal anti-inflammatory

drugs: a systematic review of observational studies. Clin Gastroenterol Hepatol 2013;11:1259–69.e10.

24. Marinangeli F, Ciccozzi A, Leonardis M, et al. Use of strong opioids in advanced cancer pain: a randomized trial. J Pain Symptom Manage 2004;27:409–16.

25. Hawley PH, Byeon JJ. A comparison of sennosides-based bowel protocols with and without docusate in hospitalized patients with cancer. J Palliat Med 2008;11: 575–81.

26. American Geriatrics Society 2012 Beers Criteria Update Expert Panel. American Geriatrics Society updated Beers Criteria for potentially inappropriate medication use in older adults. J Am Geriatr Soc 2012;60:616–31.

27. Hofman M, Ryan JL, Figueroa-Moseley CD, et al. Cancer-related fatigue: the scale of the problem. Oncologist 2007;12(Suppl 1):4–10.

28. Buss T, Modlinska A, Chelminska M, et al. Cancer related fatigue. I. Prevalence and attempt to define the problem. Pol Merkur Lekarski 2004;16:70–2 [in Polish].

29. Tsai LY, Li IF, Lai YH, et al. Fatigue and its associated factors in hospice cancer patients in Taiwan. Cancer Nurs 2007;30:24–30.

30. Cramp F, Byron-Daniel J. Exercise for the management of cancer-related fatigue in adults. Cochrane Database Syst Rev 2012;(11):CD006145.

31. van Waart H, Stuiver MM, van Harten WH, et al. Effect of low-intensity physical activity and moderate- to high-intensity physical exercise during adjuvant chemo- therapy on physical fitness, fatigue, and chemotherapy completion rates: results of the PACES randomized clinical trial. J Clin Oncol 2015;33(17):1918–27.

32. Okuyama T, Akechi T, Shima Y, et al. Factors correlated with fatigue in terminally ill cancer patients: a longitudinal study. J Pain Symptom Manage 2008;35:515–23.

33. Goedendorp MM, Gielissen MF, Verhagen CA, et al. Psychosocial interventions for reducing fatigue during cancer treatment in adults. Cochrane Database Syst Rev 2009;(1):CD006953.

34. Kirshbaum M. Cancer-related fatigue: a review of nursing interventions. Br J Community Nurs 2010;15:214–6, 218–9.

35. Ruddy KJ, Barton D, Loprinzi CL. Laying to rest psychostimulants for cancer- related fatigue? J Clin Oncol 2014;32:1865–7.

36. Paulsen O, Klepstad P, Rosland JH, et al. Efficacy of methylprednisolone on pain, fatigue, and appetite loss in patients with advanced cancer using opioids: a ran- domized, placebo-controlled, double-blind trial. J Clin Oncol 2014;32:3221–8.

37. Yennurajalingam S, Frisbee-Hume S, Palmer JL, et al. Reduction of cancer- related fatigue with dexamethasone: a double-blind, randomized, placebo- controlled trial in patients with advanced cancer. J Clin Oncol 2013;31:3076–82.

38. Gong S, Sheng P, Jin H, et al. Effect of methylphenidate in patients with cancer- related fatigue: a systematic review and meta-analysis. PLoS One 2014;9. e84391.

39. Breitbart W, Alici Y. Pharmacologic treatment options for cancer-related fatigue: current state of clinical research. Clin J Oncol Nurs 2008;12:27–36.

40. Bruera E, El Osta B, Valero V, et al. Donepezil for cancer fatigue: a double-blind, randomized, placebo-controlled trial. J Clin Oncol 2007;25:3475–81.

41. Wang YY, Li XX, Liu JP, et al. Traditional Chinese medicine for chronic fatigue syn- drome: a systematic review of randomized clinical trials. Complement Ther Med 2014;22:826–33.

42. Breitbart W, Alici Y. Agitation and delirium at the end of life: "we couldn't manage him". JAMA 2008;300:2898–910. e1.

43. Breitbart W, Alici Y. Evidence-based treatment of delirium in patients with cancer. J Clin Oncol 2012;30:1206–14.

44. Inouye SK, Westendorp RG, Saczynski JS. Delirium in elderly people. Lancet 2014;383:911–22.

45. Ely EW, Inouye SK, Bernard GR, et al. Delirium in mechanically ventilated patients: validity and reliability of the Confusion Assessment Method for the Intensive Care Unit (CAM-ICU). JAMA 2001;286:2703–10.

46. Hshieh TT, Yue J, Oh E, et al. Effectiveness of multicomponent nonpharmacological delirium interventions: a meta-analysis. JAMA Intern Med 2015;175: 512–20.

47. Derogatis LR, Morrow GR, Fetting J, et al. The prevalence of psychiatric disorders among cancer patients. JAMA 1983;249:751–7.

48. Hawthorn M. The importance of communication in sustaining hope at the end of life. Br J Nurs 2015;24:702–5.

49. Brown AJ, Shen MJ, Ramondetta LM, et al. Does death anxiety affect end-of-life care discussions? Int J Gynecol Cancer 2014;24:1521–6.

50. Tang ST, Chen JS, Chou WC, et al. Prevalence of severe depressive symptoms increases as death approaches and is associated with disease burden, tangible social support, and high self-perceived burden to others. Support Care Cancer 2015. [Epub ahead of print].

51. Janberidze E, Pereira SM, Hjermstad MJ, et al. Depressive symptoms in the last days of life of patients with cancer: a nationwide retrospective mortality study. BMJ Support Palliat Care 2015. [Epub ahead of print].

52. Evans WJ. Skeletal muscle loss: cachexia, sarcopenia, and inactivity. Am J Clin Nutr 2010;91:1123s–7s.

53. Tuca A, Jimenez-Fonseca P, Gascon P. Clinical evaluation and optimal management of cancer cachexia. Crit Rev Oncol Hematol 2013;88:625–36.

54. Suzuki H, Asakawa A, Amitani H, et al. Cancer cachexia–pathophysiology and management. J Gastroenterol 2013;48:574–94.

55. Nelson K, Walsh D, Deeter P, et al. A phase II study of delta-9-tetrahydrocannabinol for appetite stimulation in cancer-associated anorexia. J Palliat Care 1994;10:14–8.

56. Pazart L, Cretin E, Grodard G, et al. Parenteral nutrition at the palliative phase of advanced cancer: the ALIM-K study protocol for a randomized controlled trial. Trials 2014;15:370.

57. Dev R, Dalal S, Bruera E. Is there a role for parenteral nutrition or hydration at the end of life? Curr Opin Support Palliat Care 2012;6:365–70.

58. Raijmakers NJ, van Zuylen L, Costantini M, et al. Artificial nutrition and hydration in the last week of life in cancer patients. A systematic literature review of practices and effects. Ann Oncol 2011;22:1478–86.

59. Davis MP, Walsh D. Treatment of nausea and vomiting in advanced cancer. Support Care Cancer 2000;8:444–52.

60. Nystrom E, Ridderstrom G, Leffler AS. Manual acupuncture as an adjunctive treatment of nausea in patients with cancer in palliative care–a prospective, observational pilot study. Acupunct Med 2008;26:27–32.

61. Schrijvers D, van Fraeyenhove F. Emergencies in palliative care. Cancer J 2010; 16:514–20.

62. LeBlanc TW, Abernethy AP. Building the palliative care evidence base: lessons from a randomized controlled trial of oxygen vs room air for refractory dyspnea. J Natl Compr Cancer Netw 2014;12:989–92.

63. Wiese CH, Barrels UE, Graf BM, et al. Out-of-hospital opioid therapy of palliative care patients with "acute dyspnoea": a retrospective multicenter investigation. J Opioid Manag 2009;5:115–22.

64. Lopez-Saca JM, Centeno C. Opioids prescription for symptoms relief and the impact on respiratory function: updated evidence. Curr Opin Support Palliat Care 2014;8:383–90.

65. Osta BE, Palmer JL, Paraskevopoulos T, et al. Interval between first palliative care consult and death in patients diagnosed with advanced cancer at a comprehensive cancer center. J Palliat Med 2008;11:51–7.

66. Dionne-Odom JN, Azuero A, Lyons KD, et al. Benefits of early versus delayed palliative care to informal family caregivers of patients with advanced cancer: outcomes from the ENABLE III randomized controlled trial. J Clin Oncol 2015; 33:1446–52.

67. Prigerson HG, Bao Y, Shah MA, et al. Chemotherapy use, performance status, and quality of life at the end of life. JAMA Oncol 2015;1(6):778–84.

68. Beller EM, van Driel ML, McGregor L, et al. Palliative pharmacological sedation for terminally ill adults. Cochrane Database Syst Rev 2015;(1):CD010206.

Long-term Toxicity of Cancer Treatment in Older Patients

Armin Shahrokni, MD, MPH, Abraham J. Wu, MD, Jeanne Carter, PhD, Stuart M. Lichtman, MD*

KEYWORDS

- Older cancer survivors • Frailty • Cancer treatment • Toxicity • Quality of life

KEY POINTS

- The number of older cancer survivors is expected to increase in the next few decades because of the aging population, earlier cancer stage diagnosis, and proper cancer treatment.
- Although effective on cancer treatment, both chemotherapy and radiation therapy may have long-lasting negative impacts on older cancer survivors' quality of life.
- Long-term toxicities of breast and prostate cancer treatment on cognition, cardiac function, emotional wellbeing, muscle and bone health, balance and coordination, and sexual health are well known.
- In order to maintain older cancer survivors' quality of life, it is critical that primary care providers screen, diagnose, and properly manage long-term toxicities of cancer treatment.

INTRODUCTION

The number of cancer survivors is increasing in the United States. In 2014, there were 14.5 million cancer survivors. By 2024, this number is expected to increase to 19 million, with the significant portion of them being older than age 65 years.[1] Because more patients are diagnosed with earlier stages of cancer, the likelihood of cancer survivors living beyond 5 years after the initial cancer diagnosis has increased.[2] The role of primary care providers in the immediate and long-term follow-up of patients with cancer is still being defined, because there are significant differences between primary care providers' and oncologists' preferences toward follow-up care of the cancer survivors. Although 38% of primary care providers prefer shared care of the cancer

Department of Medicine, Memorial Sloan Kettering Cancer Center, 650 Commack Road, Commack, NY 11725, USA
* Corresponding author.
E-mail address: lichtmas@mskcc.org

Clin Geriatr Med 32 (2016) 63–80
http://dx.doi.org/10.1016/j.cger.2015.08.005
0749-0690/16/$ – see front matter © 2016 Elsevier Inc. All rights reserved.

geriatric.theclinics.com

survivors with the oncologists, only 16% of oncologists were in agreement with this model of care. More than half of primary care providers thought they had the necessary skills to take care of the cancer survivors, whereas this was agreed to by only 23% of the oncologists.[3] The primary care providers who were more confident in their skills to provide follow-up care for patients with cancer were more involved in the care of patients with cancer.[4]

INTERACTION BETWEEN AGING, CANCER, CANCER TREATMENT, AND THEIR IMPACT ON FRAILTY

Frailty, broadly defined, is a state of decreased (or total lack of) reserve and resistance to physical and emotional stressors, caused by continuous decline in various organ functions.[5] As patients age, they tend to become more frail, although aging and frailty do not correlate with each other all the time.[6] Patients with cancer are more likely to be frail compared with patients without cancer.[7,8] Moreover, cancer treatment can lead to frailty[9] (**Fig. 1**).

MEASURING FRAILTY AND GERIATRIC DEFICITS

Comprehensive geriatric assessment (CGA) (**Box 1**) performed by health care providers has been a useful tool to assess and manage frailty and geriatric deficits among older patients with cancer and survivors.[10,11] In the cancer setting, the data on usefulness of CGA in predicting short-term toxicities of chemotherapy,[12,13] complications and outcome after cancer surgery,[14,15] and cancer treatment decision making[16,17] are emerging.

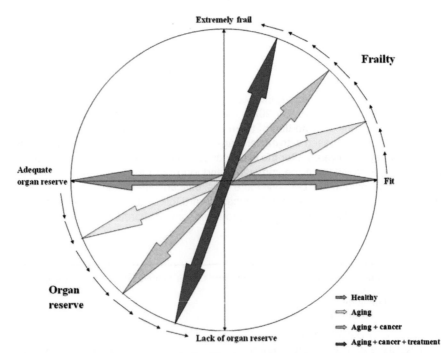

Fig. 1. Impact of aging, cancer, and cancer treatment on patients' fitness and frailty.

Box 1
Components of CGA
Activities of daily living
Instrumental activities of daily living
Cognition
Social support
Polypharmacy
Nutrition
Comorbid conditions
Emotional distress, depression

THERAPY FOR ELDERLY PATIENTS WITH CANCER

For many years, cancers were treated by surgery, chemotherapy, radiation, or hormonal treatments. Over the last 10 to 15 years, a new class of cancer treatment has emerged, which is known as targeted therapy.[18] Considering the differences with the standard and well-known chemotherapy drugs regarding their routes of administration, durations of treatment, and toxicity profiles, this class of drug is discussed separately. **Table 1** present basic facts on medical cancer treatment. This article discusses long-term toxicities of cancer treatment. **Table 2** provides information for screening, diagnosis, and management of each of the long-term toxicities.

Table 1
Basics of medical cancer treatment

		Timing	Goal
Context	Neoadjuvant	Administered before definitive surgery	To shrink the tumor so that surgery becomes feasible or easier
	Adjuvant	After definitive surgery	To treat microscopic disease, and to delay recurrence
	Palliative	Advanced cancer	Relieving symptoms (eg, pain, shortness of breath), and to slow the progression of the disease
Route	Intravenous	Most cancer treatment	
	Oral agents	Mainly targeted therapies (eg, erlotinib, lapatinib, pazopanib)	
	Subcutaneous	Very few (eg, bortezomib for multiple myeloma)	
	Intramuscular	Very few (eg, fulvestrant for breast cancer, leuprolide for prostate cancer)	
Number of agents	Multiple	Most chemotherapy regimens. At times, it is combined with targeted agents as well. In general, combined chemotherapy is more toxic than single-agent chemotherapy. Used in neoadjuvant, adjuvant, and palliative settings	
	Single	Mainly used in the palliative setting. In frail patients, it can be used in the adjuvant setting	
Dose	Standard Dose reduced	The concern over using standard doses in elderly patients is the limited number of older patients enrolled in the clinical trials. Many of those who are enrolled do not represent community-dwelling older patients with cancer	

Table 2
Long-term toxicity of cancer treatment, approach, and management

Toxicity	Diagnosis/Screening	Management
Cognitive impairment	Mini-Cog,[115] Mini Mental Status Examination,[116] Montreal Cognitive Assessment[117]	Rule out reversible causes of cognitive deficit (depression, hypothyroidism, vitamin B_{12}, and folic acid deficiency) Referral to cognitive rehabilitation,[118] when possible
Cardiotoxicity	Electrocardiogram, echocardiogram, stress test	Control other risk factors for cardiac condition (eg, hypertension management, smoking cessation, lipid control)
Depression and anxiety	Distress thermometer,[119] Geriatric Depression Scale,[120] Patient Health Questionnaire[121]	Cognitive behavior and stress management,[122] when possible Psychoeducational interventions to cope with stress[123] Selective serotonin reuptake inhibitor[124] Encouraging patients to be more physically active[125]
Ototoxicity	Hearing Handicap Inventory for the Elderly–Screening Version[126,127]	Rule out other causes of hearing impairment (cerumen impaction, chronic otitis media) Referral to audiologists and otolaryngologists to assist with the diagnosis and proper hearing aids[128]
Imbalance and lack of coordination	Mostly clinical. In rare circumstances, may consider nerve conduction velocity/electromyogram, skin and nerve biopsy to confirm the diagnosis[44]	Control other causes of neuropathy (eg, diabetes, vitamin B_{12} deficiency) Treatment with duloxetine,[42] or venlafaxine[129] Referral to physical and occupational therapy[130,131]
Osteoporosis	Bone densitometry[132] WHO Fracture Risk Assessment Tool	Lifestyle modifications: weight-bearing exercises,[133] tai chi[134] Home safety inspection[135] Vitamin D and calcium supplement[136] Starting bisphosphonates in patients with proven osteoporosis or fracture[137]
Metabolic syndrome	Assessment of weight, blood pressure, and waist circumference, measurement of glucose and lipid panels	Recommendation for smoking cessation,[138] abstinence from excessive alcohol, healthy diet,[139] and more physical activity[140]
Second malignancies	Assessment of symptoms not controlled with the conservative management Routine blood cell count Adherence to cancer screening guidelines	Referral to medical oncologist
Sexual and vaginal dysfunction	History taking (eg, erectile dysfunction, dyspareunia) and pelvic examination (eg, discomfort on examination, pelvic floor weakness)	Vulvovaginal atrophy: vaginal lubricants and moisturizers, topical or systemic estrogen therapy (for non–hormone-dependent cancers) Pelvic floor weakness: pelvic floor exercises, chronic pad use Vaginal pain or stenosis: dilators

Data from Refs.[42,44,115–140]

CHRONIC TOXICITY FROM CANCER THERAPY
Cardiotoxicity

Cardiotoxicity can present in various ways (**Table 3**). In general, patients with preexisting cardiac conditions are at highest risk for developing cardiotoxicity in the short and long terms.[19] Among patients with breast cancer, the incidence of cardiotoxicity is 3% to 35%,[20] and at times it competes with breast cancer as the leading cause of death.[21] Anthracyclines (eg, doxorubicin), frequently used chemotherapy agents in patients with breast cancer, can cause cardiotoxicity even at low doses in patients with preexisting cardiac conditions.[22] These patients are 5.4 and 6.25 times more likely to develop clinical and subclinical cardiotoxicity, respectively, compared with those who did not receive anthracycline.[23] More importantly, the risk of cardiac death was 4.94 times more compared with those who did not receive anthracycline. Older patients are at higher risk for developing cardiotoxicity, because for each 10-year increase in age, the risk of developing congestive heart disease doubles.[24]

Patients with prostate cancer on androgen deprivation therapy (ADT) may also have more cardiotoxicity than those not on ADT.[25,26] For every year's increase in age, the risk of cardiac comorbidity increases by 3%.[27] The 5-year cumulative risk of dying from cardiac causes in patients on ADT after prostatectomy reaches 5.5% compared with 2% of patients who only underwent prostatectomy.[28] Patients receiving 5-fluouracil (5-FU) are also at higher risk for cardiotoxicity. 5-FU can cause cardiotoxicity in 1.2% to 18% of patients. The toxicity is usually short term and occurs while the patient is receiving 5-FU.[29] Capecitabine, an oral derivative of 5-FU, can also cause ischemia in up to 9% of patients.[30] These toxicities are usually short term.

Emotional Effects (Depression, Anxiety)

Patients with cancer experience emotional disturbances even years after completion of the treatment. About 57% of patients with gynecologic cancer reported that they need help in dealing with cancer-related emotions; however, only 35% had received such help, and 73% thought that physicians should ask whether patients with cancer want help in dealing with emotions.[31] At least 11.6% and 17.9% of long-term cancer survivors have depression and significant levels of anxiety.[32] In extreme cases,

Table 3 Cardiotoxicity of cancer treatment		
Cardiotoxicity	**Note**	**Drugs**
Heart failure (left ventricular dysfunction)	Most common	Anthracyclines Alkylating agents (eg, cyclophosphamide) Inhibitors of microtubule polymerization (eg, paclitaxel) Monoclonal antibodies (eg, trastuzumab)
Newly induced or worsening hypertension	Class effect of VEGF inhibitors	Bevacizumab
Cardiac ischemia	—	Antimetabolites (eg, 5-FU) Inhibitors of microtubule polymerization (eg, paclitaxel) Targeted agents (eg, bevacizumab)
Arrhythmia	QT prolongation, torsades de pointes	Arsenic trioxide Most antiemetic drugs

Abbreviations: 5-FU, 5-fluouracil; VEGF, vascular endothelial growth factor.

patients may have suicidal ideation if distress and depression remain undiagnosed and untreated.[33]

Ototoxicity

Platinum agents (eg, cisplatin) can cause ototoxicity.[34] Ototoxicity can present as permanent bilateral hearing loss and/or tinnitus. Among platinum agents, cisplatin is the most common chemotherapeutic agent to cause ototoxicity, resulting in bilateral hearing loss and/or permanent tinnitus in 19% to 79% of patients.[35] Older patients with hearing difficulty are at higher risk for falls,[36] accelerated cognitive decline,[37] and poor quality of life.[38]

Balance and Coordination

Lack of balance and falls may occur in patients with cancer and can lead to injuries such as bone fracture.[39] Maintaining proper balance is a result of a complex interaction between cognition,[40] orientation to space, biomechanical changes, and sensors.[39,41] Chemotherapy-induced peripheral neurotoxicity (CIPN) may develop in 20% to 40% of patients with cancer receiving neurotoxic chemotherapy agents,[42] and can increase risk of falls and associated fractures in cancer survivors.[43] Taxanes and platinum agents are the most common drugs that can cause CIPN.[44–46] Patients with preexisting neurologic deficits such as diabetic neuropathy are at higher risk for developing CIPN.[47] Most common presenting symptoms are numbness and tingling, especially in the lower limbs, which at times is painful.[48,49] Vinca alkaloids (vincristine, vinblastine, vinorelbine) and bortezomib can also cause significant chronic neurotoxicity.[50]

Effect on Muscle and Bone Health

Cancer survivors are at higher risk for osteoporosis compared with the general population,[51] and as a result they are at higher risk for fractures.[52] Certain breast cancer treatments increase the risk of osteoporosis. Up to 70% of patients may experience menopause during adjuvant chemotherapy for breast cancer. The earlier the induced menopause occurs, the higher the risk of osteoporosis.[53] Many older patients with breast cancer receive adjuvant hormonal therapy. Although tamoxifen is associated with a decreased risk of osteoporosis if used in postmenopausal women, it may lead to an increase in the incidence of osteoporosis in premenopausal women.[54] Compared with tamoxifen, aromatase inhibitors (AIs) are associated with higher risk of low bone density and fractures.[55] Surgical or medical ovarian ablation also leads to a decrease in estrogen production resulting in bone loss.[56] Prostate cancer survivors are also at high risk for developing osteoporosis. In one study, 5 years after diagnosis of prostate cancer and receiving ADT, 19.4% of the patients had a fracture.[57] In another study, prostate cancer survivors were at least 2.49 times more likely to have osteoporosis compared with those without prostate cancer.[58] Despite higher risk for osteoporosis and fracture, one study showed that 77% of survivors with osteoporosis were undiagnosed by their primary care providers.[59] This finding has been confirmed by other studies.[58,60,61] The American Society of Clinical Oncology[62] and National Comprehensive Cancer Network[63] have proposed guidelines for the diagnosis and management of osteoporosis in patients with cancer.

Metabolic Syndrome

Metabolic syndrome (MS) is a constellation of states that increases the risk of cardiovascular events, diabetes, fatty liver, and sleep disturbances.[64] Most of the studies on incidence of MS in long-term cancer survivors have focused on testicular and early adulthood diagnosis of leukemia/lymphoma.[65,66] Two known causes of the MS are testosterone deficiency[67] and estrogen deficiency.[68] In one study, 50% of men with prostate cancer receiving long-term ADT had MS.[69] Another study on men with recurrent or locally advanced prostate cancer receiving leuprolide for 12 months showed that the mean weight, body mass index, waist circumference, and fat mass increased, whereas the percentage of lean body mass decreased compared with the baseline.[70] Breast cancer survivors are also at higher risk for development of MS. A study of 53 breast cancer survivors showed that, compared with surgery alone, patients undergoing chemotherapy are at higher risk for weight gain, increase in body fat percentage and fat mass, and decrease in lean body mass.[71] Breast cancer survivors with MS are at higher risk for cancer recurrence than those without MS.[72]

Secondary Malignancies

Cancer survivors are at high risk to develop second cancers.[73,74] This increased risk could be caused by genetic predisposition, consequence of previous cancer treatment, undergoing surveillance following first cancer treatment completion, or environmental factors.[75,76] In particular, patients who receive chemotherapy are at 4.7-fold higher risk for developing treatment-related acute myeloid leukemia (AML) compared with the general population. Nearly half of 801 cases of treatment-related AML from 1975 to 2008 occurred in breast cancer or non-Hodgkin lymphoma survivors.[77] Patients who have received topoisomerase II inhibitors (eg, doxorubicin, etoposide, irinotecan) usually develop leukemia within 5 years, and those who receive alkylating agents (eg, cyclophosphamide) develop leukemia after 5 years.[78] The incidence of leukemia also correlates with the dose of chemotherapy that patients receive.[79,80] Hodgkin lymphoma survivors are at particularly high risk for developing leukemia,[81] which is particularly related to the dose of alkylating agents. Although, with recent treatments,[82] the incidence of leukemia has been shown to have decreased, it still is worth considering when taking care of cancer survivors. In a similar fashion, patients with non-Hodgkin lymphoma are at higher risk for developing leukemia within 10 years of treatment completion.[83]

Sexual and Vaginal Dysfunction

Cancer and its associated treatment can have a major effect on vaginal health and sexuality. Disease type, stage of disease, and type of treatment can contribute or compound atrophy of the vagina and vulvar tissues, resulting in painful gynecologic examinations, sexual difficulties, and other long-term issues.[84–87] Estrogen deprivation effects include vulvovaginal atrophy (VVA), with the loss of genital tissue elasticity and lubrication, and symptoms of dryness, irritation, itching, discharge, and dyspareunia. Estrogen deprivation–associated VVA can lead to loss of sexual desire and arousal, and orgasm difficulties stemming from vaginal dryness, pain, and stenosis.[88] Older patients with cancer may mistakenly believe that sexual/vaginal changes are an inevitable result of aging rather than recognizing that cancer treatment may be a contributing factor.[89] For example, many women treated with extended endocrine therapy, specifically AIs, develop vaginal dryness, gross architectural vulvar changes, and so forth. Radiation therapy to the pelvis can cause agglutination, ulceration, stenosis, scarring, and a reduction in vaginal depth, elasticity, and sexual function. Long-term bowel issues and fear of urinary and fecal incontinence after treatment are significant concerns that can also interfere with sexual activity. Furthermore, radical vulvar excisions are significantly associated with lower sexual function and quality of life, particularly in older women. Patients have indicated a need for basic advice on the prevention and treatment of vaginal and sexual toxicities and welcome discussions on these topics with their doctors. These issues do not spontaneously resolve over time without appropriate intervention. Early identification and treatment strategies are essential in addressing these long-term challenges; physician-patient communication is imperative, and may be enhanced with the use of brief surveys and checklists.[90]

Fatigue

One of the most common long-term side effects of cancer therapy is fatigue. The symptom of fatigue that patients with cancer experience is different from the symptoms that health people experience. The feelings of fatigue that healthy people feel are often alleviated by sleep and rest. Patients who have undergone cancer treatment get fatigued after less activity than those who have not had cancer. Fatigue can affect quality of life. The cause of this symptom is multifactorial and can include the long-term effects of therapy (eg, chemotherapy, radiation, biologic therapy, surgery), anemia, nutrition, anxiety and depression, sleep disorders, and drugs. Polypharmacy, which is common in the elderly, can contribute. Specific drugs, such as anxiolytics, sleeping medicine, narcotics, and drugs that treat neuropathy (eg, gabapentin, pregabalin), contribute to this syndrome. Pharmacologic interventions have been unsuccessful unless a specific diagnosis (ie, depression) can be made.[91]

Cognitive Impairment

Many patients undergoing chemotherapy complain of cognitive changes (chemotherapy-related cognitive impairment [CRCI]).[92] These complaints are usually broad and range from distraction and lack of focus, to inability to perform daily cognitive routines (eg, paying bills).[93] Although at times subjective complaints do not correlate with the objective assessments,[94] it is vital to appreciate such complaints. Most studies on CRCI have been conducted in breast cancer survivors. In this setting, cognitive deficit usually involves certain domains of cognition (eg, verbal ability or visuospatial),[95] which could be long lasting.[96] It can develop after completion of the treatment,[97] but, in some cases, cognition may improve following completion of the treatment.[98] Hormone receptor–positive patients with breast cancer usually take antiestrogen treatments (eg, tamoxifen, exemestane), which may affect their cognition. Patients on the 5-year tamoxifen regimen reported memory complaints more than those who were not taking tamoxifen.[99] As with chemotherapy, cognitive deficit occurred in specific domains of cognition (verbal memory, verbal functioning, verbal fluency, and information processing speed).[100,101] The other common cancer is prostate cancer. Patients may require ADT, the intention being to reduce the testosterone level. About half of all patients with prostate cancer on ADT could have cognitive decline in at least 1 domain of cognition.[102,103] Like breast cancer treatment, prolonged use of ADT leads to decline in specific domains of cognition, as noted previously.[104] Patients with other types of cancer (eg, colorectal) experience the same phenomena.[105]

EFFECT OF OTHER MODALITIES
Targeted Therapies

In the past 10 to 15 years, the emergence of a new class of cancer treatment known as targeted agents has changed the spectrum of cancer treatment. In some instances, patients with metastatic disease can receive targeted agents for months or even years. In brief, targeted therapies are either monoclonal antibodies to certain proliferation or antiapoptotic proteins, or are inhibitors of pathways that signal cell proliferation.[18] These therapies are not often associated with long-term toxicities. Many of the adverse events are short lived or reversible (**Table 4**). The most common targets for these agents are epidermal growth factor receptor (EGFR), vascular endothelial growth factor (VEGF), human epidermal receptor-2 (HER2), mammalian target of rapamycin (m-TOR), and B-raf proto-oncogene, serine/threonine kinase (BRAF). Agents that target EGFR can cause skin rash, diarrhea, and electrolyte abnormalities (eg, hypomagnesemia). The toxicity of VEGF-targeted agents include hypertension, fatigue, wound healing, and thrombosis. Because of vascular toxicity they are associated with increased risk in older patients.[106] m-TOR inhibitors, especially temsirolimus, can cause hyperlipidemia and hyperglycemia. Patients who take BRAF inhibitors can develop skin cancer. Trastuzumab is associated with cardiomyopathy.

Table 4
Toxicities of targeted agents

Cancer	Name of Agent	Target	Common Side Effects
Non–small cell lung cancer	Erlotinib	EGFR	Rash, fatigue, appetite loss
	Gefitinib	EGFR	Rash, diarrhea
	Pazopanib	ALK-4	Edema, fatigue, diarrhea, visual disturbances
Renal cell carcinoma	Sunitinib	Mutikinase	Hand and foot syndrome,
	Pazopanib	Multikinase	hypertension, fatigue, rash, edema, hyperlipidemia, hyperglycemia
	Temsirolimus	m-TOR	Hypertension, fatigue, diarrhea
	Axitinib	VEGF	Hypertension, rash, diarrhea, fatigue
Colorectal cancer	Cetuximab	EGFR	Rash, diarrhea
	Panitumumab	EGFR	Rash, diarrhea
	Regorafenib	Kinase, VEGF	Hypertension, fatigue, hand and foot syndrome, proteinuria
	Aflibercept	VEGF	Hypertension, fatigue, diarrhea
Breast cancer	Trastuzumab	HER2	Heart failure
	Pertuzumab	HER2	Diarrhea, skin rash, heart failure
	Trastuzumab emtansine	HER2	Fatigue, skin rash, arthralgia, heart failure
	Lapatinib	Kinase	Skin rash, hand and foot syndrome, diarrhea
Renal cell carcinoma, hepatocellular carcinoma	Sorafenib	Multikinase	Hypertension, diarrhea, fatigue, hand and foot syndrome
Colorectal cancer, ovarian cancer	Bevacizumab	VEGF	Hypertension, thrombosis, proteinuria, delayed wound healing
Renal cell carcinoma, breast cancer	Everolimus	m-TOR	Stomatitis, diarrhea
Melanoma	Vemurafenib	BRAF kinase	Fatigue, arthralgia, skin cancer
	Dabrafenib	BRAF kinase	Fatigue, fever, arthralgia
	Ipilimumab	CTLA-4	Immune-mediated reactions (eg, diarrhea, fever, fatigue)
Chronic myeloid leukemia, GIST	Imatinib	Kinase	Edema, diarrhea, rash

Abbreviations: ALK-4, activin like kinase; CTLA4, cytotoxic T lymphocyte–associated protein 4; EGFR, epidermal growth factor receptor; GIST, gastrointestinal stromal tumors; HER, human epidermal receptor; m-TOR, mammalian target of rapamycin inhibitor.

Long-term Toxicities of Radiation

Radiation therapy has a substantial role in treating many prevalent and frequently curable malignancies, notably breast and prostate cancer. Radiotherapy can induce chronic, nonlethal changes in nonproliferating normal tissues, with fibrosis being the prototypical example. The potential late toxicities in a given patient depend on the anatomic region, volume of tissue that was irradiated, radiation dose, and use of concurrent chemotherapy. Modern tools, such as intensity-modulated radiation therapy, image-guided radiation therapy, and proton therapy, reduce the incidence and severity of late toxicity. There is also a small risk of radiation-induced secondary malignancies, typically solid tumors arising within or near the irradiated field, ten or more years after treatment.

Central nervous system

Brain radiation is most commonly used for patients with brain metastases or for gliomas. However, brain radiation is also used for less lethal tumors, such as meningioma. Studies indicate that short-term memory is the faculty most likely to be chronically impaired when radiating the brain.[107] Stereotactic radiosurgery, which can treat meningiomas, isolated brain metastases, or benign conditions such as arteriovenous malformations, also carries a risk of necrosis in the brain tissue adjacent to the target. This necrosis can cause seizures or focal neurologic deficits, months or years after treatment.[108]

Neck and upper aerodigestive tract

Radiation therapy is often used as curative or postsurgical treatment of primary head and neck tumors. Although highly effective and often allowing organ preservation, radiation therapy to this region is associated with perhaps the most frequently apparent late radiation toxicity. Permanent xerostomia caused by incidental irradiation of the parotid glands is very common and significantly affects patient quality of life. Fibrosis of the skin and connective tissue can lead to trismus and restricted range of motion in the neck. Hypothyroidism is commonly induced by head-and-neck radiotherapy, and the incidence of carotid artery stenosis after radiation has been reported to be as high as 50%.[109] Brachial plexus injury is also possible.

Thorax

Breast or chest-wall radiation for breast cancer is among the most common indications for radiation therapy and long-term survival is likely. The most common late effects include poor cosmesis (eg, skin hyperpigmentation), fibrosis limiting range of motion in the arm, and lymphedema. Radiation pneumonitis, which is a delayed inflammatory response to lung irradiation, is a subacute toxicity typically occurring within a few months to 1 year after radiotherapy. It can recur and increase the risk of radiation fibrosis, which is a chronic scarring and inactivation of lung tissue. Radiation pneumonitis is typically treated successfully with corticosteroids, but there is no established therapy for radiation-induced lung fibrosis.[110] Cardiac irradiation increases the risk of heart disease, as has been apparent from the experience with long-term survivors of Hodgkin lymphoma, and also from patients with left-sided breast cancer.[111,112]

Gastrointestinal

The largest population of gastrointestinal patients with potential late radiation toxicity is patients with rectal cancer, owing to the routine use of preoperative radiation in this prevalent and frequently cured disease. Pelvic radiation therapy can diminish bowel function, leading to chronic diarrhea, rectal bleeding, or incontinence.[113] Radiotherapy to the abdomen or pelvis also increases the risk of small bowel obstruction. Radiation for pancreatic and esophagogastric cancers increases the risk of serious mucosal injury to the stomach, duodenum, or bowel.

SUMMARY

The aging of the population and the success of cancer therapy have resulted in a large number of older cancer survivors. The chronic toxicity of therapy combined with the comorbidities seen in this population make long-term management challenging. To provide optimum care, survivorship guidelines are being formulated. These guidelines will provide oncologists, primary care physicians, and geriatricians with an organized framework to take care of these patients. In 2005, the Institute of Medicine published a report entitled *From Cancer Patient to Cancer Survivor: Lost in Transition*. This report describes recommendations for ongoing guidelines for cancer survivors, the cancer team, primary care physicians, and other health care providers. The report recommends that, at the completion of cancer treatment, clinicians provide a survivorship care plan that includes the summary of treatment delivered and a detailed plan of ongoing care, as well as surveillance guidelines, potential late effects, and potential behavioral modifications that patients can make, such as weight management, modified alcohol intake, and regular exercise.[114]

REFERENCES

1. DeSantis CE, Lin CC, Mariotto AB, et al. Cancer treatment and survivorship statistics, 2014. CA Cancer J Clin 2014;64:252–71.
2. Siegel R, Ma J, Zou Z, et al. Cancer statistics, 2014. CA Cancer J Clin 2014;64: 9–29.
3. Potosky AL, Han PK, Rowland J, et al. Differences between primary care physicians' and oncologists' knowledge, attitudes and practices regarding the care of cancer survivors. J Gen Intern Med 2011;26:1403–10.
4. Klabunde CN, Han PKJ, Earle CC, et al. Physician roles in the cancer-related follow-up care of cancer survivors. Fam Med 2013;45:463–74.
5. Rockwood K. What would make a definition of frailty successful? Age Ageing 2005;34:432–4.
6. Schuurmans H, Steverink N, Lindenberg S, et al. Old or frail: what tells us more? J Gerontol A Biol Sci Med Sci 2004;59:M962–5.
7. Mohile SG, Xian Y, Dale W, et al. Association of a cancer diagnosis with vulnerability and frailty in older Medicare beneficiaries. J Natl Cancer Inst 2009;101: 1206–15.
8. Flood KL, Carroll MB, Le CV, et al. Geriatric syndromes in elderly patients admitted to an oncology-acute care for elders unit. J Clin Oncol 2006;24: 2298–303.
9. Bylow K, Mohile SG, Stadler WM, et al. Does androgen-deprivation therapy accelerate the development of frailty in older men with prostate cancer? Cancer 2007;110:2604–13.
10. Caplan GA, Williams AJ, Daly B, et al. A randomized, controlled trial of comprehensive geriatric assessment and multidisciplinary intervention after discharge of elderly from the emergency department—the DEED II study. J Am Geriatr Soc 2004;52:1417–23.
11. Vidán M, Serra JA, Moreno C, et al. Efficacy of a comprehensive geriatric intervention in older patients hospitalized for hip fracture: a randomized, controlled trial. J Am Geriatr Soc 2005;53:1476–82.

12. Hurria A, Togawa K, Mohile SG, et al. Predicting chemotherapy toxicity in older adults with cancer: a prospective multicenter study. J Clin Oncol 2011;29: 3457–65.

13. Extermann M, Boler I, Reich RR, et al. Predicting the risk of chemotherapy toxicity in older patients: the Chemotherapy Risk Assessment Scale for High-age Patients (CRASH) score. Cancer 2012;118:3377–86.

14. Kristjansson SR, Nesbakken A, Jordhøy MS, et al. Comprehensive geriatric assessment can predict complications in elderly patients after elective surgery for colorectal cancer: a prospective observational cohort study. Crit Rev Oncol Hematol 2010;76:208–17.

15. Kristjansson SR, Jordhøy MS, Nesbakken A, et al: Which elements of a comprehensive geriatric assessment (CGA) predict post-operative complications and early mortality after colorectal cancer surgery? J Geriatr Oncol 2010;1:57–65.

16. Caillet P, Canoui-Poitrine F, Vouriot J, et al. Comprehensive geriatric assessment in the decision-making process in elderly patients with cancer: ELCAPA study. J Clin Oncol 2011;29:3636–42.

17. Chaïbi P, Magné N, Breton S, et al. Influence of geriatric consultation with comprehensive geriatric assessment on final therapeutic decision in elderly cancer patients. Crit Rev Oncol Hematol 2011;79:302–7.

18. Kelly CM, Power DG, Lichtman SM. Targeted therapy in older patients with solid tumors. J Clin Oncol 2014;32:2635–46.

19. Schmitz KH, Prosnitz RG, Schwartz AL, et al. Prospective surveillance and management of cardiac toxicity and health in breast cancer survivors. Cancer 2012; 118:2270–6.

20. Yeh ETH, Bickford CL. Cardiovascular complications of cancer therapy: incidence, pathogenesis, diagnosis, and management. J Am Coll Cardiol 2009; 53:2231–47.

21. Patnaik JL, Byers T, DiGuiseppi C, et al. Cardiovascular disease competes with breast cancer as the leading cause of death for older females diagnosed with breast cancer: a retrospective cohort study. Breast Cancer Res 2011;13:R64.

22. Ryberg M, Nielsen D, Cortese G, et al. New insight into epirubicin cardiac toxicity: competing risks analysis of 1097 breast cancer patients. J Natl Cancer Inst 2008;100:1058–67.

23. Smith L, Cornelius V, Plummer C, et al. Cardiotoxicity of anthracycline agents for the treatment of cancer: systematic review and meta-analysis of randomised controlled trials. BMC Cancer 2010;10:337.

24. Pinder M, Duan Z, Goodwin J, et al. Congestive heart failure in older women treated with adjuvant anthracycline chemotherapy for breast cancer. J Clin Oncol 2007;25:3808–15.

25. O'Farrell S, Garmo H, Holmberg L, et al. Risk and timing of cardiovascular disease after androgen-deprivation therapy in men with prostate cancer. J Clin Oncol 2015;33(11):1243–51.

26. Taylor LG, Canfield SE, Du XL. Review of major adverse effects of androgen-deprivation therapy in men with prostate cancer. Cancer 2009;115:2388–99.

27. Saigal CS, Gore JL, Krupski TL, et al. Androgen deprivation therapy increases cardiovascular morbidity in men with prostate cancer. Cancer 2007;110:1493–500.

28. Tsai HK, D'Amico AV, Sadetsky N, et al. Androgen deprivation therapy for localized prostate cancer and the risk of cardiovascular mortality. J Natl Cancer Inst 2007;99:1516–24.

29. Saif MW, Shah MM, Shah AR. Fluoropyrimidine-associated cardiotoxicity: revisited. Expert Opin Drug Saf 2009;8:191–202.

30. Curigliano G, Mayer EL, Burstein HJ, et al. Cardiac toxicity from systemic cancer therapy: a comprehensive review. Prog Cardiovasc Dis 2010;53:94–104.

31. Miller BE, Pittman B, Strong C. Gynecologic cancer patients' psychosocial needs and their views on the physician's role in meeting those needs. Int J Gynecol Cancer 2003;13:111–9.

32. Mitchell AJ, Ferguson DW, Gill J, et al. Depression and anxiety in long-term cancer survivors compared with spouses and healthy controls: a systematic review and meta-analysis. Lancet Oncol 2013;14:721–32.

33. Recklitis CJ, Zhou ES, Zwemer EK, et al. Suicidal ideation in prostate cancer survivors: Understanding the role of physical and psychological health outcomes. Cancer 2014;120:3393–400.

34. Ding D, Allman BL, Salvi R. Review: ototoxic characteristics of platinum antitumor drugs. Anat Rec (Hoboken) 2012;295:1851–67.

35. Brydøy M, Oldenburg J, Klepp O, et al. Observational study of prevalence of long-term Raynaud-like phenomena and neurological side effects in testicular cancer survivors. J Natl Cancer Inst 2009;101:1682–95.

36. Lin FR, Ferrucci L. Hearing loss and falls among older adults in the United States. Arch Intern Med 2012;172:369–71.

37. Lin FR, Yaffe K, Xia J, et al. Hearing loss and cognitive decline in older adults. JAMA Intern Med 2013;173:293–9.

38. Ciorba A, Bianchini C, Pelucchi S, et al. The impact of hearing loss on the quality of life of elderly adults. Clin Interv Aging 2012;7:159–63.

39. Ambrose AF, Paul G, Hausdorff JM. Risk factors for falls among older adults: a review of the literature. Maturitas 2013;75:51–61.

40. Muir SW, Gopaul K, Montero Odasso MM. The role of cognitive impairment in fall risk among older adults: a systematic review and meta-analysis. Age Ageing 2012;41:299–308.

41. Horak FB. Postural orientation and equilibrium: what do we need to know about neural control of balance to prevent falls? Age Ageing 2006;35:ii7–11.

42. Smith EML, Pang H, Cirrincione C, et al. Effect of duloxetine on pain, function, and quality of life among patients with chemotherapy-induced painful peripheral neuropathy: a randomized clinical trial. JAMA 2013;309:1359–67.

43. Ward PR, Wong MD, Moore R, et al. Fall-related injuries in elderly cancer patients treated with neurotoxic chemotherapy: a retrospective cohort study. J Geriatr Oncol 2014;5:57–64.

44. Grisold W, Cavaletti G, Windebank AJ. Peripheral neuropathies from chemotherapeutics and targeted agents: diagnosis, treatment, and prevention. Neuro Oncol 2012;14:iv45–54.

45. Lichtman SM, Hurria A, Cirrincione CT, et al. Paclitaxel efficacy and toxicity in older women with metastatic breast cancer: combined analysis of CALGB 9342 and 9840. Ann Oncol 2012;23:632–8.

46. Lichtman SM, Wildiers H, Chatelut E, et al. International Society of Geriatric Oncology Chemotherapy Taskforce: evaluation of chemotherapy in older patients–an analysis of the medical literature. J Clin Oncol 2007;25: 1832–43.

47. Chaudhry V, Chaudhry M, Crawford TO, et al. Toxic neuropathy in patients with pre-existing neuropathy. Neurology 2003;60:337–40.

48. Quasthoff S, Hartung HP. Chemotherapy-induced peripheral neuropathy. J Neurol 2002;249:9–17.

49. Cavaletti G, Nobile-Orazio E. Bortezomib-induced peripheral neurotoxicity: still far from a painless gain. Haematologica 2007;92:1308–10.

50. Cavaletti G, Marmiroli P. Chemotherapy-induced peripheral neurotoxicity. Curr Opin Neurol 2015;28:500–7.

51. VanderWalde A, Hurria A. Aging and osteoporosis in breast and prostate cancer. CA Cancer J Clin 2011;61:139–56.

52. Chen Z, Maricic M, Bassford TL, et al. Fracture risk among breast cancer survivors: results from the Women's Health Initiative observational study. Arch Intern Med 2005;165:552–8.

53. Gallagher JC. Effect of early menopause on bone mineral density and fractures. Menopause 2007;14:567–71.

54. Taxel P, Choksi P, Van Poznak C. The management of osteoporosis in breast cancer survivors. Maturitas 2012;73:275–9.

55. Becker T, Lipscombe L, Narod S, et al. Systematic review of bone health in older women treated with aromatase inhibitors for early-stage breast cancer. J Am Geriatr Soc 2012;60:1761–7.

56. Bines J, Oleske DM, Cobleigh MA. Ovarian function in premenopausal women treated with adjuvant chemotherapy for breast cancer. J Clin Oncol 1996;14: 1718–29.

57. Shahinian VB, Kuo Y-F, Freeman JL, et al. Risk of fracture after androgen deprivation for prostate cancer. N Engl J Med 2005;352:154–64.

58. Khan NF, Mant D, Carpenter L, et al. Long-term health outcomes in a British cohort of breast, colorectal and prostate cancer survivors: a database study. Br J Cancer 2011;105:S29–37.

59. Chen Z, Maricic M, Pettinger M, et al. Osteoporosis and rate of bone loss among postmenopausal survivors of breast cancer. Cancer 2005;104:1520–30.

60. Hoff AO, Gagel RF. Osteoporosis in breast and prostate cancer survivors. Oncology (Williston Park) 2005;19:651–8.

61. Saad F, Adachi JD, Brown JP, et al. Cancer treatment–induced bone loss in breast and prostate cancer. J Clin Oncol 2008;26:5465–76.

62. Hillner BE, Ingle JN, Chlebowski RT, et al. American Society of Clinical Oncology 2003 update on the role of bisphosphonates and bone health issues in women with breast cancer. J Clin Oncol 2003;21:4042–57.

63. Gralow JR, Biermann JS, Farooki A, et al. NCCN task force report: bone health in cancer care. J Natl Compr Canc Netw 2009;7:S1–32.

64. Grundy SM, Brewer HB, Cleeman JI, et al. Definition of metabolic syndrome: report of the National Heart, Lung, and Blood Institute/American Heart Association conference on scientific issues related to definition. Circulation 2004;109:433–8.

65. Nuver J, Smit AJ, Postma A, et al. The metabolic syndrome in long-term cancer survivors, and important target for secondary preventive measures. Cancer Treat Rev 2002;28:195–214.

66. de Haas EC, Oosting SF, Lefrandt JD, et al. The metabolic syndrome in cancer survivors. Lancet Oncol 2010;11:193–203.

67. Traish AM, Guay A, Feeley R, et al. The dark side of testosterone deficiency: I. metabolic syndrome and erectile dysfunction. J Androl 2009;30:10–22.

68. Carr MC. The emergence of the metabolic syndrome with menopause. J Clin Endocrinol Metab 2003;88:2404–11.

69. Braga-Basaria M, Dobs AS, Muller DC, et al. Metabolic syndrome in men with prostate cancer undergoing long-term androgen-deprivation therapy. J Clin Oncol 2006;24:3979–83.

70. Smith MR, Lee H, McGovern F, et al. Metabolic changes during gonadotropin-releasing hormone agonist therapy for prostate cancer: differences from the classic metabolic syndrome. Cancer 2008;112:2188–94.

71. Demark-Wahnefried W, Peterson BL, Winer EP, et al. Changes in weight, body composition, and factors influencing energy balance among premenopausal breast cancer patients receiving adjuvant chemotherapy. J Clin Oncol 2001; 19:2381–9.
72. Calip G, Malone K, Gralow J, et al. Metabolic syndrome and outcomes following early-stage breast cancer. Breast Cancer Res Treat 2014;148:363–77.
73. Demark-Wahnefried W, Aziz NM, Rowland JH, et al. Riding the crest of the teachable moment: promoting long-term health after the diagnosis of cancer. J Clin Oncol 2005;23:5814–30.
74. Aziz NM, Rowland JH. Trends and advances in cancer survivorship research: challenge and opportunity. Semin Radiat Oncol 2003;13:248–66.
75. Aziz NM. Cancer survivorship research: challenge and opportunity. J Nutr 2002; 132:3494s–503s.
76. Travis LB. Therapy-associated solid tumors. Acta Oncol 2002;41:323–33.
77. Morton LM, Dores GM, Tucker MA, et al. Evolving risk of therapy-related acute myeloid leukemia following cancer chemotherapy among adults in the United States, 1975-2008. Blood 2013;121:2996–3004.
78. Pedersen-Bjergaard J, Pedersen M, Roulston D, et al. Different genetic pathways in leukemogenesis for patients presenting with therapy-related myelodysplasia and therapy-related acute myeloid leukemia. Blood 1995;86(9):3542–52.
79. Praga C, Bergh J, Bliss J, et al. Risk of acute myeloid leukemia and myelodysplastic syndrome in trials of adjuvant epirubicin for early breast cancer: correlation with doses of epirubicin and cyclophosphamide. J Clin Oncol 2005;23:4179–91.
80. Smith RE, Bryant J, DeCillis A, et al. Acute myeloid leukemia and myelodysplastic syndrome after doxorubicin-cyclophosphamide adjuvant therapy for operable breast cancer: the National Surgical Adjuvant Breast and Bowel Project experience. J Clin Oncol 2003;21:1195–204.
81. Hodgson D, van Leeuwen F. Second malignancy risk after treatment of Hodgkin lymphoma. In: Engert A, Younes A, editors. Hodgkin Lymphoma. A Comprehensive Overview. New York: Springer International Publishing; 2015. p. 375–409.
82. Koontz MZ, Horning SJ, Balise R, et al. Risk of therapy-related secondary leukemia in Hodgkin lymphoma: the Stanford University experience over three generations of clinical trials. J Clin Oncol 2013;31:592–8.
83. Armitage JO, Carbone PP, Connors JM, et al. Treatment-related myelodysplasia and acute leukemia in non-Hodgkin's lymphoma patients. J Clin Oncol 2003;21: 897–906.
84. Palacios S, Tobar AC, Menendez C. Sexuality in the climacteric years. Maturitas 2002;43(Suppl 1):S69–77.
85. Matulonis UA, Kornblith A, Lee H, et al. Long-term adjustment of early-stage ovarian cancer survivors. Int J Gynecol Cancer 2008;18:1183–93.
86. Lindau ST, Schumm LP, Laumann EO, et al. A study of sexuality and health among older adults in the United States. N Engl J Med 2007;357:762–74.
87. Laumann EO, Paik A, Rosen RC. Sexual dysfunction in the United States: prevalence and predictors. JAMA 1999;281:537–44.
88. Carter J, Goldfrank D, Schover LR. Simple strategies for vaginal health promotion in cancer survivors. J Sex Med 2011;8:549–59.
89. Katz A: Breaking the silence on cancer and sexuality: a handbook for healthcare providers. Pittsburg (CA): Oncology Nursing Society; 2007.
90. Stabile C, Steed R, Carter J. Sexual medicine in the management of older gynecologic cancer patients. In: Lichtman SM, Audisio RA, editors. Management of gynecological cancers in older women. London: Springer; 2013. p. 349–66.

91. Mucke M, Mochamat, Cuhls H, et al. Pharmacological treatments for fatigue associated with palliative care. Cochrane Database Syst Rev 2015;(5):CD006788.

92. Tannock IF, Ahles TA, Ganz PA, et al. Cognitive impairment associated with chemotherapy for cancer: report of a workshop. J Clin Oncol 2004;22:2233–9.

93. Hess LM, Insel KC. Chemotherapy-related change in cognitive function: a conceptual model. Oncol Nurs Forum 2007;34:981–94.

94. Hutchinson AD, Hosking JR, Kichenadasse G, et al. Objective and subjective cognitive impairment following chemotherapy for cancer: a systematic review. Cancer Treat Rev 2012;38:926–34.

95. Jim HSL, Phillips KM, Chait S, et al. Meta-analysis of cognitive functioning in breast cancer survivors previously treated with standard-dose chemotherapy. J Clin Oncol 2012;30:3578–87.

96. Ganz PA, Kwan L, Castellon SA, et al. Cognitive complaints after breast cancer treatments: examining the relationship with neuropsychological test performance. J Natl Cancer Inst 2013;105(11):791–801.

97. Wefel JS, Saleeba AK, Buzdar AU, et al. Acute and late onset cognitive dysfunction associated with chemotherapy in women with breast cancer. Cancer 2010; 116:3348–56.

98. Ono M, Ogilvie JM, Wilson JS, et al. A meta-analysis of cognitive impairment and decline associated with adjuvant chemotherapy in women with breast cancer. Front Oncol 2015;5:59.

99. Paganini-Hill A, Clark L. Preliminary assessment of cognitive function in breast cancer patients treated with tamoxifen. Breast Cancer Res Treat 2000;64: 165–76.

100. Schilder CM, Seynaeve C, Beex LV, et al. Effects of tamoxifen and exemestane on cognitive functioning of postmenopausal patients with breast cancer: results from the neuropsychological side study of the tamoxifen and exemestane adjuvant multinational trial. J Clin Oncol 2010;28:1294–300.

101. Schilder CM, Eggens PC, Seynaeve C, et al. Neuropsychological functioning in postmenopausal breast cancer patients treated with tamoxifen or exemestane after AC-chemotherapy: cross-sectional findings from the neuropsychological TEAM-side study. Acta Oncol 2009;48:76–85.

102. Nelson CJ, Lee JS, Gamboa MC, et al. Cognitive effects of hormone therapy in men with prostate cancer: a review. Cancer 2008;113:1097–106.

103. Jamadar RJ, Winters MJ, Maki PM. Cognitive changes associated with ADT: a review of the literature. Asian J Androl 2012;14:232–8.

104. Jim HSL, Small BJ, Patterson S, et al. Cognitive impairment in men treated with luteinizing hormone-releasing hormone agonists for prostate cancer: a controlled comparison. Support Care Cancer 2010;18:21–7.

105. Vardy J, Dhillon HM, Pond GR, et al. Cognitive function and fatigue after diagnosis of colorectal cancer. Ann Oncol 2014;25:2404–12.

106. Sclafani F, Cunningham D. Bevacizumab in elderly patients with metastatic colorectal cancer. J Geriatr Oncol 2014;5:78–88.

107. Sun A, Bae K, Gore EM, et al. Phase III trial of prophylactic cranial irradiation compared with observation in patients with locally advanced non-small-cell lung cancer: neurocognitive and quality-of-life analysis. J Clin Oncol 2011;29: 279–86.

108. Soussain C, Ricard D, Fike JR, et al. CNS complications of radiotherapy and chemotherapy. Lancet 2009;374:1639–51.

109. Abayomi OK. Neck irradiation, carotid injury and its consequences. Oral Oncol 2004;40:872–8.

110. Graves PR, Siddiqui F, Anscher MS, et al. Radiation pulmonary toxicity: from mechanisms to management. Semin Radiat Oncol 2010;20:201–7.
111. Hancock SL, Tucker MA, Hoppe RT. Factors affecting late mortality from heart disease after treatment of Hodgkin's disease. JAMA 1993;270:1949–55.
112. Darby SC, Ewertz M, McGale P, et al. Risk of ischemic heart disease in women after radiotherapy for breast cancer. N Engl J Med 2013;368:987–98.
113. Peeters KC, van de Velde CJ, Leer JW, et al. Late side effects of short-course preoperative radiotherapy combined with total mesorectal excision for rectal cancer: increased bowel dysfunction in irradiated patients–a Dutch colorectal cancer group study. J Clin Oncol 2005;23:6199–206.
114. Available at: https://www.iom.edu/Reports/2005/From-Cancer-Patient-to-Cancer-Survivor-Lost-in-Transition.aspx. Accessed June 28, 2015.
115. Borson S, Scanlan JM, Chen P, et al. The Mini-Cog as a screen for dementia: validation in a population-based sample. J Am Geriatr Soc 2003;51:1451–4.
116. Crum RM, Anthony JC, Bassett SS, et al. Population-based norms for the Mini-Mental State Examination by age and educational level. JAMA 1993;269:2386–91.
117. Nasreddine ZS, Phillips NA, Bedirian V, et al. The Montreal Cognitive Assessment, MoCA: a brief screening tool for mild cognitive impairment. J Am Geriatr Soc 2005;53:695–9.
118. King S, Green HJ. Psychological intervention for improving cognitive function in cancer survivors: a literature review and randomized controlled trial. Front Oncol 2015;5:72.
119. Holland JC, Andersen B, Breitbart WS, et al. Distress management. J Natl Compr Canc Netw 2013;11:190–209.
120. Yesavage JA, Brink TL, Rose TL, et al. Development and validation of a geriatric depression screening scale: a preliminary report. J Psychiatr Res 1982;17:37–49.
121. Kroenke K, Spitzer RL, Williams JBW. The PHQ-9: validity of a brief depression severity measure. J Gen Intern Med 2001;16:606–13.
122. Penedo FJ, Traeger L, Dahn J, et al. Cognitive behavioral stress management intervention improves quality of life in Spanish monolingual Hispanic men treated for localized prostate cancer: results of a randomized controlled trial. Int J Behav Med 2007;14:164–72.
123. Gil K, Mishel M, Belyea M, et al. Benefits of the uncertainty management intervention for African American and white older breast cancer survivors: 20-month outcomes. Int J Behav Med 2006;13:286–94.
124. Hart SL, Hoyt MA, Diefenbach M, et al. Meta-analysis of efficacy of interventions for elevated depressive symptoms in adults diagnosed with cancer. J Natl Cancer Inst 2012;104(13):990–1004.
125. Fong DYT, Ho JWC, Hui BPH, et al. Physical activity for cancer survivors: meta-analysis of randomised controlled trials. BMJ 2012;344:e70.
126. Lichtenstein MJ, Bess FH, Logan SA. Diagnostic performance of the hearing handicap inventory for the elderly (screening version) against differing definitions of hearing loss. Ear Hear 1988;9:208–11.
127. Chou R, Dana T, Bougatsos C, et al. Screening adults aged 50 years or older for hearing loss: a review of the evidence for the U.S. Preventive Services Task Force. Ann Intern Med 2011;154:347–55.
128. Yueh B, Shapiro N, MacLean CH, et al. Screening and management of adult hearing loss in primary care: scientific review. JAMA 2003;289:1976–85.

129. Aziz MT, Good BL, Lowe DK. Serotonin-norepinephrine reuptake inhibitors for the management of chemotherapy-induced peripheral neuropathy. Ann Pharmacother 2014;48:626–32.

130. Grisold W, Vass A, Schmidhammer R, et al. Rehabilitation of neuropathies. Critical Reviews in Physical and Rehabilitation Medicine 2007;19:19–53.

131. Stubblefield MD. Cancer rehabilitation. Semin Oncol 2011;38:386–93.

132. US Preventive Services Task Force. Screening for osteoporosis in postmenopausal women: recommendations and rationale. Ann Intern Med 2002;137: 526–8.

133. Feskanich D, Willett W, Colditz G. Walking and leisure-time activity and risk of hip fracture in postmenopausal women. JAMA 2002;288:2300–6.

134. Li F, Harmer P, Fisher KJ, et al. Tai Chi and fall reductions in older adults: a randomized controlled trial. J Gerontol A Biol Sci Med Sci 2005;60:187–94.

135. Nikolaus T, Bach M. Preventing falls in community-dwelling frail older people using a home intervention team (HIT): results from the randomized falls-HIT trial. J Am Geriatr Soc 2003;51:300–5.

136. Holick MF. Vitamin D deficiency. N Engl J Med 2007;357:266–81.

137. Hadji P, Aapro MS, Body JJ, et al. Management of aromatase inhibitor-associated bone loss in postmenopausal women with breast cancer: practical guidance for prevention and treatment. Ann Oncol 2011;22:2546–55.

138. Sun K, Liu J, Ning G. Active smoking and risk of metabolic syndrome: a meta-analysis of prospective studies. PLoS One 2012;7:e47791.

139. Kastorini CM, Milionis HJ, Esposito K, et al. The effect of Mediterranean diet on metabolic syndrome and its components: a meta-analysis of 50 studies and 534,906 individuals. J Am Coll Cardiol 2011;57:1299–313.

140. Strasser B. Physical activity in obesity and metabolic syndrome. Ann N Y Acad Sci 2013;1281:141–59.

Management of Lung Cancer in the Elderly

Ajeet Gajra, MD[a],*, Syed Ali Akbar, MBBS[b], Najam Ud Din, MBBS[b]

KEYWORDS

- Lung cancer • Elderly • Geriatric assessment • Palliative care • Early stage
- Advanced stage • Metastatic • Targeted therapy

KEY POINTS

- Lung cancer is a leading cause of cancer-associated mortality and affects the elderly disproportionately.
- Despite high prevalence, high-level evidence specific to the elderly is sparse in lung cancer.
- Fit elderly patients should be offered treatment plans similar to younger patient with the same disease features and stage.
- Geriatric assessment has a predictive role for chemotherapy-associated toxicity.
- Clear communication of palliative, non-curative intent, if such is the case, should be incorporated by the oncologist early in the treatment course.

INTRODUCTION

Demographics and Scope of the Problem

Lung cancer is the leading cause of cancer-related mortality and accounts for more than one-quarter of all cancer-related deaths in both men and women in the United States. It is estimated that in 2015 there will be 221,200 new diagnoses and 158,040 deaths attributable to lung cancer. The probability of developing lung cancer increases considerably as patients age; two-thirds of all new cases will occur in patients more than 65 years of age.[1] Although there is no uniform age cutoff for classifying patients as elderly across the globe, and the World Health Organization defines elderly as patients more than 65 years old, it is reasonable to assume that at the present time age 70 years is the accepted standard for such classification in the United States.[2] Non–small cell lung cancer (NSCLC) accounts for about 80% to 85% of all lung cancers and is of particular concern in elderly patients, and this is the focus of this article.[3] It is estimated that,

[a] Upstate Cancer Center, Upstate Medical University, 750 East Adams Street, Syracuse, NY 13210, USA; [b] Department of Medicine, Upstate Medical University, 750 East Adams Street, Syracuse, NY 13210, USA
* Corresponding author.
E-mail address: gajraa@upstate.edu

Clin Geriatr Med 32 (2016) 81–95
http://dx.doi.org/10.1016/j.cger.2015.08.008
0749-0690/16/$ – see front matter © 2016 Elsevier Inc. All rights reserved.

by the year 2030, the number of adults more than 65 years of age in the United States will have doubled, leading to a dramatic increase in the incidence of this disease. It is therefore imperative to study and streamline the management of this disease in the elderly population, which has so far been understudied.

Staging

The management of lung cancer is largely dependent on staging. The American Joint Commission for Cancer (AJCC) staging principles are used by oncologists to stage lung cancer. They are:

1. Early stage: corresponds with stage I and II on the AJCC classification. These tumors are typically amenable to surgery. For tumors larger than 4 cm or with nodal involvement, postoperative adjuvant chemotherapy with cisplatin-based combinations is recommended. For patients who are medically inoperable, radiotherapy or radiosurgery with curative intent is appropriate therapy.
2. Locally advanced disease: corresponds with stage III on the AJCC classification. This stage includes patients with locally (T3–4) and/or regionally (n2/3) advanced cancer. A few patients with limited nodal involvement, good pulmonary reserve, and excellent performance status (PS) may be candidates for surgery. Most are considered inoperable and ideally are treated with concurrent chemotherapy and radiation with curative intent. For the vulnerable or frail, radiation alone with curative or palliative intent may be used.
3. Distant metastatic disease: corresponds with stage IV on the AJCC classification and includes patients with bilateral lung cancer as well as pleural involvement. However, this group accounts for more than half the patients at diagnosis. These patients are typically treated with palliative intent with chemotherapy, targeted therapy, or biologic therapy. The incidence and survival by disease stage as discerned form Surveillance, Epidemiology, and End Results (SEER) is shown in **Fig. 1**. In addition, **Table 1** provides a practical approach to discussing the management of lung cancer.

PRINCIPLES OF MANAGEMENT
Early Stage Disease

Surgery for non–small cell lung cancer
Early stage lung cancer is, by definition, surgically resectable provided the patient is able to withstand thoracotomy medically and if postresection lung function will be

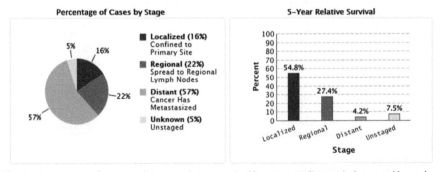

Fig. 1. Percentage of cases and 5-year relative survival by stage at diagnosis: lung and bronchus cancer. (*From* SEER Stat Fact Sheets: lung and bronchus cancer. Surveillance, Epidemiology, and End Results Program. Available at: http://seer.cancer.gov/statfacts/html/lungb.html. Accessed July 11, 2015.)

Table 1 Management principles based on stage in NSCLC		
Stage	**Ideal Treatment**	**Alternate Treatment**
Early stage (stage IA/IB)	Surgery	• Radiation/SBRT
Early stage but with limited regional spread; N1 disease (stage IIA/IIB)	Surgery followed by cisplatin-based chemotherapy	• Radiation ± chemotherapy if not a surgical candidate • After surgery if not a candidate for cisplatin, consider carboplatin-based chemotherapy
Locally and or regionally advanced disease (stage IIIA/IIIB)	Concurrent chemoradiotherapy for inoperable tumors	• Sequential radiation → chemotherapy • Radiation therapy alone (curative) • Radiation therapy (palliative)
Distant metastatic disease (stage IV)	Cytotoxic chemotherapy and/or targeted therapy	• Best supportive care

Palliative care and hospice should be involved early in the treatment course for elderly patients. Comprehensive geriatric assessment has a predictive role for chemotherapy-associated toxicity.
Abbreviation: SBRT, stereotactic body radiation therapy.

adequate without oxygen and other ventilator support. Age is reported as an independent predictor of postsurgical survival in patients with NSCLC.[4] It is also known that older patients are less likely to be offered surgical resection: only 70% of the population more than 75 years of age, compared with 92% of the younger population, was offered surgical resection ($P<.0001$). By the same token, the median survival of the different age groups was 71 months for those less than 65 years old and 28 months for patients who were more than 75 years old ($P<.0001$).[4] This result was likely based on patients' functional status and their comorbid conditions, which made them poor candidates for surgery. A more recent study, which took into account ongoing improvements in perioperative and intraoperative care in recent times, also showed that older patients are less likely to have curative surgical resection offered to them.[5] This retrospective analysis included 10,923 patients with a median age of 75 years and found that lobectomy was associated with the best long-term outcomes in elderly patients with early NSCLC compared with sublobar resection, conventional radiation, and stereotactic ablative radiotherapy (hazard ratio [HR], 0.71; confidence interval [CI], 0.45–1.12). It also showed that the percentage of patients who received lobectomy decreased with increasing age: 31% of patients 70 to 74 years old received a lobectomy compared with 18% of patients more than 80 years old ($P<.001$).[5]

Adjuvant chemotherapy in the elderly
After surgical resection, patients with large tumors (>4 cm) and/or lymph node involvement should be offered adjuvant cisplatin-based chemotherapy. Adjuvant chemotherapy in elderly patients with resected lung cancer offers many challenges. The potential improvement in survival must be weighed against the potential for immediate and long-term toxicity. The prevailing standard for stages IB to IIIA NSCLC is to treat with cisplatin-based combination chemotherapy for 4 cycles based on the results of large randomized phase III clinical trials reported over the past decade, which showed an improvement in overall survival (OS) ranging from 5% to 15%. The trials that did show a benefit for adjuvant chemotherapy include the International Adjuvant Lung

Trial (IALT), JBR.10, and Adjuvant Navelbine International Trialist Association (ANITA) trials and those that failed to show such benefit include the ALPI, BLT, and CALGB, Cancer and Leukemia Group B (CALGB) 9633 trials[6–11] (**Table 2**). The Lung Adjuvant Cisplatin Evaluation (LACE) meta-analysis reviewed results from all 5 cisplatin-containing trials and reported an OS benefit of 5.4% at 5 years.[12] Note that only 20% of patients were more than 65 years of age and 9% more than 70 years of age in these trials.[13] The CALGB 9633 trial was novel in that it was restricted to patients with stage IB disease and used a carboplatin-based regimen. However, despite an improvement in progression-free survival, there was no benefit in OS at 5 years. The proportion of subjects greater than 70 years of age was 20% in the LACE meta-analysis compared with cisplatin trials, which remains low for a disease with median age at diagnosis of 70 years. Given that clinical trials have strict eligibility criteria permitting only the fit elderly, it is reasonable to turn to population-based databases to study the impact of adjuvant chemotherapy in older adults. Using the Medicare SEER registry, an observational cohort study has been reported to address this question.[14] In this study, 3324 patients more than 65 years of age were identified as undergoing surgery to treat stage II and IIIA NSCLC with a primary end point of OS. In this group, 21% received platinum-based chemotherapy. There was an OS benefit for patients who received chemotherapy in the population less than 70 years of age (HR, 0.74; 95% CI, 0.62–0.88) and aged 70 to 79 years (HR, 0.82; 95% CI, 0.71–0.94) but not in the population more than 80 years of age (HR, 1.33; 95% CI, 0.86–2.06). The use of adjuvant chemotherapy was associated with an increased odds ratio (OR) of serious adverse events as determined by hospitalization (OR, 2.0; 95% CI, 1.5–2.6). Using the Ontario Cancer Registry, Cuffe and colleagues[15] reported an age-based breakdown in more than 6300 patients with NSCLC treated with surgery from 2001 to 2006. They used change in OS since the advent of adjuvant chemotherapy as a surrogate for benefit from, and hospitalization as a reflection of toxicity from, adjuvant

Table 2
Summary of positive trials of adjuvant chemotherapy in age-unselected patients

Trial	ANITA[1,a]	IALT[6,b]	JBR.10[8,c]	LACE[12,d]	CALGB[11,e]
Total patients (n)	840	1867	482	4584	344
Age>65–69 y; n (%)	170 (20)	328 (18)	84 (17)	901 (20)	NA
Stage	IB–IIIA	I–III	IB–II	I–IIIA	IB
PS	0–2	0–2	0, 1	NA	0–1
Cisplatin dose (mg/m^2)	400	300–400	400	150–400	NA; carboplatin AUC 6
OS increase at 5 y (%)	8.6	4.1	15	5.4	None

Abbreviations: AUC, area under the curve; LACE, Lung Adjuvant Cisplatin Evaluation; NA, not applicable; OS, overall survival.

[a] Adjuvant vinorelbine plus cisplatin versus observation in patients with completely resected stage IB to IIIA NSCLC: a randomized controlled trial.[7]

[b] Cisplatin-based adjuvant chemotherapy in patients with completely resected NSCLC.[6]

[c] Vinorelbine plus cisplatin versus observation in resected NSCLC. National Cancer Institute of Canada Clinical Trials Group, National Cancer Institute of the United States Intergroup JBR.10 Trial Investigators.[8]

[d] A pooled analysis by the LACE Collaborative Group. A meta-analysis by the NSCLC Meta-analyses Collaborative Group.[12,13]

[e] Adjuvant paclitaxel plus carboplatin compared with observation in stage IB NSCLC: CALGB 9633 with the CALGB, Radiation Therapy Oncology Group, and North Central Cancer Treatment Group Study Groups.[11]

Data from Refs.[6–8,11–13]

chemotherapy. In all, 2763 (44%) of 6304 surgical patients were 70 years of age or older. Use of adjuvant chemotherapy in this age group increased from 3.3% (2001–2003) to 16.2% (2004–2006). Among older patients, 70% received cisplatin and 28% received carboplatin-based regimens. Requirements for dose adjustments/substitutions as well as hospitalization rates were similar across age groups (28.0% for patients aged <70 years; 27.8% for patients aged ≥70 years; $P = .54$). Four-year OS of older patients increased significantly (47.1% to 49.9% for patients diagnosed 2001–2003 and 2004–2006 respectively; $P = .01$). Survival improved in all subgroups except in patients aged 80 years and older. In a recent report from the Veterans Affairs Cancer Registry of 7593 patients who underwent resection for stage IB to III NSCLC, 2897 (38%) were greater than or equal to 70 years of age.[16] The proportion of older patients who received adjuvant chemotherapy was half that of younger patients who did so (15.3% vs 31.6%; $P<.0001$). Carboplatin-based doublets were used most often in all patients (64.6%). Both younger (HR, 0.79; 95% CI, 0.72–0.86) and older patients (HR, 0.81; 95% CI, 0.71–0.92) had a lower risk of death with adjuvant chemotherapy. Further, cisplatin-based therapy was associated with a similar risk of mortality to carboplatin-based chemotherapy in the younger patients (HR for cisplatin-based therapy, 1.02; 95% CI, 0.83, 1.25). In older patients, there was a nonsignificant 12% decreased risk of deaths with cisplatin-based therapy (HR, 0.88; 95% CI, 0.59–1.30).

Locally Advanced Non–small Cell Lung Cancer

The surgical option is appropriate for a minority of patients with excellent PS and pulmonary reserve as well as limited tumor volume and minimal mediastinal nodal involvement. These patients derive significant benefit from adjuvant chemotherapy after surgery. For most patients with locally advanced NSCLC concurrent chemoradiotherapy is considered the standard treatment. However, because of a lack of prospective data and exclusion and underrepresentation of frail elderly patients from clinical trials, there is no standard of care. The gold standard for chemotherapy used for radiosensitization has long been considered to be cisplatin and etoposide at systemic doses rather than the low doses of paclitaxel and carboplatin commonly used in practice for the ease of administration. The former approach, first explored by the Southwest Oncology Group in S8805 and further studied in stage IIIB in S9019, was deemed the standard in the nonsurgical arm of the intergroup trial 0139.[17–19] In this latter intergroup trial, the median age of participants was 60 years and age was not predictive of outcomes. Its feasibility in the fit elderly has been shown with similar benefit to that obtained by younger patients, albeit at a higher toxicity than experienced by younger patients.[20] In addition, consolidation chemotherapy with docetaxel following cisplatin-based concurrent chemoradiotherapy did not add any survival benefit. The more prevalent practice of using low-dose weekly carboplatin and paclitaxel emerged from CALGB 39801.[21] A post hoc analysis of the CALGB 39801 trial identified factors predictive of decreased survival as weight loss greater than or equal to 5%, age greater than or equal to 70 years, PS of 1, and hemoglobin level less than 13 g/dL ($P<.05$).[22] Patients with greater than or equal to 2 poor prognostic factors (n = 165) had a decreased OS compared with patients with less than or equal to 1 factor (n = 166) (HR for OS was 1.88; 95% CI, 1.49–2.37; $P = .0001$; median survival times were 9 and 18 months, respectively. $P = .0001$). There is benefit to the addition of systemic doses of platinum-based chemotherapy following low-dose radiosensitization; however, this has only been tested in a phase II trial.[23] The recent results from RTOG 0617, which used this low-dose weekly paclitaxel and carboplatin regimen for radiosensitization followed by systemic doses of consolidation chemotherapy in all patients, found no benefit from escalating the dose of radio-therapy (74 Gy) compared with standard-dose (60 Gy) radiotherapy; survival times with standard radiation were better at 28.7 versus 19.5 months (P = .0007).[24] Factors predictive of less favorable OS on multivariate analysis were higher radiation dose, higher esophagitis/dysphagia grade, greater gross tumor volume, and heart volume greater than 5 Gy, but not age.

Prospective trials in the elderly

In a randomized study by the Japan Clinical Oncology Group specific to patients more than 70 years old (n = 200) with unresectable stage III NSCLC, patients were randomly assigned to chemoradiotherapy (60 Gy with concurrent low-dose carboplatin at 30 mg/m^2 per day, 5 days a week for 20 days) or radiotherapy alone with a primary end point of OS. Median OS for the chemoradiotherapy and radiotherapy alone groups were 22·4 months and 16·9 months respectively (HR, 0.68; 95.4% CI, 0.47–0.98; P = .0179). More patients had grade 3 to 4 hematological toxicity and grade 3 infections in the chemoradiotherapy group than in the radiotherapy-alone group, with no difference in rates of grade 3 to 4 pneumonitis and late lung toxicity between groups.[25] Based on pooled analyses of trials conducted with the NCCTG (North Central Cancer Treatment Group) and CALGB, older patients treated with chemoradio-therapy had improved OS compared with radiation alone but had higher rates of toxicity greater than or equal to grade 3 than patients who received radiation therapy alone.[26,27] A recent meta-analysis of 7 PRCTs (Prospective Randomized Control Trial) (1205 patients) comparing concurrent with sequential chemoradiotherapy in stage III NSCLC reported a significant benefit of concomitant chemoradiotherapy on OS (HR, 0.84; 95% CI, 0.74–0.95; P = .004), with an absolute benefit of 5.7% (18.1%–23.8%) at 3 years and 4.5% at 5 years.[28] Concomitant chemoradiotherapy increased acute esophageal toxicity (grade 3–4) from 4% to 18% with a relative risk of 4.9 (95% CI, 3.1–7.8; P<.001). This analysis included 459 (38%) patients greater than or equal to 65 years old and 16% greater than or equal to 70 years old. However, no differences in efficacy outcomes were evident based on age. Thus, older adults fit enough to meet eligibility for prospective randomized studies were as likely to derive survival benefit from concurrent chemoradiotherapy as younger patients.

Results from population databases

Using the SEER registry, a recent study evaluated the prevalence and effectiveness of radiation therapy alone in stage III NSCLC. Of the 10,376 cases identified that were not treated with chemotherapy, 62% received radiation therapy alone. Radiotherapy was associated with improved OS (HR, 0.76; 95% CI, 0.74–0.79), albeit with increased risk of hospitalization for pneumonitis and esophagitis.[29] Another study using the SEER registry reported that in locally advanced NSCLC only 66% of older adults received any treatment (based on cases diagnosed 1997–2009). Of those that were treated, only 45% received combined chemoradiotherapy, which is considered the standard of care for this group of patients.[30] Recent single-institution retrospective reviews sug-gest that outcomes in the elderly are associated with PS rather than chronologic age alone. In one such study of 189 patients, those greater than or equal to 70 years old (n = 86) were more likely to have Eastern Cooperative Oncology Group (ECOG) PS greater than or equal to 2 (P<.05) and receive palliative intent treatment (P<.05), and less likely to receive concurrent chemoradiotherapy (P<.05) and cisplatin (P<.05).[31] Median survival was 10.3 months for the elderly compared with 17.2 months for younger patients (P<.05). On multivariate analysis, older age was not associated (P = .43) with increased risk of death, whereas poor ECOG PS ($\geq$2) was significantly associated with death ($P<.05$). In elderly patients, definitive treatment ($P<.05$), chemotherapy administration ($P<.05$), and ECOG PS of 0 to 1 ($P<.05$) were associated with improved outcome. In another study of 389 patients, the elderly group (≥ 75 years old), had a median survival of 19.9 months in the combined modality group versus 7.8 months in the other treatments group ($P = .0048$), suggesting that elderly patients likely derive benefit from combined modality therapy if their PS is adequate.[32] Better methods of risk stratification for these elderly are therefore needed.

Advanced Disease: Management Principles

Importance of histology and molecular markers

It is imperative to classify lung cancer beyond small cell or non–small cell histologies. Within NSCLC, it is important to determine squamous versus adenocarcinoma histology. Two of the commonly used agents in NSCLC are not used in the squamous subtype (pemetrexed because of lack of efficacy and bevacizumab because of higher risk of toxicity). Further, adenocarcinoma tumors should be tested for molecular markers that offer options for treatment with targeted agents, especially mutations in the epidermal growth factor receptor (EGFR) and the EML-ALK genes (echinoderm microtubule-associated protein-like 4 [EML4] - anaplastic lymphoma kinase [ALK]). Those with proven mutations can be treated with tyrosine kinase inhibitors like erlotinib or afatinib and crizotinib or ceritinib for EGFR and EML-ALK mutations respectively. Thus, cytotoxic chemotherapy can be delayed in these patients in favor of these oral agents. About 10% to 15% of patients with adenocarcinoma may harbor such actionable mutations, with the likelihood being highest in nonsmokers. Commonly used oral agents with frequently encountered adverse events are listed in **Table 3**.

Cytotoxic chemotherapy in advanced disease

The standard of care for most patients with advanced, recurrent, or metastatic NSCLC is platinum-based combination chemotherapy. There is no specific age cutoff for the use of combination therapy but the use is generally restricted to patients with PS of 0 to 1. Toxicity associated with chemotherapy is higher with combination regimens and typically increases with age because of the decline in physiologic function with age as well as the increase in comorbidity burden. Thus, whether to treat an older patient with advanced lung cancer with a platinum-based combination regimen to maximize efficacy versus single-agent chemotherapy to minimize toxicity and maintain function and quality of life (QoL) is a question commonly encountered in clinical practice. Elderly patients have largely been excluded from practice-changing studies in

Table 3
Targeted therapies in lung cancer

Mutation	Prevalence (%)	Treatment Options	Common Side Effects
EGFR (exon 21 and L858R)	15	Erlotinib, gefitinib, afatinib	Diarrhea, acneiform rash, ocular toxicity, pulmonary toxicity (dyspnea, ILD)
ALK	5	Crizotinib, ceritinib	Myelosuppression, QTc prolongation, bradycardia, hepatotoxicity, pulmonary toxicity (ILD)
ROS1	1–2	Crizotinib	Myelosuppression, QTc prolongation, bradycardia, hepatotoxicity, pulmonary toxicity (ILD)

Abbreviations: ALK, anaplastic lymphoma kinase; ILD, interstitial lung disease; ROS1, proto-oncogene tyrosine-protein kinase reactive oxygen species.

advanced NSCLC. Among the 100 most cited trials between 1980 and 2010, 33% specifically excluded elderly patients in their trial design (age exclusion ranged from >65 to >75 years of age). The average patient median age reported in these trials was 60.9 years. The average age for trials that did not exclude elderly patients was not significantly different at 61.0 ($P = .97$). The average median age of patients was 61 years (95% CI, 60.4–61.6) in all trials. There have been several clinical trials and subset analyses that have been reported over the past decade to address this issue. The Elderly Lung Cancer Vinorelbine Italian Study (ELVIS) randomized 161 patients greater than or equal to 70 years of age with stage IIIB or IV NSCLC (PS, 0–2) to single-agent vinorelbine or best supportive care. Vinorelbine-treated patients scored better than control patients on QoL functioning scales, and they reported fewer lung cancer–related symptoms but reported worse toxicity-related symptoms. There was a statistically significant (2-sided $P = .03$) survival advantage for patients receiving vinorelbine; median survival increased from 21 to 28 weeks in the vinorelbine-treated group. The relative hazard of death for vinorelbine-treated patients was 0.65 (95% CI, 0.45–0.93).[33] This study established the role of palliative single-agent chemotherapy in advanced NSCLC. The follow-up study, the MILES (Multicenter Italian Lung Cancer in the Elderly Study) trial, assessed the superiority of a nonplatinum chemotherapy combination compared with single agents in a 3-arm phase III design in patients aged 70 years or older.[34] A total of 698 patients were randomized to vinorelbine, gemcitabine, or a combination of gemcitabine and vinorelbine administered up to a maximum of 6 cycles. There was no statistically significant difference between the 3 arms in terms of median OS (36 weeks for vinorelbine, $P = .93$; 28 weeks for gemcitabine, $P = .65$) compared with the combination median OS of 30 weeks but with higher toxicity in the combination arm. The Southern Italy Cooperative Oncology Group (SICOG) similarly randomized 120 patients (>70 years old) to vinorelbine or a combination of gemcitabine and vinorelbine on days 1 and 8 every 3 weeks for a maximum of 6 cycles. Median survival was better with the combination (29 vs 18 weeks; $P<.01$), with higher QoL scores for the combination arm, albeit with 3 toxic deaths in the combination arm compared with 1 in the vinorelbine arm.[35] The West Japan Thoracic Oncology Group Trial (WJTOG 9904) was a phase III trial that compared 2 single agents. Patients aged more than 70 years (n = 182) with stage IIIB/IV NSCLC were randomized to docetaxel (60 mg/m^2 every 21 days) or vinorelbine (25 mg/m^2 on days 1 and 8 of a 21-day cycle).[36] Response rates were significantly higher for docetaxel (22.7% vs 9.9%). Median survival was 14.3 months for docetaxel and 9.9 months for vinorelbine ($P = .138$). Grade 3 or 4 neutropenia was higher in the docetaxel arm, but there was no difference in grade 3 or febrile neutropenia or infection. Docetaxel was associated with an improved symptom score compared with vinorelbine. In addition, in a recent randomized phase III study, 451 patients (aged 70–89 years; PS, 0–2) with advanced NSCLC were randomized to single-agent gemcitabine (1150 mg/m^2 days 1 and 8 every 21 days), single-agent vinorelbine (25 mg/m^2 days 1 and 8 every 21 days), or carboplatin (area under the curve, 6) plus paclitaxel (90 mg/m^2) on days 1, 8, and 15 every 28 days.[37] Five cycles of single-agent or 4 cycles of combination therapy were allowed. Median survival was better with the combination (10.4 vs 6.2 months; $P = .0001$). Although there were more hematologic toxicities in the combination arm (54.1% vs 17.9%), there was no difference in early deaths.

Use of Targeted Therapy

Bevacizumab is a monoclonal antibody to the vascular endothelial growth factor that has been shown to improve OS when combined with paclitaxel and carboplatin in patients with advanced (nonsquamous) NSCLC compared with the same chemotherapy alone. The median survival was 12.3 months in the group assigned to chemotherapy plus bevacizumab, compared with 10.3 months in the chemotherapy-alone group (HR for death, 0.79; $P = .003$). In a post hoc subset analysis of patients greater than or equal to 70 years old (n = 224; 26%), there was a trend toward higher response rate (29% vs 17%; $P = .067$) and progression-free survival (5.9 vs 4.9 months; $P = .063$) with bevacizumab compared with chemotherapy alone, although OS (11.3 months and 12.1 months, respectively; $P = .4$) was similar. However, grade 3 or worse adverse events, which included a greater number of deaths, were noted in 87% of elderly patients treated with bevacizumab versus 61% who were not ($P>.001$).[38] Other retrospective analyses limited to the elderly have also found no improvement in OS with the addition of bevacizumab to chemotherapy.[39–41]

Erlotinib is a tyrosine kinase inhibitor against the EGFR receptor pathway that has shown efficacy in patients with EGFR mutations. The elderly seem to gain as much benefit from this agent in terms of response and survival as younger patients but are most likely to have adverse events, especially rash, diarrhea, and dehydration, which can lead to earlier discontinuation of this agent.[42] Other common tumor-associated complications seen in patients with advanced lung cancer and their management are listed in **Table 4**.

Table 4
Commonly encountered complications in patients with advanced lung cancer

Complications of Lung Cancer	Incidence (%)	Symptoms/Signs	Management Outline
Brain metastasis	45–65 (over the course of patients with advanced lung cancer)	• Altered mental status • Seizures • Weakness and/or numbness	• Steroids • Radiation therapy and/or surgery • Can consider chemotherapy for asymptomatic brain metastasis with extensive systemic disease
Malignant pleural effusion	10–15	• Dyspnea • Cough • Chest pain	• Therapeutic thoracentesis • For patients with rapid accumulation: indwelling pleural catheter • Chemical pleurodesis alone or with an indwelling catheter
Superior vena cava syndrome	2–4 (more common in SCLC) Often related to central venous access devices	• Dyspnea • Facial/arm swelling • Distension of the veins in the neck and on the chest wall • Facial plethora	SCLC: chemotherapy NSCLC: • Radiation • Use of endovascular stents • Removal of central venous access devices if present, followed by anticoagulation

Abbreviation: SCLC, small cell lung cancer.

Risk Stratification Using Geriatric Assessment

Geriatric assessment (GA) has been used to a limited extent in NSCLC. Maione and colleagues[43] reported on the prognostic value for OS of baseline assessment of functional status, comorbidity, and QoL in 566 elderly patients with advanced NSCLC enrolled in the phase III randomized Multicenter Italian Lung Cancer in the Elderly Study (MILES). Functional status was measured as activities of daily living (ADL) and instrumental ADL (IADL). Comorbidity was summarized using the Charlson scale. Better values of baseline QoL ($P = .0003$) and IADL ($P = .04$) were significantly associated with better prognosis, whereas ADL ($P = .44$) and Charlson score ($P = .66$) had no prognostic value in this study. In the recent French study that evaluated the prognostic value of ADL, Mini–Mental State Examination, and Charlson Comorbidity Index, the investigators reported that a normal activities of daily living score was a significant independent favorable prognostic factor, whereas the Mini–Mental State Examination and Charlson Index were not prognostically useful.[37] In a novel Dutch study, 181 patients greater than or equal to 70 years old, PS of 0 to 2 with stage III to IV NSCLC were treated with 2 different carboplatin-based doublets.[44] The primary end point was change in global QoL from baseline compared with week 18. A pretreatment comprehensive GA and mini-GA during and after treatment were undertaken. A principal component (PC) analysis was performed to determine the underlying dimensions of CGA and QoL and was subsequently related to survival. There were no changes in QoL after treatment. CGA items were associated with neuropsychiatric toxicity. The PC analysis derived from CGA and QoL items had only 1 dominant underlying dimension, which had significant prognostic value. Physical and role functioning, frailty, and depression were the most prominent elements of this underlying structure. More recently the Cancer and Aging Research Group (CARG) incorporated CGA with patient-related and tumor-related factors to develop a composite score that is predictive of chemotherapy-associated toxicity in the elderly across tumor types and stages (**Fig. 2**).[45,46] In a study from China, 120 patients with lung cancer who were greater than or equal to 65 years of age were classified based on their CARG scores. Toxicity varied significantly among the risk groups ($P<.001$), but the incidence of toxicity did not vary significantly among the Karnofsky Performance Status (KPS)–based risk groups ($P = .322$), suggesting a better utility of this toxicity tool in predicting the risks

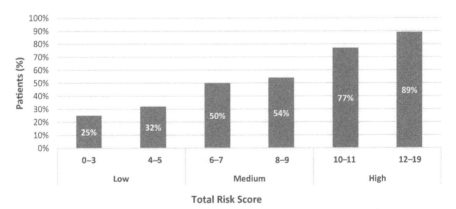

Fig. 2. Ability of CARG risk score to predict grade 3 to 5 chemotherapy toxicity. (*Adapted from* Hurria A, Togawa K, Mohile SG, et al. Predicting chemotherapy toxicity in older adults with cancer: a prospective multicenter study. J Clin Oncol 2011;29:3463.)

of chemotherapy toxicity compared with KPS for older patients with lung cancer.[47] Because the elderly are particularly vulnerable to toxicity, it is vital to have the ability to assess the risk for toxicity before initiating therapy. The CARG retrospectively studied the factors associated with early discontinuation of chemotherapy (defined as chemotherapy duration of ≤ 6 weeks) in patients greater than or equal to 65 years old with stage IV NSCLC (n = 100). On multivariate analysis, factors independently associated with early discontinuation included second or higher line of chemotherapy (OR, 5.93; 95% CI, 2.25–15.61) and lower Medical Outcomes Study physical score of less than 70 (OR, 4.19; 95% CI, 1.56–11.29), the latter being a measure of physical function.[48] A potential paradigm for decision making in the clinic is presented in **Fig. 3**.

Patients' Preferences and Understanding of Goals of Therapy

Older patients may have goals or expectations that are different from those of younger patients, and this may be particularly true in the setting of a lethal disease such as lung cancer. In a novel study conducted in patients with advanced lung cancer after at least 1 cycle of chemotherapy, the median survival threshold for accepting chemotherapy was 4.5 months for mild toxicity and 9 months for severe toxicity. When given the choice between supportive care and chemotherapy, only 22% of patients chose chemotherapy for a survival benefit of 3 months; 68% of patients chose chemotherapy if it substantially reduced symptoms without prolonging life. Older patients tended to demand greater benefit before accepting chemotherapy and were more likely to accept supportive care instead of chemotherapy than younger patients.[49] A national, prospective, observational cohort study that included 1193 patients with newly diagnosed advanced lung or colorectal cancers treated with palliative intent chemotherapy sought to characterize the prevalence of the expectation that chemotherapy might be curative in these patients.[50] Of the 710 patients with lung cancer, 69% gave answers that were not consistent with understanding that chemotherapy was very unlikely to cure their cancer. In multivariable logistic regression, factors that were associated with a greater likelihood of this apparent misunderstanding were nonwhite race or

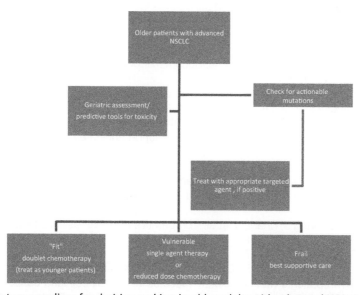

Fig. 3. Future paradigm for decision making in older adults with advanced NSCLC.

ethnic group compared with white race (OR for Hispanic patients, 2.82; 95% CI, 1.51–5.27; OR for black patients, 2.93; 95% CI, 1.80–4.78). Educational level, functional status, and the patient's role in decision making were not associated with inaccurate beliefs about chemotherapy. There was a strong trend of worse understanding with age (OR 1.68 for patients in the age group 70–79 years; 95% CI, 1.10–2.59). Thus, goals of chemotherapy need to be conveyed clearly to patients and there is a high prevalence of misconceptions about the role of chemotherapy, with minority ethnic groups and older patients being at the greatest risk for such misunderstanding.

The Role of Palliative Care

A recent prospective randomized controlled study evaluated the effect of early palliative care after the diagnosis of metastatic NSCLC on patient-reported outcomes and end-of-life care among ambulatory patients with newly diagnosed disease. Of the 151 patients who underwent randomization, 27 died by 12 weeks and 107 (86% of the remaining patients) completed assessments.[51] Patients assigned to early palliative care had a better QoL than the patients assigned to standard care (mean score on the FACT-L (Functional Assessment of Cancer Therapy- Lung) scale [in which scores range from 0 to 136, with higher scores indicating better QoL], 98.0 vs 91.5; $P = .03$). In addition, fewer patients in the palliative care group than in the standard care group had depressive symptoms (16% vs 38%; $P = .01$). Despite there being fewer patients in the early palliative care group than in the standard care group receiving aggressive end-of-life care (33% vs 54%; $P = .05$), median survival was longer among patients receiving early palliative care (11.6 months vs 8.9 months; $P = .02$).

SUMMARY

Lung cancer is a disease of the elderly. Older patients with good functional status and PS can be treated similarly to younger patients, although data for octogenarians are scant. Integration of GA can help with better risk stratification of patients and improve clinical decision making in these patients.

REFERENCES

1. Siegel R, Jamal A. Cancer facts and figures 2015. Available at: http://www.cancer.org/acs/groups/content/@editorial/documents/document/acspc-044552.pdf. Accessed July 11, 2015.
2. World Health Organization. Available at: http://www.who.int/healthinfo/survey/ageingdefnolder/en/. Accessed July 11, 2015.
3. American Cancer Society. Available at: http://www.cancer.org/cancer/lungcancer-non-smallcell/detailedguide/non-small-cell-lung-cancer-key-statistics. Accessed July 11, 2015.
4. Mery C, Pappas A, Bueno R, et al. Similar long term survival of elderly patients with non-small cell lung cancer treated with lobectomy or wedge resection within the Surveillance, Epidemiology, and End Results database. Chest 2005;128: 237–45.
5. Shrivani S, Jiang J, Chang J, et al. Comparative effectiveness of 5 treatment strategies for early-stage non-small cell lung cancer in the elderly. Int J Radiat Oncol Biol Phys 2012;84:1060–70.
6. Arriagada R, Bergman B, Dunant A, et al. Cisplatin-based adjuvant chemotherapy in patients with completely resected non-small-cell lung cancer. N Engl J Med 2004;350:351–60.

7. Douillard JY, Rosell R, De Lena M, et al. Adjuvant vinorelbine plus cisplatin versus observation in patients with completely resected stage IB-IIIA non-small-cell lung cancer (Adjuvant Navelbine International Trialist Association [ANITA]): a randomised controlled trial. Lancet Oncol 2006;7:719–27.

8. Winton T, Livingston R, Johnson D, et al. Vinorelbine plus cisplatin vs. observation in resected non-small-cell lung cancer. N Engl J Med 2005;352:2589–97.

9. Waller D, Peake MD, Stephens RJ, et al. Chemotherapy for patients with non-small cell lung cancer: the surgical setting of the Big Lung Trial. Eur J Cardio-thorac Surg 2004;26:173–82.

10. Scagliotti GV, Fossati R, Torri V, et al. Randomized study of adjuvant chemotherapy for completely resected stage I, II, or IIIA non-small-cell lung cancer. J Natl Cancer Inst 2003;95:1453–61.

11. Strauss GM, Herndon JE, Maddaus MA, et al. Adjuvant paclitaxel plus carboplatin compared with observation in stage IB non-small-cell lung cancer: CALGB 9633 with the Cancer and Leukemia Group B, Radiation Therapy Oncology Group, and North Central Cancer Treatment Group Study Groups. J Clin Oncol 2008;26:5043–51.

12. Pignon JP, Tribodet H, Scagliotti GV, et al. Lung adjuvant cisplatin evaluation: a pooled analysis by the LACE Collaborative Group. J Clin Oncol 2008;26:3552–9.

13. NSCLC Meta-analyses Collaborative Group, Arriagada R, Auperin A, et al. Adjuvant chemotherapy, with or without postoperative radiotherapy, in operable non-small-cell lung cancer: two meta-analyses of individual patient data. Lancet 2010; 375:1267–77.

14. Wisnivesky J, Smith C, Packer S, et al. Survival and risk of adverse events in older patients receiving postoperative adjuvant chemotherapy for resected stages II-IIIA lung cancer: observational cohort study. BMJ 2011;343:d4013.

15. Cuffe S, Booth CM, Peng Y, et al. Adjuvant chemotherapy for non-small-cell lung cancer in the elderly: a population-based study in Ontario, Canada. J Clin Oncol 2012;30:1813–21.

16. Ganti AK, Williams CD, Gajra A, et al. Effect of age on the efficacy of adjuvant chemotherapy for resected non-small cell lung cancer. Cancer 2015. http://dx.doi.org/10.1002/cncr.29360.

17. Albain KS, Rusch VW, Crowley JJ, et al. Concurrent cisplatin/etoposide plus chest radiotherapy followed by surgery for stages IIIA(N2) and IIIB non–small cell lung cancer: Mature results of Southwest Oncology Group Phase II Study 8805. J Clin Oncol 1995;13:1880–92.

18. Albain KS, Crowley JJ, Turrisi AT 3rd, et al. Concurrent cisplatin, etoposide, and chest radiotherapy in pathologic stage IIIB non-small-cell lung cancer: a Southwest Oncology Group phase II study, SWOG 9019. J Clin Oncol 2002;20(16): 3454–60.

19. Albain KS, Swann RS, Rusch VW, et al. Radiotherapy plus chemotherapy with or without surgical resection for stage III non-small-cell lung cancer: a phase III randomised controlled trial. Lancet 2009;374(9687):379–86.

20. Jalal SI, Riggs HD, Melnyk A, et al. Updated survival and outcomes for older adults with inoperable stage III non-small-cell lung cancer treated with cisplatin, etoposide, and concurrent chest radiation with or without consolidation docetaxel: analysis of a phase III trial from the Hoosier Oncology Group (HOG) and US Oncology. Ann Oncol 2012 Jul;23(7):1730–8.

21. Vokes EE, Herndon JE 2nd, Kelley MJ, et al, Cancer and Leukemia Group B. Induction chemotherapy followed by chemoradiotherapy compared with chemoradiotherapy alone for regionally advanced unresectable stage III non-

small-cell lung cancer: Cancer and Leukemia Group B. J Clin Oncol 2007;25(13): 1698–704.

22. Stinchcombe TE, Hodgson L, Herndon JE 2nd, et al, Cancer and Leukemia Group B. Treatment outcomes of different prognostic groups of patients on cancer and leukemia group B trial 39801: induction chemotherapy followed by chemoradiotherapy compared with chemoradiotherapy alone for unresectable stage III non-small cell lung cancer. J Thorac Oncol 2009;4(9):1117–25.

23. Belani CP, Choy H, Bonomi P, et al. Combined chemoradiotherapy regimens of paclitaxel and carboplatin for locally advanced non-small-cell lung cancer: a randomized phase II locally advanced multi-modality protocol. J Clin Oncol 2005; 23(25):5883–91 [Erratum appears in J Clin Oncol 2006;24(12):1966].

24. Bradley JD, Paulus R, Komaki R, et al. Standard-dose versus high-dose conformal radiotherapy with concurrent and consolidation carboplatin plus paclitaxel with or without cetuximab for patients with stage IIIA or IIIB non-small-cell lung cancer (RTOG 0617): a randomised, two-by-two factorial phase 3 study. Lancet Oncol 2015;16(2):187–99.

25. Atagi S, Kawahara M, Yokoyama A, et al. Japan Clinical Oncology Group Lung Cancer Study Group. Thoracic radiotherapy with or without daily low-dose carboplatin in elderly patients with non-small-cell lung cancer: a randomised, controlled, phase 3 trial by the Japan Clinical Oncology Group (JCOG0301). Lancet Oncol 2012;13(7):671–8.

26. Schild SE, Mandrekar SJ, Jatoi A, et al. The value of combined-modality therapy in elderly patients with stage III nonsmall cell lung cancer. Cancer 2007;110: 363–8.

27. Rocha Lima CM, Herndon JE II, Kosty M, et al. Therapy choices among older patients with lung carcinoma: an evaluation of two trials of the Cancer and Leukemia Group B. Cancer 2002;94:181–7.

28. Aupérin A, Le Péchoux C, Rolland E, et al. Meta-analysis of concomitant versus sequential radiochemotherapy in locally advanced non-small-cell lung cancer. J Clin Oncol 2010;28:2181–90.

29. Sigel K, Lurslurchachai L, Bonomi M, et al. Effectiveness of radiation therapy alone for elderly patients with unresected stage III non-small cell lung cancer. Lung Cancer 2013;82:266–70.

30. Davidoff AJ, Gardner JF, Seal B, et al. Population-based estimates of survival benefit associated with combined modality therapy in elderly patients with locally advanced non-small cell lung cancer. J Thorac Oncol 2011;6:934–41.

31. Aridgides PD, Janik A, Bogart JA, et al. Radiotherapy for stage III non-small-cell lung carcinoma in the elderly (age ≥ 70 years). Clin Lung Cancer 2013;14:674–9.

32. Pirapati H, Karlin NJ, Schild SE, et al. Multimodality therapy improves survival in elderly patients with locally advanced non-small cell lung cancer–A retrospective analysis. J Geriatr Oncol 2012;3:104–10.

33. Effects of vinorelbine on quality of life and survival of elderly patients with advanced non-small-cell lung cancer. The Elderly Lung Cancer Vinorelbine Italian Study Group. J Natl Cancer Inst 1999;91:66–72.

34. Gridelli C, Perrone F, Gallo C, et al. Chemotherapy for elderly patients with advanced non-small-cell lung cancer: the Multicenter Italian Lung Cancer in the Elderly Study (MILES) phase III randomized trial. J Natl Cancer Inst 2003; 95:362–72.

35. Frasci G, Lorusso V, Panza N, et al. Gemcitabine plus vinorelbine versus vinorelbine alone in elderly patients with advanced non-small-cell lung cancer. J Clin Oncol 2000;18:2529–36.

36. Kudoh S, Takeda K, Nakagawa K, et al. Phase III study of docetaxel compared with vinorelbine in elderly patients with advanced non-small-cell lung cancer: results of the West Japan Thoracic Oncology Group Trial (WJTOG 9904). J Clin Oncol 2006; 24:3657–63.

37. Quoix E, Zalcman G, Oster JP, et al. Carboplatin and weekly paclitaxel doublet chemotherapy compared with monotherapy in elderly patients with advanced non-small-cell lung cancer: IFCT-0501 randomised, phase 3 trial. Lancet 2011; 378:1079–88.

38. Sandler A, Gray R, Perry MC, et al. Paclitaxel-carboplatin alone or with bevacizumab in non-small-cell lung cancer. N Engl J Med 2006;355:2542–50.

39. Ramalingam SS, Dahlberg SE, Langer CJ, et al. Outcomes for elderly, advanced-stage non-small cell lung cancer patients treated with bevacizumab in combination with carboplatin and paclitaxel: analysis of Eastern Cooperative Oncology Group Trial 4599. J Clin Oncol 2008;26:60–5.

40. Leighl NB, Zatlouka P, Mezger J, et al. Efficacy and safety of bevacizumab-based therapy in elderly patients with advanced or recurrent nonsquamous non-small cell lung cancer in the phase III BO17704 study (AVAiL). J Thorac Oncol 2010; 5:1970–6.

41. Laskin J, Crino L, Felip E, et al. Safety and efficacy of first-line bevacizumab in elderly patients with advanced or recurrent nonsquamous non-small cell lung cancer: safety of Avastin in lung trial (MO19390). J Thorac Oncol 2012;7:203–11.

42. Wheatley-Price P, Ding K, Seymour L, et al. Erlotinib for advanced non-small cell lung cancer in the elderly: an analysis of the National Cancer Institute of Canada Clinical Trials Group Study BR.21. J Clin Oncol 2008;26:2350–7.

43. Maione P, Perrone F, Gallo C, et al. Pretreatment quality of life and functional status assessment significantly predict survival of elderly patients with advanced non-small-cell lung cancer receiving chemotherapy: a prognostic analysis of the multicenter Italian Lung Cancer in the Elderly study. J Clin Oncol 2005;23: 6865–72.

44. Biesma B, Wymenga AN, Vincent A, et al. Quality of life, geriatric assessment and survival in elderly patients with non-small-cell lung cancer treated with carboplatin-gemcitabine or carboplatin-paclitaxel: NVALT-3 a phase III study. Ann Oncol 2011;22:1520–7.

45. Hurria A, Cirrincione CT, Muss HB, et al. Implementing a geriatric assessment in cooperative group clinical cancer trials: CALGB 360401. J Clin Oncol 2011;29: 1290–6.

46. Hurria A, Togawa K, Mohile SG, et al. Predicting chemotherapy toxicity in older adults with cancer: a prospective multicenter study. J Clin Oncol 2011;29: 3457–65.

47. Nie X, Liu D, Li Q, et al. Predicting chemotherapy toxicity in older adults with lung cancer. J Geriatr Oncol 2013;4:334–9.

48. Gajra A, Tew WP, Hardt M, et al. Predictors of early discontinuation of chemotherapy (EDC) in patients (pts) age 65 or older with stage IV non-small cell lung cancer (NSCLC). J Clin Oncol 2012;30(Suppl) [abstract: e18133].

49. Silvestri G, Pritchard R, Welch HG. Preferences for chemotherapy in patients with advanced non-small cell lung cancer: descriptive study based on scripted interviews. BMJ 1998;317:771–5.

50. Weeks JC, Catalano PJ, Cronin A, et al. Patients' expectations about effects of chemotherapy for advanced cancer. N Engl J Med 2012;367:1616–25.

51. Temel JS, Greer JA, Muzikansky A, et al. Early palliative care for patients with metastatic non-small-cell lung cancer. N Engl J Med 2010;363:733–42.

Management of Colorectal Cancer in Older Adults

Joleen M. Hubbard, MD

KEYWORDS

- Colon cancer treatment • Rectal cancer treatment • Geriatric oncology

KEY POINTS

- Assess each colorectal cancer patient for their degree of fitness and tailor the aggressiveness of the treatment appropriately.
- The goals of care, curative versus palliative, should guide therapeutic management.
- Employ strategies such as intermittent oxaliplatin or omission of bolus 5-fluorouracil to improve chemotherapy tolerance for older adults.

INTRODUCTION

Globally, colorectal cancer (CRC) is the third leading cause of cancer among men and the second leading cause of cancer among women.[1] Approximately 60% of CRC diagnoses occur in patients 65 years of age or older, 36% of new cases are in patients 75 years of age or older, and 12% in patients 84 years or older.[2] Therefore, as the population ages, the prevalence of older adults with CRC will also increase.

Mortality rates from CRC in the United States have been on the decline. From 1990 to 2005, CRC mortality in the United States has decreased by 32% for men and 28% for women. This decrease has been attributed to improved screening methods and better treatment strategies. However, it is unclear whether older patients with CRC are achieving the same degree of benefit from newer treatment strategies as younger patients. Older adults with CRC are less likely to be referred to a medical oncologist, and those patients who are referred to oncology are less likely to receive chemotherapy.[3] Elderly patients are less likely to receive the standard of care for CRC treatment and their treatment is more likely to be discontinued early.[4,5]

The challenge in treating older adults with CRC is that it is often difficult to determine which patients are at increased risk for adverse events from systemic therapy. Because adverse events occur with increased frequency in older age, clinicians

Financial Disclosure: Dr J.M. Hubbard receives research support for clinical trials from Genentech, Bayer, Boston Biomedical Inc, and Senhwa Biosciences Inc. Advisory board for Bayer (Honorarium to Mayo Clinic).
Department of Oncology, Mayo Clinic, 200 First Street Southwest, Rochester, MN 55902, USA
E-mail address: Hubbard.Joleen@mayo.edu

Clin Geriatr Med 32 (2016) 97–111
http://dx.doi.org/10.1016/j.cger.2015.08.002
0749-0690/16/$ – see front matter © 2016 Elsevier Inc. All rights reserved.

have very valid concerns about the tolerance of treatment. In fact, a study on barriers to treating older adults with cancer revealed the most common challenge clinicians noted was dealing with treatment toxicity.[6] With the aging patient, the art of oncology is finding a way to balance effective treatment strategies while minimizing toxicity to preserve quality of life during treatment. This article focuses on the risks and benefits of CRC treatment in the elderly, as well as ways to tailor therapy to the individual older patient.

At all points in CRC management, older adults should be presented with the opportunity to participate in clinical trials investigating novel therapeutics, novel regimens, and novel treatment modalities. In addition, there may be trials designed specifically for the older CRC patient or trials investigating supportive care interventions that attempt to improve the tolerability of cancer therapy.

COLORECTAL CANCER SCREENING

Although more than one-third of CRC cases occur in patients 75 years or older, the age at which colon cancer screening should be discontinued remains an area of debate. The U.S. Preventative Services Task Force recommends against the routine use of screening colonoscopy among patients aged 76 to 85, and recommends against any CRC screening in patients over 85 years.[7] This is owing to the increased risks of colonoscopy, including perforation, gastrointestinal bleeding, and cardiopulmonary complications, as well as the diminishing extension of life expectancy with CRC screening in this older adult population. Special consideration for colonoscopy may need to be given for patients aged 76 to 85 with above average health and life expectancy.

SURGERY

More than 70% of CRC cases are diagnosed at early stages (I–III) and therefore amenable to operative resection.[8] Surgery for CRC is usually well-tolerated among the elderly, especially with advances in laparoscopic colectomy, which result in similar postoperative complications (death, anastomotic leak, and postoperative ileus) among younger and older patients.[9] Excellent survival results can be achieved even among the oldest patients. A recent analysis of the Surveillance, Epidemiology and End Results Medicare database showed 93% survival at 90 days after surgery and 85.7% survival at 1 year among patients 80 years of age or older undergoing colectomy for colon cancer.[10]

As with any elective surgery for an older patient, those with higher degrees of frailty are at risk for postoperative complications from CRC surgery. There have been tools developed to assess risk in the preoperative setting, including the Elderly Physiologic and Operative Severity Score for the Enumeration of Mortality and Morbidity (POSSUM). The Elderly POSSUM can predict both morbidity and mortality in older adults undergoing CRC surgery.[11]

A small subset of patients presents with metastatic CRC (mCRC) and may undergo operative resection with curative intent. The metastatic sites are limited typically to a small number of pulmonary and/or hepatic lesions. Older patients should be evaluated for surgical resection in this setting as well. Two retrospective studies evaluating CRC metastatectomies in older patients both demonstrated no difference in postoperative morbidity or mortality between younger and older patients.[12,13]

Alternatives to Surgery

For older adults who are not candidates for CRC surgery, other management modalities may be used to extend duration of life and/or preserve quality of life.

Colonic stents

If a patient is unable to undergo surgery or systemic chemotherapy or radiation therapy (in the case of rectal cancer), an advancing lesion in the colon or rectum may eventually lead to bowel obstruction. The use of colonic or rectal stents can help to maintain an adequate lumen diameter to prevent this complication and help to extend patients' lives in the palliative setting.

Radiofrequency ablation

Radiofrequency ablation is appropriate for those patients with a small number and size (<3–4 cm) of liver metastases. A recent analysis of 2 European clinical trials involving patients with CRC liver metastases demonstrated similar local recurrence rates with surgical resection and radiofrequency ablation.[14] Radiofrequency ablation is a good treatment modality to address limited metastatic lesions for patients who are either not candidates for operative intervention or are seeking less invasive management options, and therefore gaining widespread use in the older adult population.

RECTAL CANCER

The current standard of care in the management of locally advanced rectal cancer, including lesions that have invaded through the muscularis propria and/or lymph node positive disease found on either pelvic MRI or rectal endoscopic ultrasonography, is for neoadjuvant chemotherapy with a fluoropyrimidine followed by operative resection plus 4 more months of additional chemotherapy.[15] Patients over 75 years of age are at risk of early termination of treatment, treatment interruptions, and dose reduction.[16] Less fit patients may be good candidates for short-course radiation therapy (1 week) because this does not seem to compromise recurrence rates when compared with the standard radiation course given over 5.5 weeks.[17] The surgical and adjuvant therapy management follow the same principles as for colon cancer.

SYSTEMIC THERAPY FOR COLORECTAL CANCER

The use of systemic chemotherapy improves survival after operative resection of CRC (adjuvant setting) as well as when surgery is unable to be performed (palliative setting). Multiple studies have shown that older adults with CRC are undertreated in both the adjuvant as well as the metastatic setting.[5,18,19] Undertreating older adults with systemic chemotherapy may decrease survival outcomes in this age group. Several database studies have shown that older patients with CRC who receive adjuvant therapy do have a survival benefit, and those who receive a longer duration of therapy have decreased mortality.[20,21]

Even though patients 65 years of age or older make up the majority of patients with CRC, older adults have been underrepresented in clinical trials.[22] This has undoubtedly contributed to our lack of knowledge on the tolerability and survival benefits of newly developed regimens in older adults. Much of the available data on systemic therapy for CRC in the elderly population come from database studies, subset analyses of randomized trials, or pooled analyses using data from multiple clinical trials. **Table 1** lists the available agents used in the management of CRC.

Adjuvant Chemotherapy for Older Adults

The fluoropyrimidines (5-fluoruracil and capecitabine)

Adjuvant chemotherapy with 5-fluorouracil (5-FU)–based therapy became the standard of care in the early 1990s after Moertel and colleagues[23] reported the results of a randomized phase III clinical trial demonstrating a 41% decrease in tumor

Table 1
Systemic chemotherapies approved for use for colorectal cancer

Drug	Brand Name	Adjuvant	Metastatic	Common Side Effects
5-flurouracil	Adrucil	+	+	Mucositis, cytopenias, nausea, vomiting, diarrhea, anorexia
Capecitabine	Xeloda	+	+	Stomatitis, nausea, vomiting, diarrhea, hand-foot syndrome
Oxaliplatin	Eloxatin	+	+	Acute cold sensory and chronic peripheral neuropathy, neutropenia, thrombocytopenia, anemia, nausea, vomiting, fatigue
Irinotecan	Camptosar	—	+	Alopecia, cytopenias, nausea, vomiting, diarrhea, hepatotoxicity, hypersensitivity
Bevacizumab	Avastin	—	+	Bleeding, hypertension, proteinuria, epistaxis, headache, rhinitis, thromboembolic events
Aflibercept	Zaltrap	—	+ (second line)	Leukopenia, diarrhea, neutropenia, proteinuria, elevated transaminases, stomatitis, fatigue, thrombocytopenia, hypertension, weight loss, anorexia, epistaxis, abdominal pain, dysphonia, creatinine increase, headache
Ramicurimab	Cyramza	—	+ (second line)	Diarrhea, neutropenia, anorexia, epistaxis, stomatitis
Regorafenib	Stivarga	—	+ (third line)	Asthenia/fatigue, anorexia, hand–foot skin reaction, diarrhea, mucositis, weight loss, infection, hypertension, dysphonia
Cetuximab	Erbitux	—	+	Rash, pruritus, and nail changes, headache, diarrhea, and infection
Panitumumab	Vectibix	—	+	Diarrhea, stomatitis, paronychia, anorexia, hypomagnesemia, hypokalemia, rash, pruritus, and dry skin

recurrence for patients who received 5-FU after surgery for stage II or III colon cancer compared with patients who received surgery alone. Final results of this study demonstrated a 33% reduction in mortality.[24]

The survival benefit of adjuvant 5-FU–based therapy was shown to apply to older patients with resected colon cancer as well. Several retrospective analyses showed improved survival rates among older patients who received adjuvant 5-FU–based therapy, compared with older adults who received no additional treatment after resection of colon cancer.[25–27] Among these was a pooled analysis of 7 phase III randomized controlled trials evaluating adjuvant 5-FU–based therapy, which demonstrated the disease-free survival (DFS) benefit was consistent across all age groups.[26] The overall survival (OS) benefit from adjuvant therapy decreased as patients aged, likely a result of competing causes of death. Tolerance of chemotherapy did not differ among older and younger patients with the exception of leukopenia in 1 study.

Older patients enrolled in clinical trials often represent the most healthy and robust subset of individuals in this population and may not be representative of the average older patient with CRC. However, there is evidence to suggest that even patients with comorbidities do benefit from adjuvant treatment. A Surveillance, Epidemiology and End Results database study evaluated 5330 older patients with stage III colon cancer.[28] Patients with heart failure, chronic obstructive pulmonary disease, and diabetes were less likely to receive chemotherapy, but among patients with those comorbidities who did receive adjuvant therapy, all had a significant reduction in mortality compared with those with the same comorbidity who did not receive chemotherapy. In addition, there was no difference in the probability of all-cause, condition-specific, or toxicity-related hospitalization associated with adjuvant therapy among patients with comorbidities compared with those who were untreated.

The Xeloda in Adjuvant Colon Cancer Therapy (X-ACT) clinical trial showed that adjuvant therapy with oral capecitabine was equivalent in terms of efficacy as 5-FU/leucovorin (LV), establishing it as a convenient alternative for chemotherapy after resection of colon cancer.[29] A subset analysis evaluating outcomes in older patients on this trial showed they have similar survival benefits as younger patients with the use of capecitabine.[30] Side effects among patients receiving capecitabine including diarrhea, stomatitis, nausea/vomiting, alopecia, and neutropenia, were significantly less than patients who received 5-FU/LV ($P<.001$), but more patients experienced hand–foot syndrome with capecitabine than those receiving 5-FU/LV. However, this trial used the bolus form of 5-FU/LV (aka the Mayo Clinic regimen), which has been replaced by an infusional 5-FU/LV regimen that is less toxic. Therefore, the oral fluoropyrimidine capecitabine may not necessarily be better tolerated option for adjuvant therapy. In fact, a study of capecitabine versus 5-FU/LV in the metastatic setting demonstrated higher rates of toxicity and lower quality of life with capecitabine compared with 5-FU.[31]

The decision of whether to use intravenous 5-FU/LV versus oral capecitabine requires careful consideration of the risks and benefits associated with each regimen outlined in **Table 2** .[32]

Oxaliplatin plus a fluoropyrimidine

In 2004, the results of the Multicenter International Study of Oxaliplatin/5-Fluorouracil/Leucovorin in the Adjuvant Treatment of Colon Cancer (MOSAIC) trial led to a new standard of care of the adjuvant treatment of high-risk stage II and III colon cancer.[33] In this trial patients were randomized to receive 6 months of adjuvant therapy with 5-FU plus LV plus oxaliplatin or 5-FU/LV alone. Patients in the oxaliplatin arm had a 5.3% improvement in 3-year DFS over the 5-FU/LV–only arm (78.2% and 72.9% respectively; $P = -.002$), which led to a 4.2% improvement in OS in the oxaliplatin plus 5-FU/LV arm compared with 5-FU/LV alone (72.9% and 68.7%, respectively; $P = .023$).[34] The DFS benefits of oxaliplatin plus a fluoropyrimidine were confirmed by 2 additional randomized phase III trials, one of which evaluated the use of capecitabine combined with oxaliplatin.[35,36]

In contrast with the studies of older patients having similar benefit as younger patients with the use of 5-FU in the adjuvant setting, the benefits of adding oxaliplatin to a fluoropyrimidine in the adjuvant setting in the older patient population are less clear. Although subgroup analyses of older patients within the MOSAIC and National Surgical Adjuvant Breast and Bowel Project (NASBP) C-07 trials[33,36] did not show a significant DFS benefit with the addition of oxaliplatin to 5-FU/LV in older patients, the trial comparing 5-FU/LV to a combination of capecitabine and oxaliplatin (XELOX) did show that elderly patients received a benefit in 3-year DFS (OS data still maturing).[35]

Table 2
5-Fluorouracil versus capecitabine in older adults

Drug	Advantages	Disadvantages
5-Fluorouracil	Less likely to cause hand-foot syndrome, diarrhea, nausea, or vomiting[31] Less expensive May be used in patients with renal and liver dysfunction	Administered via an ambulatory pump over 46 h; may pose a challenge for patients with mobility issues
Capecitabine	Oral administration	Increased incidence of adverse events including hand–foot syndrome, diarrhea, nausea, and vomiting[1] Caution with liver and kidney dysfunction Drug interaction with warfarin Oral medications associated with lower rates of compliance[32] Patients may have high copayment depending on prescription drug coverage

Data from Seymour MT, Thompson LC, Wasan HS, et al. Chemotherapy options in elderly and frail patients with metastatic colorectal cancer (MRC FOCUS2): an open-label, randomised factorial trial. Lancet 2011;377:1749–59; and MacLaughlin EJ, Raehl CL, Treadway AK, et al. Assessing medication adherence in the elderly: which tools to use in clinical practice? Drugs Aging 2005;22:231–55.

A subsequent pooled analysis of these 3 trials as well as 4 other adjuvant trials including data on 14,528 patients, of which 2575 were 70 years of age or older, was performed to address the question of whether older patients benefit from oxaliplatin combined with a fluoropyrimidine in the adjuvant setting for colon cancer.[37] Results of this analysis did not show a DFS or OS benefit with the use of oxaliplatin in the older adult population. However, there was lack of significant effect modification by age for these end points, suggesting age does not impact the efficacy of oxaliplatin-based adjuvant therapy.

In another analysis of 4 adjuvant colon cancer trials, investigators evaluated the impact of age and comorbidity on treatment outcomes in resected stage III colon cancer.[38] Patients were categorized by age (<70 or ≥70 years), Charlson comorbidity index (≤1 or >1), or National Cancer Institute comorbidity index (≤1 or >1). Regardless of age or comorbidity index, patients in each category had a significant improvement in both DFS and OS. Thus, for older adults healthy enough to be considered for these clinical trials, it seems that they achieved the same benefit with the addition of oxaliplatin to a fluoropyrimidine in the adjuvant setting.

Population-based studies have tried to shed light on the benefits of oxalipatin in a more "real-world" setting. One Surveillance, Epidemiology and End Results–Medicare study evaluated 814 patients older than 65 years who received oxaliplatin-based adjuvant therapy for stage III colon cancer compared with 3581 patients who received 5-FU/LV alone. The investigators found that oxaliplatin-based therapy was associated with improved OS (hazard ratio [HR], 0.73; 95% CI, 0.62–0.86; $P<.001$) and CRC-specific survival (HR, 0.39; 95% CI, 0.28–0.55; $P<.001$) when compared with 5-FU/LV alone. This benefit was seen in patients age 66 to 79, but not for those 80 years or older. Another study including 4 databases showed a small benefit with the use of oxaliplatin in the adjuvant setting among patients greater than 75 years that was not consistently significant between the databases.[20] Although these population-based studies suggest older adults do benefit from combining oxaliplatin with a fluoropyrimidine in the adjuvant setting, they are subject to selection bias because healthier older adults are the ones more likely to receive more aggressive treatment regimens.

Tolerance of oxaliplatin in the elderly
An analysis of pooled data from several clinical trials in both the adjuvant and metastatic setting evaluated the safety of using combination 5-FU/LV and oxaliplatin (FOLFOX).[39] Among 3742 patients with CRC receiving FOLFOX, 614 were 70 years of age or older. Older patients did not have a higher incidence of severe adverse events than younger patients overall. The only differences in toxicity were related to cytopenias: older adults were more likely to have neutropenia (49% vs 43% in younger adults; $P = .04$) and thrombocytopenia (5% vs 2% in younger adults; $P = .04$). Other toxicities including neurotoxicity, diarrhea, nausea/vomiting, and infection were not different between younger and older patients. The fact that infection rates were not higher suggests that the increased rate of neutropenia may not be significant clinically. Older patients received fewer chemotherapy cycles than younger patients, but the dose intensity did not differ between the 2 groups. This study suggests oxaliplatin can be well-tolerated in older adults undergoing treatment for CRC.

Summary: Tailoring Adjuvant Therapy for the Older Adult with Colorectal Cancer
Older adults should be referred to a medical oncologist for a discussion regarding management after resection of their colon cancer. The evaluation by the medical oncologist should include an assessment of the patient's overall physical function, comorbidities, cognition, mental health, concurrent medications, and degree of social support. The following categories help to determine the best management option of the individual patient: very fit older adults, moderately fit older adults, and unfit older adults.

Very fit older adults
Older patients who have few comorbidities and maintain an active lifestyle may be considered for combination fluoropyrimidine plus oxaliplatin therapy. Because the data on the use of oxaliplatin combined with a fluoropyrimidine for older adults in the adjuvant setting are not entirely clear, a careful discussion explaining there are no robust data to confirm the same degree of benefit applies to patients 70 years or older, as well as the adverse effects of oxaliplatin, should be conducted with the individual older patient. The peripheral neuropathy resulting from oxaliplatin can affect older patients' independence by limiting their ability to perform activities of daily living (ie, securing buttons while dressing) and by contributing to falls.

Moderately fit older adults
Patients in this category often have several coexisting medical conditions as well as multiple medications for chronic medical conditions. In addition, their physical activity levels have declined and/or they have preexisting neuropathy or gait abnormalities where a neurotoxic agent may impact their independence significantly. This subset of patients should still be considered for adjuvant therapy, but are more appropriate for single agent chemotherapy with a fluoropyrimidine (either 5-FU or capecitabine) alone.

Unfit older adults
Patients with very advanced medical conditions or very poor physical, cognitive, or mental health status are unlikely to benefit from adjuvant therapy. Patients and families

may still want to discuss an observation plan to monitor for cancer recurrence with an oncologist. Patients who have severe complications from colorectal surgery such as abscesses, nonhealing surgical wounds, and lack of independence in activities of daily living may fall into this category as well. If complications have not improved enough by 12 weeks after surgery, then adjuvant therapy should not be administered.[40]

Advanced/Metastatic Disease in Older Adults

Approximately 20% of patients with CRC present with metastatic disease.[41] As with all patients, the most crucial step in the management of older patients with mCRC is to establish the goals of care. The status of the patient's metastatic disease falls into 3 categories determined by a multidisciplinary team of radiologists, surgeons, and medical oncologists: resectable, borderline resectable, and palliative care.

Resectable
Both the primary lesion and/or metastatic disease are amenable to curative resection. These patients are often treated with perioperative chemotherapy with combination of oxaliplatin and fluoropyrimidine, followed by surgical resection, followed by 3 additional months of the same chemotherapy. Because this approach is with curative intent, there is a general acceptance of a higher toxicity risk with more aggressive combination therapy in exchange for the potential of curing the disease.

Borderline resectable
These patients' metastatic disease and/or primary lesion are potentially resectable if enough of a response is achieved with systemic therapy. The decision to be aggressive with this approach depends on the overall health of the patient, taking into account the patient's underlying comorbidities, functional status, and social support going through treatment. These patients receive combination chemotherapy with or without a biologic agent to try to enhance the disease response. Patients are treated until their disease becomes resectable, and then continue chemotherapy after surgery for a goal total of 6 months of perioperative therapy.

Palliative treatment
Patients in this category present with metastatic disease that will never be amenable to surgical resection. The goal of treatment in patients in this category is to help them live the best quality of life as possible while living with mCRC. With the use of available systemic therapies, the median OS among all patients in this category is 29 months.[42]

Systemic Therapy for Older Adults with Metastatic Colorectal Cancer

The following discussion outlines the available systemic therapy agents with activity in mCRC. Strategies and considerations for use of these agents will be discussed (see **Table 1**).

Combination cytotoxic chemotherapy
Oxaliplatin plus fluoropyrimidine The combination of oxaliplatin and 5-FU/LV became a standard of care after the randomized, controlled trial N9741 demonstrated a 4.5-month improvement in OS with FOLFOX over an irinotecan/5-FU combination regimen and an 8-month improvement over the historical survival outcome with 5-FU/LV alone (19.5, 15.0, and 11.5 months, respectively).[43] In contrast with the conflicting data on whether the use of oxaliplatin combined with a flouropyrimidine provides a survival benefit in the adjuvant setting, the survival benefits for using oxaliplatin in older adults with mCRC are clear. Data from multiple clinical trials have demonstrated that this combination improves outcomes in this patient

population.[29,44–46] As mentioned in the section on adjuvant therapy, the oxaliplatin/fluoropyrimidine combination can be well-tolerated in the fit older adult population.[38,39] Oxaliplatin combined with capecitabine has also been shown to be safe and effective in the older adult population.[47,48]

The results of the FOCUS2 trial provide valuable information on the management of older and/or frail adults with mCRC.[31] Patients deemed not to be candidates for full-dose combination therapy with a fluorpyrimidine and oxaliplatin by their physician were randomized in a 2 × 2 design to receive capecitabine or 5-FU/LV with or without oxaliplatin at a decreased dose (20%). The 5-FU/LV and capecitabine arms had similar efficacy; however, toxicity was greater and quality of life was lower in the capecitabine arm. Patients who received reduced-dose oxaliplatin did not have greater toxicity, but there was no improvement in survival outcomes. The results of this trial indicate that, if an oncologist does not feel the patient can tolerate full-dose oxaliplatin, the dual cytotoxic approach may not provide a survival benefit, and the patient may be better suited for single agent therapy with or without a biologic agent (see below).

Irinotecan plus 5-Fluoracil Irinotecan combined with 5-FU/LV became a standard of care after the combination demonstrated a 4.2-month improvement in OS over 5-FU/LV alone (14.8 vs 12.6 months, respectively; $P = .04$). Currently, irinotecan and 5-FU/LV are administered as the FOLFIRI regimen. From data on fit, older patients enrolled in clinical trials, FOLFIRI has similar efficacy and toxicity as seen in younger patients. Analysis of 4 randomized clinical trials comparing irinotecan + 5-FU/LV to 5-FU/LV alone reported no interaction between efficacy and age for response rates, progression-free survival, or OS. There was an interaction between toxicity and age for nausea and hepatic toxicity, which disappeared when age was used as a continuous variable.[49]

In a study of patients 75 years of age or older undergoing first-line treatment for mCRC, patients were randomized to receive FOLFIRI or 5-FU/LV alone.[50] Patients in the FOLFIRI arm did not have a significant difference in progression-free survival or OS. In addition, FOLFIRI was associated with a 76.3% severe toxicity rate compared with 52.2% with 5-FU/LV alone, with most common toxicities of neutropenia (38.5% vs 5.2%), diarrhea (22.2% vs 5.2%), and febrile neutropenia (6.7% vs 0.7%). Risk factors for toxicity were a mini-mental status examination of 27 or fewer out of 30 points and impaired activities of daily living. Thus, similar to combination therapy with FOLFOX, less fit older patients may not be appropriate candidates for combination irinotecan plus 5-FU/LV.

Minimizing toxicity with chemotherapy

Intermittent oxaliplatin administration The major toxicity of concern with oxaliplatin is neurotoxicity, which occurs in 2 forms: (1) acute, cold sensory neuropathy that leads to numbness, tingling, and/or pain when exposed to cold, especially in the extremities and with swallowing, and (2) chronic peripheral neuropathy, which occurs in a stocking–glove distribution and is cumulative over time. Neuropathy can lead to decreased proprioception and increase risk of falls. One strategy to minimize the degree of neuropathy is to use the intermittent oxaliplatin administration, or OPTIMOX, strategy. After 6 to 8 cycles of FOLFOX, patients can transition to maintenance 5-FU or capecitabine. Oxaliplatin can be reintroduced upon progression on maintenance therapy. This strategy results in the same survival as continuous FOLFOX administration, but reduces the incidence of grade 3/4 neurotoxicity.[51]

Omission of 5-fluoracil bolus The main toxicities of 5-FU are nausea/vomiting, diarrhea, and cytopenias. These effects are more likely to occur with bolus administration of 5-FU than the infusional form. Both forms are used in the FOLFOX regimen. However, it seems that in the palliative setting, survival times are similar with omission of the 5-FU bolus, although toxicities are less.[52] Thus, this is an excellent strategy to reduce toxicity but maintain efficacy in the palliative setting of mCRC management.

Biologic agents
In the past 2 decades, several classes of biologic agents have been approved for the treatment of mCRC. These agents can be used in combination with cytotoxic chemotherapy and some can be used as single agents.

The vascular endothelial growth factor therapies Three agents (bevacizumab, aflibercept, ramucirumab) target the vascular endothelial growth factor (VEGF) pathway. Bevacizumab, a monoclonal antibody (mAb) directed against VEGF-A ligand, combined with chemotherapy leads to survival benefits in the first- and second-line treatment setting of mCRC.[53–55] Aflibercept is a fusion protein targeting the VEGF-A and -B ligands that leads to a 1.4-month improvement in OS when combined with FOLFIRI in the second-line treatment of mCRC over FOLFIRI alone.[56] Comparing adverse effects of aflibercept to trials using bevacizumab, aflibercept seems to have increased risk for toxicity with no clear survival advantage, and therefore has not gained widespread use in mCRC. Ramucirumab, a mAb against the VEGF-A receptor, also improves survival by 1.6 months in combination with FOLFIRI in the second-line setting for mCRC over FOLFIRI alone.[57] Given that ramucirumab has just recently gained FDA approval, limited data are available on its use in the elderly, but it is likely that the extremely high cost of this drug will limit its use in mCRC.

Most of the data on VEGF target therapy in older patients come from studies on bevacizumab. Bevacizumab is remarkably well-tolerated, with most common adverse effects consisting of bleeding, hypertension, proteinuria, and arterial and venous thrombotic events; rare but serious events include wound healing complications, fistula or abscess, gastrointestinal perforation, and congestive heart failure. Owing to the toxicity profile, there was much concern over administering bevacizumab in the elderly population. However, when pooled data of bevacizumab from clinical trials was evaluated, arterial thrombotic events are the toxicity that occurs with increased frequency in older adults compared with the younger population.[58,59] There was no increased risk of gastrointestinal bleeding/perforation or hypertension in older patients receiving bevacizumab compared with younger patients. Older adults should be counseled on the increased risk of arterial thrombotic events, and for those over 75 with prior arterial thrombotic event, bevacizumab is contraindicated.

In general, bevacizumab is well-tolerated in the elderly and associated with very manageable adverse effects when combined with cytotoxic therapy. The Avastin in Elderly with Xeloda (AVEX) trial evaluated the combination of bevacizumab in patients 70 years or older who were not felt to be candidates for combination cytotoxic chemotherapy.[60] Patients who received capecitabine plus bevacizumab had a median OS of 20.7 months, which is approaching the survival of fit older adults able to receive chemotherapy doublets plus biologic agents. Thus, bevacizumab combined with a fluoropyrimidine is a potentially well-tolerated alternative to more aggressive regimens for less fit, older adults.

The epidermal growth factor receptor–targeted agents Two antibodies with efficacy in mCRC, cetuximab and panitumumab, target the epidermal growth factor receptor (EGFR). Panitumumab is a humanized mAb and therefore has less chance of causing an allergic/anaphylactic reaction than cetuximab, which is a chimeric mAb. Both EGFR therapies have shown to improve survival outcomes when combined with cytotoxic chemotherapy and as single agents in mCRC.[61–64] Thus, for older, frail adults who are not candidates for more aggressive cytotoxic chemotherapy regimens, either EGFR inhibitor administered as a single agent is an alternative. Cetuximab seems to have similar efficacy and tolerability in older adults as younger patients.[65,66] Patients whose mCRC harbors a RAS mutation are not eligible to receive EGFR inhibitor treatment. The main side effects from EGFR inhibitors include an acneiform rash, hypomagnesemia, diarrhea, and allergic reactions. The rash may be ameliorated by topical steroid creams and a macrolide antibiotic.[67]

Regorafenib, a multikinase inhibitor Regorafenib is approved for use in the third-line setting of mCRC after failure or intolerance of oxaliplatin and irinotecan-based regimens. A randomized, placebo-controlled, phase III trial showed a survival benefit of 1.4 months compared with placebo.[68] The majority of patients are unable to tolerate the approved starting dose, owing to side effects of hand–foot skin reaction, fatigue, diarrhea, hypertension, and rash or desquamation, and therefore dose reductions are often used upfront. Limited data are available on the tolerance of regorafenib in the older patient population. The decision to use regorafenib in the elderly patient must weigh the minimal survival benefit with the toxicity profile.

Summary: Tailoring Therapy for the Older Adult with Metastatic Colorectal Cancer

Very fit older adults
Robust older adults may be candidates for dual cytotoxic chemotherapy such as FOLFOX or FOLFIRI combined with a biologic agent in both the first and second line treatment setting. Strategies such as omitting the 5-FU bolus and intermittent oxaliplatin administration may improve tolerance for these patients.

Moderately fit older adults
This subset of patients may benefit from less aggressive regimens such as single agent cytotoxic chemotherapy with a biologic agent. This strategy still provides an improvement in survival, but is less likely to cause adverse effects that limit patients' ability to remain independent.

Unfit older adults
These adults may still be considered for a trial single agent therapy, such as low-dose capecitabine or single agent panitumumab (if RAS wild type). With good social support, these regimens may have very low side effect profile and extend survival by months.

REFERENCES

1. Torre LA, Bray F, Siegel RL, et al. Global cancer statistics, 2012. CA Cancer J Clin 2015;65:87–108.
2. McCleary NJ, Dotan E, Browner I. Refining the chemotherapy approach for older patients with colon cancer. J Clin Oncol 2014;32:2570–80.
3. Luo R, Giordano SH, Freeman JL, et al. Referral to medical oncology: a crucial step in the treatment of older patients with stage III colon cancer. Oncologist 2006;11:1025–33.
4. Abrams TA, Brightly R, Mao J, et al. Patterns of adjuvant chemotherapy use in a population-based cohort of patients with resected stage II or III colon cancer. J Clin Oncol 2011;29:3255–62.
5. Ho C, Ng K, O'Reilly S, et al. Outcomes in elderly patients with advanced colorectal cancer treated with capecitabine: a population-based analysis. Clin Colorectal Cancer 2005;5:279–82.

6. Wan-Chow-Wah D, Monette J, Monette M, et al. Difficulties in decision making regarding chemotherapy for older cancer patients: a census of cancer physicians. Crit Rev Oncol Hematol 2011;78:45–58.

7. U.S. Preventive Services Task Force. Screening for colorectal cancer: U.S. Preventive Services Task Force recommendation statement. Ann Intern Med 2008; 149:627–37.

8. Korc-Grodzicki B, Downey RJ, Shahrokni A, et al. Surgical considerations in older adults with cancer. J Clin Oncol 2014;32:2647–53.

9. Grailey K, Markar SR, Karthikesalingam A, et al. Laparoscopic versus open colorectal resection in the elderly population. Surg Endosc 2013;27:19–30.

10. Neuman HB, Weiss JM, Leverson G, et al. Predictors of short-term postoperative survival after elective colectomy in colon cancer patients >/= 80 years of age. Ann Surg Oncol 2013;20:1427–35.

11. Tran Ba Loc P, du Montcel ST, Duron JJ, et al. Elderly POSSUM, a dedicated score for prediction of mortality and morbidity after major colorectal surgery in older patients. Br J Surg 2010;97:396–403.

12. Cook EJ, Welsh FK, Chandrakumaran K, et al. Resection of colorectal liver metastases in the elderly: does age matter? Colorectal Dis 2012;14:1210–6.

13. Cannon RM, Martin RC, Callender GG, et al. Safety and efficacy of hepatectomy for colorectal metastases in the elderly. J Surg Oncol 2011;104:804–8.

14. Tanis E, Nordlinger B, Mauer M, et al. Local recurrence rates after radiofrequency ablation or resection of colorectal liver metastases. Analysis of the European Organisation for Research and Treatment of Cancer #40004 and #40983. Eur J Cancer 2014;50:912–9.

15. Sauer R, Becker H, Hohenberger W, et al. Preoperative versus postoperative chemoradiotherapy for rectal cancer. N Engl J Med 2004;351:1731–40.

16. Margalit DN, Mamon HJ, Ancukiewicz M, et al. Tolerability of combined modality therapy for rectal cancer in elderly patients aged 75 years and older. Int J Radiat Oncol Biol Phys 2011;81:e735–41.

17. Ngan SY, Burmeister B, Fisher RJ, et al. Randomized trial of short-course radiotherapy versus long-course chemoradiation comparing rates of local recurrence in patients with T3 rectal cancer: Trans-Tasman Radiation Oncology Group trial 01.04. J Clin Oncol 2012;30:3827–33.

18. Kahn KL, Adams JL, Weeks JC, et al. Adjuvant chemotherapy use and adverse events among older patients with stage III colon cancer. JAMA 2010;303: 1037–45.

19. Schrag D, Cramer LD, Bach PB, et al. Age and adjuvant chemotherapy use after surgery for stage III colon cancer. J Natl Cancer Inst 2001;93:850–7.

20. Sanoff HK, Carpenter WR, Sturmer T, et al. Effect of adjuvant chemotherapy on survival of patients with stage III colon cancer diagnosed after age 75 years. J Clin Oncol 2012;30:2624–34.

21. Neugut AI, Matasar M, Wang X, et al. Duration of adjuvant chemotherapy for colon cancer and survival among the elderly. J Clin Oncol 2006;24:2368–75.

22. Hurria A, Dale W, Mooney M, et al. Designing therapeutic clinical trials for older and frail adults with cancer: U13 conference recommendations. J Clin Oncol 2014;32:2587–94.

23. Moertel CG, Fleming TR, Macdonald JS, et al. Levamisole and fluorouracil for adjuvant therapy of resected colon carcinoma. N Engl J Med 1990;322:352–8.

24. Moertel CG, Fleming TR, Macdonald JS, et al. Fluorouracil plus levamisole as effective adjuvant therapy after resection of stage III colon carcinoma: a final report. Ann Intern Med 1995;122:321–6.

25. Jessup JM, Stewart A, Greene FL, et al. Adjuvant chemotherapy for stage III colon cancer: implications of race/ethnicity, age, and differentiation. JAMA 2005; 294:2703–11.
26. Sargent DJ, Goldberg RM, Jacobson SD, et al. A pooled analysis of adjuvant chemotherapy for resected colon cancer in elderly patients. N Engl J Med 2001;345:1091–7.
27. Sundararajan V, Mitra N, Jacobson JS, et al. Survival associated with 5-fluorouracil-based adjuvant chemotherapy among elderly patients with node-positive colon cancer. Ann Intern Med 2002;136:349–57.
28. Gross CP, McAvay GJ, Guo Z, et al. The impact of chronic illnesses on the use and effectiveness of adjuvant chemotherapy for colon cancer. Cancer 2007; 109:2410–9.
29. Twelves C, Wong A, Nowacki MP, et al. Capecitabine as adjuvant treatment for stage III colon cancer. N Engl J Med 2005;352:2696–704.
30. Scheithauer W, McKendrick J, Begbie S, et al. Oral capecitabine as an alternative to i.v. 5-fluorouracil-based adjuvant therapy for colon cancer: safety results of a randomized, phase III trial. Ann Oncol 2003;14:1735–43.
31. Seymour MT, Thompson LC, Wasan HS, et al. Chemotherapy options in elderly and frail patients with metastatic colorectal cancer (MRC FOCUS2): an open-label, randomised factorial trial. Lancet 2011;377:1749–59.
32. MacLaughlin EJ, Raehl CL, Treadway AK, et al. Assessing medication adherence in the elderly: which tools to use in clinical practice? Drugs Aging 2005;22: 231–55.
33. Andre T, Boni C, Mounedji-Boudiaf L, et al. Oxaliplatin, fluorouracil, and leucovorin as adjuvant treatment for colon cancer. N Engl J Med 2004;350:2343–51.
34. Andre T, Boni C, Navarro M, et al. Improved overall survival with oxaliplatin, fluorouracil, and leucovorin as adjuvant treatment in stage II or III colon cancer in the MOSAIC trial. J Clin Oncol 2009;27:3109–16.
35. Haller DG, Tabernero J, Maroun J, et al. Capecitabine plus oxaliplatin compared with fluorouracil and folinic acid as adjuvant therapy for stage III colon cancer. J Clin Oncol 2011;29:1465–71.
36. Kuebler JP, Wieand HS, O'Connell MJ, et al. Oxaliplatin combined with weekly bolus fluorouracil and leucovorin as surgical adjuvant chemotherapy for stage II and III colon cancer: results from NSABP C-07. J Clin Oncol 2007;25:2198–204.
37. McCleary NJ, Meyerhardt JA, Green E, et al. Impact of age on the efficacy of newer adjuvant therapies in patients with stage II/III colon cancer: findings from the ACCENT database. J Clin Oncol 2013;31:2600–6.
38. Haller DG, O'Connell MJ, Cartwright TH, et al. Impact of age and medical comorbidity on adjuvant treatment outcomes for stage III colon cancer: a pooled analysis of individual patient data from four randomized, controlled trials. Ann Oncol 2015;26:715–24.
39. Goldberg RM, Tabah-Fisch I, Bleiberg H, et al. Pooled analysis of safety and efficacy of oxaliplatin plus fluorouracil/leucovorin administered bimonthly in elderly patients with colorectal cancer. J Clin Oncol 2006;24:4085–91.
40. Hershman D, Hall MJ, Wang X, et al. Timing of adjuvant chemotherapy initiation after surgery for stage III colon cancer. Cancer 2006;107:2581–8.
41. Siegel RL, Miller KD, Jemal A. Cancer statistics, 2015. CA Cancer J Clin 2015;65: 5–29.
42. Venook AP, Niedzwiecki D, Lenz H-J, et al. CALGB/SWOG 80405: phase III trial of irinotecan/5-FU/leucovorin (FOLFIRI) or oxaliplatin/5-FU/leucovorin (mFOLFOX6) with bevacizumab (BV) or cetuximab (CET) for patients (pts) with KRAS

wild-type (wt) untreated metastatic adenocarcinoma of the colon or rectum (MCRC). Report of the proceedings of the American Society of Clinical Oncology Meeting Abstracts 2014;32:LBA3.

43. Goldberg RM, Sargent DJ, Morton RF, et al. A randomized controlled trial of fluorouracil plus leucovorin, irinotecan, and oxaliplatin combinations in patients with previously untreated metastatic colorectal cancer. J Clin Oncol 2004;22:23–30.

44. Berretta M, Cappellani A, Fiorica F, et al. FOLFOX4 in the treatment of metastatic colorectal cancer in elderly patients: a prospective study. Arch Gerontol Geriatr 2011;52:89–93.

45. Rosati G, Cordio S, Tucci A, et al. Phase II trial of oxaliplatin and tegafur/uracil and oral folinic acid for advanced or metastatic colorectal cancer in elderly patients. Oncology 2005;69:122–9.

46. de Gramont A, Figer A, Seymour M, et al. Leucovorin and fluorouracil with or without oxaliplatin as first-line treatment in advanced colorectal cancer. J Clin Oncol 2000;18:2938–47.

47. Grande C, Quintero G, Candamio S, et al. Biweekly XELOX (capecitabine and oxaliplatin) as first-line treatment in elderly patients with metastatic colorectal cancer. J Geriatr Oncol 2013;4:114–21.

48. Twelves CJ, Butts CA, Cassidy J, et al. Capecitabine/oxaliplatin, a safe and active first-line regimen for older patients with metastatic colorectal cancer: post hoc analysis of a large phase II study. Clin Colorectal Cancer 2005;5:101–7.

49. Folprecht G, Seymour MT, Saltz L, et al. Irinotecan/fluorouracil combination in first-line therapy of older and younger patients with metastatic colorectal cancer: combined analysis of 2,691 patients in randomized controlled trials. J Clin Oncol 2008;26:1443–51.

50. Aparicio T, Jouve JL, Teillet L, et al. Geriatric factors predict chemotherapy feasibility: ancillary results of FFCD 2001-02 phase III study in first-line chemotherapy for metastatic colorectal cancer in elderly patients. J Clin Oncol 2013;31: 1464–70.

51. Tournigand C, Cervantes A, Figer A, et al. OPTIMOX1: a randomized study of FOLFOX4 or FOLFOX7 with oxaliplatin in a stop-and-go fashion in advanced colorectal cancer–a GERCOR study. J Clin Oncol 2006;24:394–400.

52. Yoshida Y, Hasegawa J, Nishimura J, et al. Clinical significance of bolus 5-fluorouracil for recurrent or metastatic colorectal cancer treated with FOLFOX+ Bevacizumab Therapy. Gan To Kagaku Ryoho 2011;38:1293–6 [In Japanese].

53. Hurwitz H, Fehrenbacher L, Novotny W, et al. Bevacizumab plus irinotecan, fluorouracil, and leucovorin for metastatic colorectal cancer. N Engl J Med 2004;350: 2335–42.

54. Saltz LB, Clarke S, Diaz-Rubio E, et al. Bevacizumab in combination with oxaliplatin-based chemotherapy as first-line therapy in metastatic colorectal cancer: a randomized phase III study. J Clin Oncol 2008;26:2013–9.

55. Giantonio BJ, Catalano PJ, Meropol NJ, et al. Bevacizumab in combination with oxaliplatin, fluorouracil, and leucovorin (FOLFOX4) for previously treated metastatic colorectal cancer: results from the Eastern Cooperative Oncology Group Study E3200. J Clin Oncol 2007;25:1539–44.

56. Van Cutsem E, Tabernero J, Lakomy R, et al. Addition of aflibercept to fluorouracil, leucovorin, and irinotecan improves survival in a phase III randomized trial in patients with metastatic colorectal cancer previously treated with an oxaliplatin-based regimen. J Clin Oncol 2012;30:3499–506.

57. Tabernero J, Yoshino T, Cohn AL, et al. Ramucirumab versus placebo in combination with second-line FOLFIRI in patients with metastatic colorectal carcinoma

that progressed during or after first-line therapy with bevacizumab, oxaliplatin, and a fluoropyrimidine (RAISE): a randomised, double-blind, multicentre, phase 3 study. Lancet Oncol 2015;16:499–508.

58. Kozloff MF, Berlin J, Flynn PJ, et al. Clinical outcomes in elderly patients with metastatic colorectal cancer receiving bevacizumab and chemotherapy: results from the BRiTE observational cohort study. Oncology 2010;78:329–39.

59. Scappaticci FA, Skillings JR, Holden SN, et al. Arterial thromboembolic events in patients with metastatic carcinoma treated with chemotherapy and bevacizumab. J Natl Cancer Inst 2007;99:1232–9.

60. Cunningham D, Lang I, Marcuello E, et al. Bevacizumab plus capecitabine versus capecitabine alone in elderly patients with previously untreated metastatic colorectal cancer (AVEX): an open-label, randomised phase 3 trial. Lancet Oncol 2013;14:1077–85.

61. Cunningham D, Humblet Y, Siena S, et al. Cetuximab monotherapy and cetuximab plus irinotecan in irinotecan-refractory metastatic colorectal cancer. N Engl J Med 2004;351:337–45.

62. Jonker DJ, O'Callaghan CJ, Karapetis CS, et al. Cetuximab for the treatment of colorectal cancer. N Engl J Med 2007;357:2040–8.

63. Van Cutsem E, Peeters M, Siena S, et al. Open-label phase III trial of panitumumab plus best supportive care compared with best supportive care alone in patients with chemotherapy-refractory metastatic colorectal cancer. J Clin Oncol 2007;25:1658–64.

64. Bokemeyer C, Van Cutsem E, Rougier P, et al. Addition of cetuximab to chemotherapy as first-line treatment for KRAS wild-type metastatic colorectal cancer: pooled analysis of the CRYSTAL and OPUS randomised clinical trials. Eur J Cancer 2012;48:1466–75.

65. Jehn CF, Boning L, Kroning H, et al. Cetuximab-based therapy in elderly comorbid patients with metastatic colorectal cancer. Br J Cancer 2012;106:274–8.

66. Bouchahda M, Macarulla T, Spano JP, et al. Cetuximab efficacy and safety in a retrospective cohort of elderly patients with heavily pretreated metastatic colorectal cancer. Crit Rev Oncol Hematol 2008;67:255–62.

67. Lacouture ME, Mitchell EP, Piperdi B, et al. Skin toxicity evaluation protocol with panitumumab (STEPP), a phase II, open-label, randomized trial evaluating the impact of a pre-emptive skin treatment regimen on skin toxicities and quality of life in patients with metastatic colorectal cancer. J Clin Oncol 2010;28:1351–7.

68. Grothey A, Van Cutsem E, Sobrero A, et al. Regorafenib monotherapy for previously treated metastatic colorectal cancer (CORRECT): an international, multicentre, randomised, placebo-controlled, phase 3 trial. Lancet 2013;381:303–12.

Management of Prostate Cancer in the Elderly

Kae Jack Tay, MBBS, MRCS(Ed), MCI[a], Judd W. Moul, MD[a],
Andrew J. Armstrong, MD, ScM[b],*

KEYWORDS

- Prostate cancer • Elderly • Geriatric • Localized • Metastatic • Oncology • Surgery
- Radiation

KEY POINTS

- The impact of prostate cancer in the elderly depends largely on the aggressiveness of the disease and the time horizon over which prostate cancer morbidity and mortality may occur.
- Comorbidity and quality-of-life concerns are the key considerations when deciding whether treatment is necessary or the type of treatment modality to be used in prostate cancer in the elderly.
- In the elderly with metastatic prostate cancer, exercise and vitamin D serve to improve bone health and functional status to offset complications from hormonal therapy.

INTRODUCTION

Because of the stabilization of birth rates, better medical care, and improved living standards, the number of older persons worldwide tripled in the latter half of the twentieth century; this number is projected to triple again in the next 50 years.[1] In the United States, the proportion of the population aged older than 65 years has increased by 15% in the last decade alone.[2] Prostate cancer, currently the most incident cancer and the second highest cause of cancer death among men in the United States, is notably diagnosed in the later years of life.[3] The incidence of clinically detected prostate cancer in the United States between 2009 and 2011 was noted to be 1 in 304 for men younger than 49 years, 1 in 44 for men aged 55 to 59 years, 1 in 16 for men aged 60 to 69 years, and 1 in 9 for men 70 years and older.

Despite concerns regarding overdiagnosis of indolent disease, advanced and lethal prostate cancer are also more likely among older men.[4–6] The median age of death

[a] Division of Urology, Duke University Medical Center, DUMC Box 103861, Durham, NC 27710, USA; [b] Department of Medical Oncology, Duke University Medical Center, DUMC Box 103861, Durham, NC 27710, USA
* Corresponding author. Department of Medical Oncology, Duke University Medical Center, 905 La Salle Street, GSRB1 Room 3006, Durham, NC 27710.
E-mail address: andrew.armstrong@dm.duke.edu

Clin Geriatr Med 32 (2016) 113–132
http://dx.doi.org/10.1016/j.cger.2015.08.001
0749-0690/16/$ – see front matter © 2016 Elsevier Inc. All rights reserved.

from prostate cancer is 77 years, with men surviving to 90 years of age having a nearly 1 in 5 probability of dying of prostate cancer (**Fig. 1**). Although age definitions for the geriatric population may differ, it is clear that the prevalence of prostate cancer increases with age and older men are disproportionately affected by lethal prostate cancer. The authors discuss here the impact of prostate cancer and its treatment in the elderly and review the best available evidence with which clinicians may formulate management strategies.

CLINICALLY LOCALIZED PROSTATE CANCER
Deciding Who Needs to be Treated

Autopsy studies show that the prevalence of indolent prostate cancer is high and that this increases with age.[7] In 1997, Johansson and colleagues[8] reported on a 15-year follow-up of a Swedish cohort of 300 men with rectally detected early stage prostate cancer who were generally older than 60 years, finding a similar adjusted survival rate among men who received treatment and those who did not. These findings prompted controversy over the necessity for localized prostate cancer to be treated. With longer follow-up, however, it seems that the time horizon for disease progression is a critical factor. From follow-up reports at the 20- and 30-year intervals of the Johansson series, it has become apparent that local tumor progression and aggressive metastatic disease may occur in the long-term, even for men considered low risk at diagnosis.[9,10]

Two other natural history studies reported by Albertsen and colleagues[11] (767 men aged 55–74 years) and Cuzick and colleagues[12] (2333 men with a maximum age of 76 years) identified the Gleason score and prostate-specific antigen (PSA) as predictors

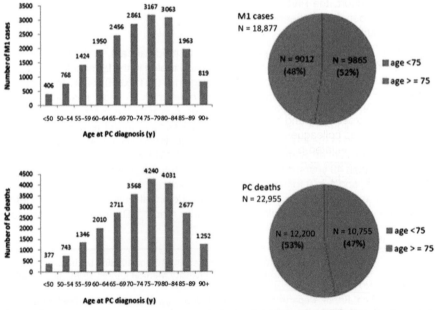

Fig. 1. The contribution of different age groups to the pool of patients who had prostate cancer (PC) with metastatic disease (M1) at diagnosis and PC deaths is illustrated. (*From* Scosyrev E, Messing EM, Mohile S, et al. Prostate cancer in the elderly: frequency of advanced disease at presentation and disease-specific mortality. Cancer 2012;118(12):3065; with permission.)

of disease progression. Albertsen and colleagues[11] also reported that men with Gleason 8 to 10 prostate cancer were highly likely to die of prostate cancer within the first 10 years of cancer diagnosis. The prognostic factors of serum PSA, biopsy Gleason score, and clinical stage have since been validated as prognosticators for prostate cancer and are commonly grouped using the D'Amico risk classification system into low, intermediate, and high risk.[13]

The time horizon for morbidity and mortality to occur, or the life expectancy, thus, seems more important than chronologic age in dictating treatment of localized disease and, regardless of age, men with low-risk prostate cancer and a life expectancy of greater than 10 to 15 years and men with intermediate- to high-risk prostate cancer and a life expectancy of 5 to 10 years should be considered candidates for treatment. In the Scandinavian randomized trial on radical prostatectomy versus watchful waiting in prostate cancer (SPCG-4), which found a benefit with prostatectomy with a 44% relative risk reduction in deaths, the benefits were maximal in men younger than 65 years, illustrating the point that treatment advantages are apparent to those with a longer life expectancy.[14] On the contrary, the Prostate Intervention versus Observation Trial (PIVOT), randomizing men to radical prostatectomy or active surveillance, could not detect an overall survival benefit with prostatectomy, though a small advantage was seen in the intermediate-risk subgroup; this may be partly attributed to the fact that 40% of men in both arms died by the study conclusion date at 10 years, raising concerns that the group had an overall lower life expectancy than normal.[15] It is important to note that SPCG-4 was conducted in the pre-PSA screening era when most tumors, though localized, were clinically T2 and digitally palpable, whereas in PVIOT, most tumors were clinically T1c, impalpable, and detected by PSA screening, suggesting that with sufficient interval to overcome the lead time over the SPCG-4 cohort, the PIVOT group may have demonstrated a larger, detectable magnitude of benefit. Furthermore, in SPCG-4, though men older than 65 years did not have a survival advantage, they did experience a 32% relative risk reduction for the development of metastasis; in PIVOT, an overall 60% risk reduction in the development of bone metastasis was observed. In a paradigm of localized disease preceding metastasis and metastasis preceding death, this again emphasizes the chronologically distant impact of prostate cancer treatment.

The most favorable outcome for the elderly man can, thus, only be attained through balancing life expectancy and disease aggressiveness. In a decision-analytic Markov model, Alibhai and colleagues[16] showed that treatment of men up to 75 years old with moderately differentiated prostate cancers, and men up to 80 years old with poorly differentiated prostate cancers, produced gains in both life expectancy and quality-adjusted life expectancy.

Estimating Life Expectancy

Life-expectancy estimation is discussed by Li and colleagues, Dale and colleagues and, Wingfield and colleagues.[17–19] In short, according to the 2010 period actuarial life table published by the Social Security Administration, the average US man at 70 years of age has a 14-year life expectancy and at 80 years of age, an 8.1-year life expectancy.[20] Although national actuarial estimates alone remained the best estimators of life expectancy, predictive models co-opting a range of comorbidities may be more consistent and accurate than physician estimates.[21]

The competing risk of death conferred by comorbidities has been addressed elegantly by Daskivich and colleagues[22] in a report from the Prostate Cancer Outcomes Study, a cohort of 3183 men with localized prostate cancer. When men were classified by comorbidity count, older men were found to have a higher absolute risk of other-cause mortality at the 14-year follow-up, with a proportional increase in other-cause mortality with the number of comorbidities present (**Fig. 2**). On the other hand, a higher D'Amico risk status was associated with a higher likelihood of dying of prostate cancer. One criticism of the study is the equal analytical weightage given to debatably less serious comorbidities, such as arthritis, inflammatory bowel disease, or Crohn disease, as more life-threatening comorbidities, such as stroke and myocardial infarction. Nonetheless, this study demonstrates that the number of comorbidities matter; their impact increases with age; and that these should be accounted for in clinical decision making around definitive therapy versus active surveillance in older men.

Beyond comorbidity, frailty is often subjectively assessed by clinicians using the eyeball test. The extent of independence in daily activities predicts survival in the elderly.[23] Cognitive impairment is also linked to shorter survival as well as worse postoperative outcomes, including complications and longer hospital stays.[23,24] The degree of frailty, when comprehensively measured by the geriatric status scale including independence in activities of daily living, bowel/urinary continence, and the presence of cognitive impairment, has also been found to impact survival.[25] Frailty and poor survival are in turn associated with poor nutritional status.[26,27] Incorporating these factors, the International Society of Geriatric Oncology Prostate Cancer Task Force has recommended that

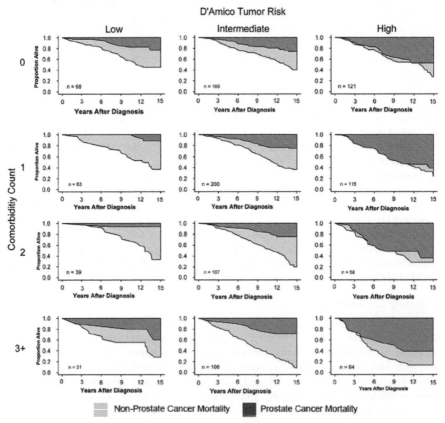

Fig. 2. Mortality by comorbidity count and D'Amico risk status in men aged greater than 70 years. (*From* Daskivich TJ, Fan KH, Koyama T, et al. Prediction of long-term other-cause mortality in men with early-stage prostate cancer: results from the Prostate Cancer Outcomes Study. Urology 2015;85(1):98; with permission.)

elderly men with prostate cancer undergo a comprehensive assessment for comorbidities using the cumulative illness score rating–geriatrics (CISR-G), dependence status, and nutritional status to determine whether they undergo oncologic treatment (**Fig. 3**).[28]

Ultimately, the aim of treatment of prostate cancer in the elderly man is to maintain a life free of the complications of local progression or systemic disease and avoiding prostate cancer–related mortality by obtaining oncological control *when necessary*. Solely relying on physician estimates may lead to an underestimation of life expectancy with resultant undertreatment of even high-risk categories of prostate cancer.[29] The use of geriatric assessment tools may better stratify elderly men for treatment or observation and reduce risks of therapy-associated morbidity.[30]

Expectant Management: Watchful Waiting or Active Surveillance?

Watchful waiting is a strategy of clinical observation, with interventions reserved for symptoms when they develop.[31] With this strategy, it is generally accepted that local progression and/or metastases may develop at some point and that these will be treated with palliative measures. Active surveillance, on the other hand, is a proactive process of close monitoring for disease progression over time with the aim of deferring but preserving the option for definitive therapy. Traditional surveillance regimes include men with low-risk cancer and recommend at least one rebiopsy within 12 to 18 months with subsequent biopsies dependent on PSA or other clinical triggers.[32] In a large cohort of men undergoing active surveillance, Klotz and colleagues[33] reported that 75.7% of men avoided intervention at 5 years, 63.5% at 10 years, and 55.5% at 15 years, with a metastasis rate of 2.8% and a prostate cancer–related mortality rate of 1.5%.

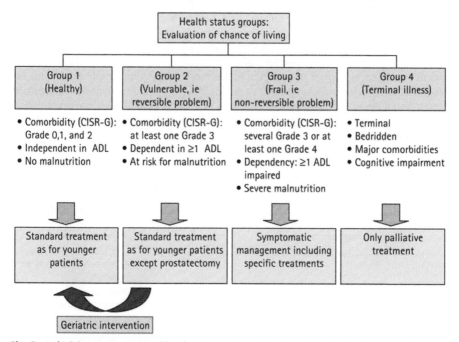

Fig. 3. A decision tree proposed by the International Society of Geriatric Oncology for treating patients with localized disease based on comorbidity and functional status. ADL, activities of daily living. (*From* Droz JP, Balducci L, Bolla M, et al. Management of prostate cancer in older men: recommendations of a working group of the International Society of Geriatric Oncology. BJU Int 2010;106(4):464; with permission.)

Watchful waiting is, thus, considered suitable for elderly men with organ-confined prostate cancer when life expectancy is shorter than 5 to 10 years as they are unlikely to experience symptoms of disease progression or to die of prostate cancer.[8] Active surveillance is considered more appropriate in older men with prostate cancer when the disease is low risk and life expectancy is greater than 10 to 15 years.

However, both expectant management strategies are hampered by prostate cancer risk underclassification resulting from the use of random biopsies with high rates of sampling error. This underclassification, whereby intermediate- or high-risk cancers are erroneously classified as low risk, has been observed at a rate of 30% to 50% in prostatectomy studies, which, by avoiding sampling error, are the reference standard for accurate cancer risk classification.[34] In active surveillance series following men with biopsy-proven low-risk prostate cancer, up to 28% have a Gleason score upgrading at the first surveillance rebiopsy at 12 to 18 months, which is, arguably, given the short time frame, a result of underclassification in the first place.[32] In elderly men older than 65 years, more pathologic upgrading and upstaging occurred compared with younger men in the Prostate Research International: Active Surveillance study.[35] Delaying treatment in such men with underclassified cancer results in adverse outcomes.[36] Indeed, in the Klotz series, those eventually subjected to treatment had post-treatment biochemical recurrence rates as high as 53%, highlighting the limitations of the current selection criteria.[33]

Furthermore, periodic rebiopsies during active surveillance are significant sources of morbidity with attendant risks of bleeding and urosepsis that may be amplified in the elderly.[37] Staging saturation biopsies may improve the accuracy of risk classification before embarking on active surveillance, but there are no long-term data to support reducing the number of subsequent biopsies during the course of active surveillance.[38] Similarly, outcomes of modern protocols using multi-parametric MRI, fusion biopsies, and molecular markers that may potentially reduce subsequent follow-up or biopsy intensity because of better initial risk classification are awaited.[34] Nonetheless, some form of surveillance that is more active than simply watchful waiting should be implemented in a healthy elderly man with ostensibly low-risk prostate cancer and a life expectancy of 10 to 15 years or more (**Table 1**). At some point during surveillance, it is reasonable to consider switching to a more passive form of expectant management as life expectancy reduces.

Table 1
Contemporary guideline recommendations for low-risk disease

Guideline	Condition	Recommendation
NCCN	Life expectancy ≤10 y	Observation
	Life expectancy >10 y	Active surveillance as an option
AUA	All men	Active surveillance as an option
EAU	Short life expectancy	Observation
	>10 y life expectancy and low volume disease (≤2 cores positive cores, ≤50% core involvement)	Active surveillance as an option

Abbreviations: AUA, American Urological Association; EAU, European Association of Urology; NCCN, National Comprehensive Cancer Network.

Adapted from National Comprehensive Cancer Network Clinical Practice Guidelines in Oncology (Prostate Cancer) version 1.2015; American Urological Association Guideline for the Management of Clinically Localized Prostate Cancer (2007, up to date as of 2011); and European Association of Urology Guidelines on Prostate Cancer(updated March 2015).

Deciding on What Type of Treatment, If Treatment is Necessary

Treatment is necessary in the fit elderly man with high-volume intermediate- or high-risk disease and a life expectancy of more than 5 to 10 years. Although there are no randomized trials comparing the major treatment modalities of surgery or radiation, it is generally accepted that their efficacy is comparable across different risk groups. Compared with nonextirpative modalities, detection of recurrence after surgery is more well defined using PSA.[39] Data from the PCOS study suggest that both surgery and radiation are associated with a similar decline in sexual, urinary, and bowel symptom scores at the long-term 10- to 15-year follow-up, with most men experiencing erectile dysfunction.[40] Thus, treatment selection largely depends on the side-effect profile of each modality.

Radical prostatectomy in the elderly

Complete surgical extirpation is the gold standard for cure in clinically localized prostate cancer. Radical prostatectomy has undergone significant evolution in the last 2 decades with refinement of the original open techniques and the adoption of minimally invasive techniques. In particular, robot-assisted procedures in organ-confined prostate cancer have resulted in reduced blood loss while maintaining anatomic nerve and sphincter-sparing dissections through improved visualization and dexterity.[41,42] However, reduced cardiorespiratory reserves in the elderly raise concerns regarding the additional morbidity of pneumoperitoneum.[43,44] In general, perioperative mortality rates in prostatectomy cohorts have been less than 1% and complications rates less than 2%, though this may reflect a high degree of patient selection.[45]

Elderly men should be counseled that younger age is significantly associated with the return of continence and potency at 1 year after radical prostatectomy and men older than 70 years have a significantly longer time to reach continence.[46,47] On the other hand, the incidence of symptomatic bladder outlet obstruction increases with age; men with concurrent obstructive urinary symptoms benefit from both a better flow rate and cure of cancer with radical prostatectomy. An analysis of long-term functional outcomes in the SPCG-4 cohort showed that those undergoing radical prostatectomy had a 30% risk reduction in the incidence of poor flow and a 21% risk reduction in the incidence of nocturia at a median follow-up of 12 years.[48] It is also known that the degree of improvement in urinary symptoms is closely related to patient-perceived satisfaction with treatment.[49]

Radiation therapy in the elderly

Radiation therapy has been the mainstay of definitive prostate cancer treatment in the elderly, particularly in those deemed requiring treatment but unfit for surgical intervention. External beam radiation therapy has evolved to boost delivery and minimize collateral damage culminating in modern intensity-modulation (intensity-modulated radiation therapy [IMRT]), stereotactic (stereotactic body radiation therapy), and proton beam techniques. IMRT, the workhorse of radiation therapy, typically involves 8 to 9 weeks of daily Monday-to-Friday fractionation schemes, delivering doses of 78 Gy. The effects of collateral radiation remain the main concern following radiation therapy. Although high-grade early rectal and urinary radiation toxicity are rare, the incidence of late toxicity is notable for urinary frequency, diarrhea, radiation cystitis and proctitis, urethral strictures, and a small long-term risk of secondary malignancy.[50] Wallis and colleagues[51] showed in a propensity-matched analysis that the complication rates of radiation are similar to prostatectomy at 1 year but diverge at 3 years, with radiation having twice the complications. In an elderly man, the probability of suffering these consequences would increase with the length of life expectancy.

On the other hand, interstitial brachytherapy using radioactive iodine or palladium isotopes seek to overcome the problems of collateral radiation by achieving cell-kill through gradual emission of low-penetrance alpha radiation. The main toxicity is to the urethra, with almost all patients experiencing some form of urinary irritation in the early post-treatment period and some early series reporting a urethral stricture rate of up to 10% to 12%.[52,53] Careful dosimetric considerations can reduce the risk of acute urinary toxicity, and contemporary stricture rates are closer to 5% to 6%.[52,54]

In men with high-risk prostate cancer, Jones and colleagues[55] showed that short-term androgen deprivation therapy (ADT) combined with radiation improved overall survival compared with radiation alone in a cohort of men with a median age of 71 years. Bolla and colleagues[56] demonstrated that 3 years of ADT was better than 6 months when combined with radiation therapy in men with a median age of 70 years. On the other hand, D'Amico and colleagues[57] showed that the beneficial effect of adjuvant ADT was not seen in men with moderate to severe comorbidities. In particular, one brachytherapy study showed that adjuvant ADT increased mortality in men with underlying cardiovascular disease.[58] These factors should be taken into account before subjecting the elderly man with high-risk prostate cancer to radiotherapy. In high-risk localized disease, successful surgical resection may help men avoid ADT. One alternative to addition of ADT to external beam radiation is a 2-fraction high-dose–rate radiation boost.

Thermal ablation in the elderly
Thermal ablation with high-intensity focused ultrasound (HIFU) and cryotherapy has been used as a minimally invasive method to treat prostate cancer. Many studies have been done in older men, and thermal ablation is limited by the need for downsizing with ADT in large prostates. Crouzet and colleagues,[59] reporting on a cohort of 1002 men with a mean age of 72 years undergoing primary whole-gland HIFU, found the biochemical recurrence-free rate at 8 years to be 76%, 63%, and 57% for low-, intermediate-, and high-risk men, respectively, with an early complication rate of up to 18.0% and a late complication rate of 9.4%.

Cryotherapy is another form of thermal ablation with advantages of better estimation of treatment extent by visualizing the edge of the expanding ice ball. In an analysis by Dhar and colleagues[60] on 860 men aged greater than 75 years from the Cryo On-Line Data registry, the biochemical recurrence-free survival rate at 5 years was found to be 82.4%, 78.3%, and 77.6% for low-, intermediate-, and high-risk prostate cancer. Early complications were seen in 6% and late complications in 0.1%. Incontinence was noted in 0.9% of patients. Similar to other contemporary cryotherapy reports, the rate of potency after treatment was low at 11%.

Focal therapy
Focal therapy is an experimental treatment in prostate cancer.[61] In the elderly, selective ablation of one or 2 lesions that are intermediate or high grade, may down-classify men back into the active surveillance or conservative management pool.[62] Although this is an attractive proposition, the feasibility and long-term outcomes of this strategy are unknown and represent an active area of research.

ADVANCED PROSTATE CANCER
Locally Advanced Prostate Cancer: Sequencing Multimodality Treatment in Elderly Patients

Men with locally advanced prostate cancer are at high risk of positive surgical margins and nodal and systemic microdissemination and are likely to require multimodality treatment, encompassing various combinations of surgery, radiation, and hormonal therapy.[63] In very fit elderly men, the advantage of surgery in this setting is to preserve radiation and hormonal therapy as subsequent salvage options in view that salvage prostatectomy has markedly more complications and poorer functional outcomes than primary prostatectomy.[64] Radiation with adjuvant hormonal therapy is otherwise a reasonable therapeutic strategy. In men who are unfit even for radiation, hormonal therapy, discussed in detail later, may be used to palliate symptoms as a monotherapy.

Metastatic Prostate Cancer in the Elderly

Elderly men may be susceptible to more aggressive prostate cancer. A Surveillance, Epidemiology, and End Results database study spanning 1998 to 2007 found that men older than 75 years were more likely to present with metastatic disease than their younger counterparts and had a greater risk of death of prostate cancer despite having higher death rates from competing comorbidities.[6] The mainstay of treatment of metastatic prostate cancer is ADT.[65] Additionally, particularly fit elderly men with high-volume metastatic prostate cancer may benefit from an induction regime of 6 cycles of docetaxel for a survival benefit of 13 to 17 months as found in the ECOG CHAARTED trial (the Eastern Cooperative Oncology Group Chemo-Hormonal Therapy versus Androgen Ablation Randomized Trial for Extensive Disease in Prostate Cancer).[66]

Androgen deprivation therapy

Early androgen deprivation is recommended for men with asymptomatic M1 disease based on findings from the UK Medical Research Council trial that men with ADT deferred until symptomatic were twice as likely to develop pathologic fractures, spinal cord compression, ureteric obstruction, and extraskeletal metastasis.[67] Before starting ADT, though, one should be cognizant that it has not been shown to improve cancer-specific survival and only impacts overall survival marginally at 10 years.[68]

ADT can be achieved using medical or surgical means. Surgical castration with bilateral orchiectomy results in the most rapid reduction in serum testosterone.[69] It results in better quality of life and is particularly useful in elderly men who are unlikely to be compliant to follow-up.[70] On the other hand, medical castration, typically with a luteinizing hormone-releasing hormone (LHRH) agonist, allows for the use of intermittent ADT and is suitable for men who are reluctant for orchiectomy.[71] Although several types and formulations of LHRH agonists (1, 3, and 6 monthly depot injections) exist, their clinical efficacy is considered to be similar.[72] At initial administration, LHRH agonists may produce a surge in testosterone resulting in a clinical flare in patients with extensive metastasis.[73] To prevent this, a peripheral antiandrogen is usually used in combination for 1 to 4 weeks during the first dose of the LHRH agonist.[74] Degarelix, currently the only Food and Drug Administration–approved LHRH antagonist, does not have the flare problem but may cause more hot flashes and is available only in 1-month depot formulations. Combined androgen blockade with the long-term addition of an antiandrogen to medical or surgical castration has not been found to have a meaningful impact on overall survival and cannot be recommended in the elderly man.[75]

ADT is associated with significant morbidities that may be exacerbated in elderly men.[76] These morbidities include fatigue, anemia, sexual dysfunction leading to loss of sexual intimacy, increased insulin resistance, and an increased risk of diabetes mellitus by 16% to 44%, increased arterial stiffness, increased triglycerides, and the eventual development of metabolic syndrome. ADT has been inconsistently linked to an increase in cardiovascular events; but in these studies, other traditional risk factors have been significant confounders, and a link to cardiovascular *mortality* remains elusive. The further implications of metabolic changes in body fat composition, reduced muscle mass, and bone mineral density loss are a decrease in physical strength and endurance. In a group of men older than 70 years on ADT for 3 months, a 56% reduction in physical function and a 22% incidence of falls were reported.[77] Although the subsequent fates of these men are unknown, falls are generally linked to a high subsequent readmission rate and a 1-year mortality rate of 33%.[78] ADT has also been linked, albeit inconsistently, to cognitive decline, which is pertinent to the elderly man.[79]

There are several strategies to ameliorate these adverse effects. Intermittent ADT improves quality of life with reported benefits in vasomotor symptoms, sexual function, physical well-being, and weight management.[80] A systematic review of 7 phase III randomized trials with 4675 cumulative patients indicates that it is oncologically noninferior to continuous ADT.[81] A nadir PSA of less than 4 ng/mL after initiation of ADT has been found to identify a group of men with a longer survival during which the adverse effects of ADT may be experienced.[82] Intermittent ADT may thus be suited to the educated elderly man with a good prognosis, advanced or low-volume metastatic prostate cancer, and a desire for a break from therapy with the caveat that he is compliant to follow-up and recognizes the potential for a small increased risk of cancer progression and death. Close monitoring with resumption of ADT based on an increase in PSA to 10 to 20 should mitigate this risk in most men.

Vitamin D and calcium are commonly recommended for use in men on ADT based on their benefits in bone mineral density preservation and fracture risk reduction in trials of patients with osteoporosis. Fracture risk can be calculated using the FRAX risk calculator in order to provide an individual assessment of risk. Bisphosphonates have been shown to significantly improve lumbar and femoral bone mineral density, reduce osteoporosis by 61%, and reduce the risk of fractures by 20%.[83] However, bisphosphonates are not without adverse effects themselves and have been commonly reported to cause bone pain, fatigue, and anemia.[84] These effects depend on renal clearance, which is often decreased in the elderly. The most serious complication of bisphosphonate, osteonecrosis of the jaw, is thought to be related to dental caries, another significant risk in the elderly, and may be reduced by the use of dental preventative measures.[85] Denosumab, a monoclonal antibody that inhibits osteoclast maturation, has been shown to improve bone mineral density and reduce the vertebral fracture rate by 62% in men with nonmetastatic prostate cancer on ADT when given every 6 months.[86] In a trial evaluating denosumab against zoledronic acid in men with castrate-resistant prostate cancer, although denosumab was superior in the prevention of skeletal-related events, it also resulted in a greater incidence of hypocalcemia, which may produce nonspecific symptoms in the elderly.[87]

Gabapentin and medroxyprogesterone have proven efficacy in treating vasomotor symptoms, and data from case series suggest that acupuncture may be helpful.[88–90] Resistance exercises improve upper- and lower-body strength.[91] A combination of metformin and aerobic exercise has been shown to reduce abdominal girth, weight, and body mass index.[92] Given the higher risk of falls in the elderly and the evidence of ADT-induced sarcopenia and muscle loss, regular exercise at least 30 minutes 3 to 5 times per week is recommended to all men undergoing ADT. Exercise may also maintain sexual activity in men undergoing ADT.[93] Finally, in men who are unable to tolerate the side effects of ADT, bicalutamide 150 mg monotherapy, which is less efficacious than castration but has a more acceptable side-effect profile, may be used after proper counseling.[94]

Castrate-Resistant Prostate Cancer

The morbidity of castrate-resistant prostate cancer (CRPC) is substantial except in the most infirm. The median disease-specific survival in the patients with CRPC is 12 to 15 months. The management of CRPC is both complex and costly.[95] In the elderly, particular attention should be paid to underlying comorbidities, which place them at higher risk of adverse treatment effects, and financial toxicity, which may affect them disproportionately.

Secondary hormonal manipulation

Enzalutamide is a multistep inhibitor of the androgen receptor, from nuclear translocation to DNA binding and coactivator recruitment, thus increasing its potency over traditional antiandrogens. The efficacy of enzalutamide was demonstrated in 2 randomized controlled trials: first in the castration-resistant postchemotherapy setting (AFFIRM) and in then in the prechemotherapy setting (PREVAIL).[96,97] In both trials, diarrhea, fatigue, and hot flashes seemed to be the major adverse effects. Although there was an initial concern with seizures (0.6% incidence in AFFIRM [A Study Evaluating the Efficacy and Safety of the Investigational Drug MDV3100]), the incidence was later found to be lower in PREVAIL (0.1%). A post hoc analysis in AFFIRM (median age 69 years) comparing those aged greater than 75 years with those younger showed a similar efficacy and side-effect profile.[98] However, emerging data suggest more falls in men older than 75 years, which may be related to the impact of potent AR blockade in muscular tissue.[99] This finding emphasizes the importance of exercise and conditioning during a potent hormonal therapy, such as enzalutamide, which is being further investigated in the ongoing EXTEND (Safety and Efficacy of EXercise Training in Men Receiving ENzalutamide in Combination With Conventional Androgen Deprivation Therapy for Hormone Naïve Prostate Cancer) trial (NCT02256111).

Abiraterone acetate is a CYP17 (Cytochrome P450 17alpha hydroxylase/17,20 lyase) inhibitor targeting adrenal androgen synthesis. In men with CRPC, abiraterone was shown in the COU-AA-301 trial after chemotherapy and in the COA-AA-302 chemotherapy-naïve trial to improve survival compared with placebo.[100,101] Side effects of abiraterone are largely secondary to its mechanism resulting in a secondary mineralocorticoid excess, which can be managed with a mineralocorticoid receptor antagonist.[102] In both trials, the median age of the participants was 69 to 72 years. Given that abiraterone is given together with prednisolone and both undergo hepatic metabolism, liver function should be monitored in elderly patients receiving them. Data to date have not suggested differential increased toxicity in elderly patients with abiraterone. However, long-term use of corticosteroids may impact bone mineral density and risk of infection with immunosuppression, induce steroid skin changes such as purpura, and cause metabolic syndrome and insulin resistance, which are adverse effects that may burden elderly men.

Immunotherapy

Sipuleucel T is an autologous cellular immunotherapy, whereby antigen-presenting cells are exposed to PSA and prostatic acid phosphatase fused to colony-stimulating factor before reintroduction into the patients. The IMPACT trial (Immunotherapy for Prostate Adenocarcinoma Treatment), involving 512 men at a median age of 71 years, demonstrated a 22% reduction in death, translating to a 4.1-month median survival benefit in the treatment arm.[103] Similar to findings from smaller, prior randomized trials, no improvement was seen in progression-free survival.[104,105] This finding was attributed to a delayed antitumor response relative to the progression, which was noted to be early in the entire IMPACT cohort. This lack of short-term benefit carries importance when considering treatment for palliative purposes in the elderly. The most common adverse events occurring in the treatment group compared with the control group were chills, fever, and headache. There are presently no data to suggest a differential efficacy or toxicity in elderly men, as overall this is a well-tolerated therapy that is completed in a 4-week treatment period. However, there is a need for a central venous catheter in up to 25% of patients with poor intravenous access.

Radioisotopes

Radium 223 is a calcium-mimetic that is absorbed by osteoblasts in areas of high-bone turnover.[106] It then emits short-range alpha-radiation targeting areas of metastasis, while relatively sparing the bone marrow because of its limited penetration. The ALSYMPCA trial (Alpharadin in Symptomatic Prostate Cancer Patients) randomized men with CRPC who declined or were not eligible for docetaxel to radium 223 or placebo and best available care, finding a 3.6-month overall survival benefit and a 5.8-month longer time to first skeletal event with radium 223.[107] The median age in this cohort was 71 years, with less adverse events reported in the radium 223 group compared with placebo. Side effects include low risks of and gastrointestinal (GI) toxicity due to GI excretion. In addition to survival, secondary benefits may include pain response and delay in spinal cord compression over time. However, PSA declines are not commonly seen with this agent. Radium 223 is appropriate for symptomatic patients with metastatic CRPC who have bone metastatic-predominant disease, no liver metastases, and adequate bone marrow reserve but are too frail to receive docetaxel chemotherapy or who wish to receive docetaxel at a later time. Concurrent use of palliative radiation, hormonal therapy, corticosteroids, and ADT is permitted.

Cytotoxic chemotherapy

Docetaxel, a microtubule inhibitor, is the first cytotoxic agent to prolong survival in men with CRPC. Two randomized trials, SWOG 9916 (Southwest Oncology Group trial 9916) and TAX-327, compared docetaxel against the standard of care, mitoxantrone, and found a 1.8- to 2.4-month survival benefit.[108,109] TAX-327 (XRP6258 Plus Prednisone Compared to Mitoxantrone Plus Prednisone in Hormone Refractory Metastatic Prostate Cancer) further established the superiority of docetaxel administered every 3 weeks versus a weekly dose.[109] The median age in the SWOG trial was 70 years and 68 years in TAX-327, with 20% of the patients aged 75 years and older. In both trials, the docetaxel arm experienced significantly more grade 3 to 4 neutropenic fevers, fatigue, neuropathy, stomatitis, and lower limb edema. In TAX-327, the docetaxel arm had fewer cardiovascular events, whereas, in the SWOG trial, the reverse was observed. This finding may be due to the combined use of estramustine in the latter trial. In subsequent analyses, the benefits of every-3-weeks docetaxel on survival was found to be independent of age, as men older than 65 years had a similar survival benefit as younger men, provided they had adequate functional status.[110] Secondary benefits of docetaxel include a high rate of PSA decline, radiographic responses, and preserved quality of life due to delayed disease progression and pain progression. Reduced dosing or use of alternative schedules may reduce adverse effects in the elderly.

Cabazitaxel, a taxane with similar mechanism of action to docetaxel, is approved for use in docetaxel-refractory tumors at 25 mg/m^2 every 3 weeks with prednisone. The TROPIC trial, comparing cabazitaxel with mitoxantrone in this setting, showed a 30% reduction in risk of death, translating to an overall survival advantage of 1.4 months.[111] Febrile neutropenia and diarrhea were the most common adverse events noted. These adverse events may be addressed with prophylactic use of granulocyte colony-stimulating factor (G-CSF) and dose reductions to 20 mg/m^2.

Sequencing treatments in castrate-resistant prostate cancer

The proliferation of novel agents in CRPC has led to much debate regarding the sequencing of treatments.[112] To further complicate matters, the overlap in targeting of the androgen receptor pathway by novel agents and taxanes could limit the efficacy

Table 2
Treatment options for CRPR

Agent	Benefit	Toxicity	Other Considerations	Cost[a]
Enzalutamide	Prechemotherapy: 2.2-mo median survival benefit, 70%–80% radiographic PFS, 17-mo delay to chemotherapy Postchemotherapy: 5.2-mo median survival benefit, better QOL and longer time to PSA/radiological progression	Falls (>75-year-old subgroup), diarrhea, fatigue, hot flashes, seizures (0.1%–0.6%)	An exercise/ physical conditioning program may be beneficial to reduce muscular effects of potent androgen suppression	$7500/mo
Abiraterone	Prechemotherapy: 3.9-mo survival benefit Postchemotherapy: 25% reduction in all-cause mortality	Hypertension, hyperkalemia, edema, side effects of prednisolone	Needs to be on prednisolone Hepatic metabolism Liver function monitoring recommended	$5800/mo
Sipuleucel T	4.1-mo survival benefit	—	No PSA response seen May need central venous access	$93,000 per course of 3 treatments
Radium 223	3.6-mo survival benefit, 5.8 mo longer to first skeletal event	Myelosuppression (<10%), GI toxicity (low-grade diarrhea/nausea)	Use in bone-predominant metastasis Hepatic metabolism	$75,000 per course of 6 treatments
Docetaxel	2-mo survival benefit	Neutropenic fever, neuropathy, fatigue, stomatitis, lower limb edema	Consider reduced dosing or alternative schedules to reduce adverse effects	$2300 per cycle[b]
Cabazitaxel	1.4-mo survival advantage	Neutropenic fever, diarrhea	Consider prophylactic G-CSF or dose reductions to reduce adverse effects	$50,000 per course of 6 cycles

Cost-benefit table for secondary agents in CRPC.
Abbreviations: PFS, progression-free survival; QOL, quality of life.
[a] Cost derived from Lew and colleagues,[95] in US dollars.
[b] Estimated cost based on docetaxel (Taxotere).

of treatments used later in the sequence.[113] Cross-resistance observed between enzalutamide and abiraterone acetate may also limit clinical benefit from sequential oral-oral therapy.[114] In the elderly, it is prudent to choose a treatment based on its side-effect profile and tolerability, accounting for comorbidity and physiologic reserves (**Table 2**). It is also important to note that the response to treatment may not be immediate, and sufficient time should be allowed to elapse before declaring a treatment inadequate.[115]

SUMMARY

The goal of treating prostate cancer in the elderly is to maximize survival and quality of life while minimizing treatment-related morbidity. Life expectancy, comorbid conditions, and physiologic reserve are critical considerations in choosing therapeutic modalities in order to achieve these goals.

REFERENCES

1. Population Division, Department of economic and social affairs, United Nations. World population aging 2013. Available at: http://www.un.org/en/development/desa/population/publications/ageing/WorldPopulationAgeing2013.shtml. Accessed April 27, 2015.
2. US Census Bureau. 2010 census brief 2010. Available at: http://www.census.gov/prod/cen2010/briefs/c2010br-03.pdf. Accessed April 27, 2015.
3. American Cancer Society. Cancer facts and figures 2015. Atlanta (GA): American Cancer Society; 2015.
4. Soos G, Tsakiris I, Szanto J, et al. The prevalence of prostate carcinoma and its precursor in Hungary: an autopsy study. Eur Urol 2005;48(5):739–44.
5. Sun L, Caire AA, Robertson CN, et al. Men older than 70 years have higher risk prostate cancer and poorer survival in the early and late prostate specific antigen eras. J Urol 2009;182(5):2242–8.
6. Scosyrev E, Messing EM, Mohile S, et al. Prostate cancer in the elderly: frequency of advanced disease at presentation and disease-specific mortality. Cancer 2012;118(12):3062–70.
7. Bell KJ, Del Mar C, Wright G, et al. Prevalence of incidental prostate cancer: a systematic review of autopsy studies. Int J Cancer 2015;137(7):1749–57.
8. Johansson JE, Holmberg L, Johansson S, et al. Fifteen-year survival in prostate cancer. A prospective, population-based study in Sweden. JAMA 1997;277(6):467–71.
9. Johansson JE, Andren O, Andersson SO, et al. Natural history of early, localized prostate cancer. JAMA 2004;291(22):2713–9.
10. Popiolek M, Rider JR, Andrén O, et al. Natural history of early, localized prostate cancer: a final report from three decades of follow-up. Eur Urol 2013;63(3):428–35.
11. Albertsen PC, Hanley JA, Fine J. 20-year outcomes following conservative management of clinically localized prostate cancer. Jama 2005;293(17):2095–101.
12. Cuzick J, Fisher G, Kattan MW, et al. Long-term outcome among men with conservatively treated localised prostate cancer. Br J Cancer 2006;95(9):1186–94.
13. D'Amico AV, Whittington R, Malkowicz SB, et al. Biochemical outcome after radical prostatectomy, external beam radiation therapy, or interstitial radiation therapy for clinically localized prostate cancer. JAMA 1998;280(11):969–74.

14. Bill-Axelson A, Holmberg L, Garmo H, et al. Radical prostatectomy or watchful waiting in early prostate cancer. N Engl J Med 2014;370(10):932–42.

15. Wilt TJ, Brawer MK, Jones KM, et al. Radical prostatectomy versus observation for localized prostate cancer. N Engl J Med 2012;367(3):203–13.

16. Alibhai SMH, Naglie G, Nam R, et al. Do older men benefit from curative therapy of localized prostate cancer? J Clin Oncol 2003;21(17):3318–27.

17. Li D, de Glas NA, Hurria A. Cancer and Aging-General Principles, Biology, and Geriatric Assessment. Clin Geriatr Med 2015, in press.

18. Dale W, Chow S, Sajid S. Socioeconomic Considerations and Shared-Care Models of Cancer-Care for Older Adults. Clin Geriatr Med 2015, in press.

19. Wingfield SA, Heflin MT. Cancer Screening in Older Adults. Clin Geriatr Med 2015, in press.

20. Social Security Administration. 2010 Actuarial life tables 2010. Available at: http://www.socialsecurity.gov/OACT/STATS/table4c6.html. Accessed April 28, 2015.

21. Sammon JD, Abdollah F, D'Amico A, et al. Predicting life expectancy in men diagnosed with prostate cancer. Eur Urol 2015. [Epub ahead of print].

22. Daskivich TJ, Fan K-H, Koyama T, et al. Prediction of long-term other-cause mortality in men with early-stage prostate cancer: results from the prostate cancer outcomes study. Urology 2015;85(1):92–100.

23. Stineman MG, Xie D, Pan Q, et al. All-cause 1-, 5-, and 10-year mortality in elderly people according to activities of daily living stage. J Am Geriatr Soc 2012;60(3):485–92.

24. Robinson TN, Wu DS, Pointer LF, et al. Preoperative cognitive dysfunction is related to adverse postoperative outcomes in the elderly. J Am Coll Surg 2012;215(1):12–7 [discussion: 7–8].

25. Rockwood K, Stadnyk K, MacKnight C, et al. A brief clinical instrument to classify frailty in elderly people. Lancet 1999;353(9148):205–6.

26. Blanc-Bisson C, Fonck M, Rainfray M, et al. Undernutrition in elderly patients with cancer: target for diagnosis and intervention. Crit Rev Oncol Hematol 2008;67(3):243–54.

27. Bartali B, Frongillo EA, Bandinelli S, et al. Low nutrient intake is an essential component of frailty in older persons. J Gerontol A Biol Sci Med Sci 2006; 61(6):589–93.

28. Droz J-P, Balducci L, Bolla M, et al. Management of prostate cancer in older men: recommendations of a working group of the International Society of Geriatric Oncology. BJU Int 2010;106(4):462–9.

29. Bratt O, Folkvaljon Y, Hjalm Eriksson M, et al. Undertreatment of men in their seventies with high-risk nonmetastatic prostate cancer. Eur Urol 2015;68(1):53–8.

30. Decoster L, Van Puyvelde K, Mohile S, et al. Screening tools for multidimensional health problems warranting a geriatric assessment in older cancer patients: an update on SIOG recommendations. Ann Oncol 2015;26(2):288–300.

31. Jones GW. Prospective, conservative management of localized prostate cancer. Cancer 1992;70(Suppl 1):307–10.

32. Dall'Era MA, Albertsen PC, Bangma C, et al. Active surveillance for prostate cancer: a systematic review of the literature. Eur Urol 2012;62(6):976–83.

33. Klotz L, Vesprini D, Sethukavalan P, et al. Long-term follow-up of a large active surveillance cohort of patients with prostate cancer. J Clin Oncol 2015;33(3): 272–7.

34. Tay KJ, Mendez M, Moul JW, et al. Active surveillance for prostate cancer: can we modernize contemporary protocols to improve patient selection and outcomes in the focal therapy era? Curr Opin Urol 2015;25(3):185–90.

35. Busch J, Magheli A, Leva N, et al. Higher rates of upgrading and upstaging in older patients undergoing radical prostatectomy and qualifying for active surveillance. BJU Int 2014;114(4):517–21.

36. Abern MR, Aronson WJ, Terris MK, et al. Delayed radical prostatectomy for intermediate-risk prostate cancer is associated with biochemical recurrence: possible implications for active surveillance from the search database. Prostate 2013;73(4):409–17.

37. van den Heuvel S, Loeb S, Zhu X, et al. Complications of initial prostate biopsy in a European randomized screening trial. Am J Clin Exp Urol 2013; 1(1):66–71.

38. Abouassaly R, Lane BR, Jones JS. Staging saturation biopsy in patients with prostate cancer on active surveillance protocol. Urology 2008;71(4):573–7.

39. Cookson MS, Aus G, Burnett AL, et al. Variation in the definition of biochemical recurrence in patients treated for localized prostate cancer: the American Urological Association Prostate Guidelines for Localized Prostate Cancer Update Panel report and recommendations for a standard in the reporting of surgical outcomes. J Urol 2007;177(2):540–5.

40. Resnick MJ, Koyama T, Fan KH, et al. Long-term functional outcomes after treatment for localized prostate cancer. N Engl J Med 2013;368(5):436–45.

41. Novara G, Ficarra V, Rosen RC, et al. Systematic review and meta-analysis of perioperative outcomes and complications after robot-assisted radical prostatectomy. Eur Urol 2012;62(3):431–52.

42. Sood A, Jeong W, Peabody JO, et al. Robot-assisted radical prostatectomy: inching toward gold standard. Urol Clin North Am 2014;41(4):473–84.

43. Ramly E, Kaafarani HM, Velmahos GC. The effect of aging on pulmonary function: implications for monitoring and support of the surgical and trauma patient. Surg Clin North Am 2015;95(1):53–69.

44. Martin RS, Farrah JP, Chang MC. Effect of aging on cardiac function plus monitoring and support. Surg Clin North Am 2015;95(1):23–35.

45. Tewari A, Sooriakumaran P, Bloch DA, et al. Positive surgical margin and perioperative complication rates of primary surgical treatments for prostate cancer: a systematic review and meta-analysis comparing retropubic, laparoscopic, and robotic prostatectomy. Eur Urol 2012;62(1):1–15.

46. Mandel P, Graefen M, Michl U, et al. The effect of age on functional outcomes after radical prostatectomy. Urol Oncol 2015;33(5):203.e11–8.

47. Kumar A, Samavedi S, Bates AS, et al. Continence outcomes of robot assisted radical prostatectomy in patients with adverse urinary continence risk factors. BJU Int 2015. [Epub ahead of print].

48. Johansson E, Steineck G, Holmberg L, et al. Long-term quality-of-life outcomes after radical prostatectomy or watchful waiting: the Scandinavian Prostate Cancer Group-4 randomised trial. Lancet Oncol 2011;12(9):891–9.

49. Yamamoto S, Masuda H, Urakami S, et al. Patient-perceived satisfaction after definitive treatment for men with high-risk prostate cancer: radical prostatectomy vs. intensity-modulated radiotherapy with androgen deprivation therapy. Urology 2015;85(2):407–13.

50. Ataman F, Zurlo A, Artignan X, et al. Late toxicity following conventional radiotherapy for prostate cancer: analysis of the EORTC trial 22863. Eur J Cancer 2004;40(11):1674–81.

51. Wallis CJ, Herschorn S, Saskin R, et al. Complications after radical prostatectomy or radiotherapy for prostate cancer: results of a population-based, propensity score-matched analysis. Urology 2015;85(3):621–7.

52. Merrick GS, Butler WM, Tollenaar BG, et al. The dosimetry of prostate brachytherapy-induced urethral strictures. Int J Radiat Oncol Biol Phys 2002; 52(2):461–8.
53. Zelefsky MJ, Wallner KE, Ling CC, et al. Comparison of the ear outcome and morbidity of three-dimensional conformal radiotherapy versus transperineal permanent iodine-125 implantation for early-stage prostatic cancer. J Clin Oncol 1999;17(2):517–22.
54. Hathout L, Folkert MR, Kollmeier MA, et al. Dose to the bladder neck is the most important predictor for acute and late toxicity after low-dose-rate prostate brachytherapy: implications for establishing new dose constraints for treatment planning. Int J Radiat Oncol Biol Phys 2014;90(2):312–9.
55. Jones CU, Hunt D, McGowan DG, et al. Radiotherapy and short-term androgen deprivation for localized prostate cancer. N Engl J Med 2011;365(2):107–18.
56. Bolla M, de Reijke TM, Van Tienhoven G, et al. Duration of androgen suppression in the treatment of prostate cancer. N Engl J Med 2009;360(24):2516–27.
57. D'Amico AV, Chen MH, Renshaw AA, et al. Androgen suppression and radiation vs radiation alone for prostate cancer: a randomized trial. JAMA 2008;299(3): 289–95.
58. Nanda A, Chen MH, Moran BJ, et al. Cardiovascular comorbidity and mortality in men with prostate cancer treated with brachytherapy-based radiation with or without hormonal therapy. Int J Radiat Oncol Biol Phys 2013;85(5):e209–15.
59. Crouzet S, Chapelon JY, Rouviere O, et al. Whole-gland ablation of localized prostate cancer with high-intensity focused ultrasound: oncologic outcomes and morbidity in 1002 patients. Eur Urol 2014;65(5):907–14.
60. Dhar N, Ward JF, Cher ML, et al. Primary full-gland prostate cryoablation in older men (> age of 75 years): results from 860 patients tracked with the COLD Registry. BJU Int 2011;108(4):508–12.
61. Polascik TJ. Focal therapy of prostate cancer: making steady progress toward a first-line image-guided treatment modality. Curr Opin Urol 2015;25(3):183–4.
62. Klotz L, Polascik TJ. Low-risk and very-low-risk prostate cancer: is there a role for focal therapy in the era of active surveillance? Yes, the two approaches complement each other. Oncology (Williston Park) 2014;28(11):950-c3.
63. Messing EM, Manola J, Yao J, et al. Immediate versus deferred androgen deprivation treatment in patients with node-positive prostate cancer after radical prostatectomy and pelvic lymphadenectomy. Lancet Oncol 2006;7(6):472–9.
64. Stephenson AJ, Eastham JA. Role of salvage radical prostatectomy for recurrent prostate cancer after radiation therapy. J Clin Oncol 2005;23(32): 8198–203.
65. Huggins C, Hodges CV. Studies on prostatic cancer: I. The effect of castration, of estrogen and of androgen injection on serum phosphatases in metastatic carcinoma of the prostate. Cancer Res 1941;1:293.
66. Sweeney C, Chen YH, Carducci MA, et al. Impact on overall survival (OS) with chemohormonal therapy versus hormonal therapy for hormone-sensitive newly metastatic prostate cancer (mPrCa): an ECOG-led phase III randomized trial. J Clin Oncol 2014;32(15).
67. Immediate versus deferred treatment for advanced prostatic cancer: initial results of the Medical Research Council Trial. The Medical Research Council Prostate Cancer Working Party Investigators Group. Br J Urol 1997;79(2):235–46.
68. Nair B, Wilt T, MacDonald R, et al. Early versus deferred androgen suppression in the treatment of advanced prostatic cancer. Cochrane Database Syst Rev 2002;(1):CD003506.

69. Oefelein MG, Feng A, Scolieri MJ, et al. Reassessment of the definition of castrate levels of testosterone: implications for clinical decision making. Urology 2000;56(6):1021–4.

70. Potosky AL, Knopf K, Clegg LX, et al. Quality-of-life outcomes after primary androgen deprivation therapy: results from the prostate cancer outcomes study. J Clin Oncol 2001;19(17):3750–7.

71. Fontana D, Mari M, Martinelli A, et al. 3-month formulation of goserelin acetate ('Zoladex' 10.8-mg depot) in advanced prostate cancer: results from an Italian, open, multicenter trial. Urol Int 2003;70(4):316–20.

72. Pagliarulo V, Bracarda S, Eisenberger MA, et al. Contemporary role of androgen deprivation therapy for prostate cancer. Eur Urol 2012;61(1):11–25.

73. Bubley GJ. Is the flare phenomenon clinically significant? Urology 2001;58(2 Suppl 1):5–9.

74. Labrie F, Dupont A, Belanger A, et al. Flutamide eliminates the risk of disease flare in prostatic cancer patients treated with a luteinizing hormone-releasing hormone agonist. J Urol 1987;138(4):804–6.

75. Maximum androgen blockade in advanced prostate cancer: an overview of the randomised trials. Prostate Cancer Trialists' Collaborative Group. Lancet 2000; 355(9214):1491–8.

76. Nguyen PL, Alibhai SMH, Basaria S, et al. Adverse effects of androgen deprivation therapy and strategies to mitigate them. Eur Urol 2015;67(5):825–36.

77. Bylow K, Dale W, Mustian K, et al. Falls and physical performance deficits in older patients with prostate cancer undergoing androgen deprivation therapy. Urology 2008;72(2):422–7.

78. Ayoung-Chee P, McIntyre L, Ebel BE, et al. Long-term outcomes of ground-level falls in the elderly. J Trauma Acute Care Surg 2014;76(2):498–503 [discussion].

79. Green HJ, Pakenham KI, Headley BC, et al. Altered cognitive function in men treated for prostate cancer with luteinizing hormone-releasing hormone analogues and cyproterone acetate: a randomized controlled trial. BJU Int 2002; 90(4):427–32.

80. Abrahamsson PA. Potential benefits of intermittent androgen suppression therapy in the treatment of prostate cancer: a systematic review of the literature. Eur Urol 2010;57(1):49–59.

81. Sciarra A, Abrahamsson PA, Brausi M, et al. Intermittent androgen-deprivation therapy in prostate cancer: a critical review focused on phase 3 trials. Eur Urol 2013;64(5):722–30.

82. Hussain M, Tangen CM, Higano C, et al. Absolute prostate-specific antigen value after androgen deprivation is a strong independent predictor of survival in new metastatic prostate cancer: data from Southwest Oncology Group trial 9346 (INT-0162). J Clin Oncol 2006;24(24):3984–90.

83. Serpa Neto A, Tobias-Machado M, Esteves MAP, et al. Bisphosphonate therapy in patients under androgen deprivation therapy for prostate cancer: a systematic review and meta-analysis. Prostate Cancer Prostatic Dis 2012;15(1):36–44.

84. Parker CC. The role of bisphosphonates in the treatment of prostate cancer. BJU Int 2005;95(7):935–8.

85. Ripamonti CI, Maniezzo M, Campa T, et al. Decreased occurrence of osteonecrosis of the jaw after implementation of dental preventive measures in solid tumour patients with bone metastases treated with bisphosphonates. The experience of the National Cancer Institute of Milan. Ann Oncol 2009;20(1):137–45.

86. Smith MR, Egerdie B, Toriz NH, et al. Denosumab in men receiving androgen-deprivation therapy for prostate cancer. N Engl J Med 2009;361(8):745–55.

87. Fizazi K, Carducci M, Smith M, et al. Denosumab versus zoledronic acid for treatment of bone metastases in men with castration-resistant prostate cancer: a randomised, double-blind study. Lancet 2011;377(9768):813–22.

88. Loprinzi CL, Dueck AC, Khoyratty BS, et al. A phase III randomized, double-blind, placebo-controlled trial of gabapentin in the management of hot flashes in men (N00CB). Ann Oncol 2009;20(3):542–9.

89. Irani J, Salomon L, Oba R, et al. Efficacy of venlafaxine, medroxyprogesterone acetate, and cyproterone acetate for the treatment of vasomotor hot flushes in men taking gonadotropin-releasing hormone analogues for prostate cancer: a double-blind, randomised trial. Lancet Oncol 2010;11(2):147–54.

90. Lee MS, Kim KH, Shin BC, et al. Acupuncture for treating hot flushes in men with prostate cancer: a systematic review. Support Care Cancer 2009;17(7):763–70.

91. Segal RJ, Reid RD, Courneya KS, et al. Resistance exercise in men receiving androgen deprivation therapy for prostate cancer. J Clin Oncol 2003;21(9):1653–9.

92. Nobes JP, Langley SEM, Klopper T, et al. A prospective, randomized pilot study evaluating the effects of metformin and lifestyle intervention on patients with prostate cancer receiving androgen deprivation therapy. BJU Int 2012;109(10):1495–502.

93. Cormie P, Newton RU, Taaffe DR, et al. Exercise maintains sexual activity in men undergoing androgen suppression for prostate cancer: a randomized controlled trial. Prostate Cancer Prostatic Dis 2013;16(2):170–5.

94. Tyrrell CJ, Kaisary AV, Iversen P, et al. A randomised comparison of 'Casodex' (bicalutamide) 150 mg monotherapy versus castration in the treatment of metastatic and locally advanced prostate cancer. Eur Urol 1998;33(5):447–56.

95. Lew I. Managed care implications in castration-resistant prostate cancer. Am J Manag Care 2013;19(Suppl 18):s376–81.

96. Scher HI, Fizazi K, Saad F, et al. Increased survival with enzalutamide in prostate cancer after chemotherapy. N Engl J Med 2012;367(13):1187–97.

97. Beer TM, Armstrong AJ, Rathkopf DE, et al. Enzalutamide in metastatic prostate cancer before chemotherapy. N Engl J Med 2014;371(5):424–33.

98. Sternberg CN, de Bono JS, Chi KN, et al. Improved outcomes in elderly patients with metastatic castration-resistant prostate cancer treated with the androgen receptor inhibitor enzalutamide: results from the phase III AFFIRM trial. Ann Oncol 2014;25(2):429–34.

99. Graff JN, Baciarello G, Armstrong AJ, et al. Clinical outcomes and safety in men ≥75 and <75 years with metastatic castration-resistant prostate cancer (mCRPC) treated with enzalutamide in the phase 3 PREVAIL trial. J Clin Oncol 2015;33(Suppl 7):200.

100. de Bono JS, Logothetis CJ, Molina A, et al. Abiraterone and increased survival in metastatic prostate cancer. N Engl J Med 2011;364(21):1995–2005.

101. Ryan CJ, Smith MR, de Bono JS, et al. Abiraterone in metastatic prostate cancer without previous chemotherapy. N Engl J Med 2013;368(2):138–48.

102. Attard G, Reid AH, Yap TA, et al. Phase I clinical trial of a selective inhibitor of CYP17, abiraterone acetate, confirms that castration-resistant prostate cancer commonly remains hormone driven. J Clin Oncol 2008;26(28):4563–71.

103. Kantoff PW, Higano CS, Shore ND, et al. Sipuleucel-T immunotherapy for castration-resistant prostate cancer. N Engl J Med 2010;363(5):411–22.

104. Small EJ, Schellhammer PF, Higano CS, et al. Placebo-controlled phase III trial of immunologic therapy with sipuleucel-T (APC8015) in patients with metastatic,

asymptomatic hormone refractory prostate cancer. J Clin Oncol 2006;24(19): 3089–94.

105. Kantoff PW, Schuetz TJ, Blumenstein BA, et al. Overall survival analysis of a phase II randomized controlled trial of a poxviral-based PSA-targeted immunotherapy in metastatic castration-resistant prostate cancer. J Clin Oncol 2010; 28(7):1099–105.

106. Henriksen G, Breistol K, Bruland OS, et al. Significant antitumor effect from bone-seeking, alpha-particle-emitting (223)Ra demonstrated in an experimental skeletal metastases model. Cancer Res 2002;62(11):3120–5.

107. Parker C, Nilsson S, Heinrich D, et al. Alpha emitter radium-223 and survival in metastatic prostate cancer. N Engl J Med 2013;369(3):213–23.

108. Petrylak DP, Tangen CM, Hussain MH, et al. Docetaxel and estramustine compared with mitoxantrone and prednisone for advanced refractory prostate cancer. N Engl J Med 2004;351(15):1513–20.

109. Tannock IF, de Wit R, Berry WR, et al. Docetaxel plus prednisone or mitoxantrone plus prednisone for advanced prostate cancer. N Engl J Med 2004; 351(15):1502–12.

110. Berthold DR, Pond GR, Soban F, et al. Docetaxel plus prednisone or mitoxantrone plus prednisone for advanced prostate cancer: updated survival in the TAX 327 study. J Clin Oncol 2008;26(2):242–5.

111. de Bono JS, Oudard S, Ozguroglu M, et al. Prednisone plus cabazitaxel or mitoxantrone for metastatic castration-resistant prostate cancer progressing after docetaxel treatment: a randomised open-label trial. Lancet 2010;376(9747): 1147–54.

112. Fitzpatrick JM, Bellmunt J, Fizazi K, et al. Optimal management of metastatic castration-resistant prostate cancer: highlights from a European Expert Consensus Panel. Eur J Cancer 2014;50(9):1617–27.

113. Van Soest RJ, Van Royen ME, De Morrée ES, et al. Cross-resistance between taxanes and new hormonal agents abiraterone and enzalutamide may affect drug sequence choices in metastatic castration-resistant prostate cancer. Eur J Cancer 2013;49(18):3821–30.

114. Zhang T, Dhawan MS, Healy P, et al. Exploring the clinical benefit of docetaxel or enzalutamide after disease progression during abiraterone acetate and prednisone treatment in men with metastatic castration-resistant prostate cancer. Clin Genitourin Cancer 2015;13(4):392–9.

115. Merseburger AS, Bellmunt J, Jenkins C, et al. Perspectives on treatment of metastatic castration-resistant prostate cancer. Oncologist 2013;18(5):558–67.

Approach and Management of Breast Cancer in the Elderly

Meghan Karuturi, MD[a], Noam VanderWalde, MD[b], Hyman Muss, MD[c],*

KEYWORDS

- Curative surgery • Axillary staging • Endocrine therapy • Adjuvant chemotherapy
- Adjuvant radiation • Palliative chemotherapy

KEY POINTS

- The population of patients aged 65 years and older is growing rapidly, with breast cancer representing a common disease in older women.
- The treatment decision processes in older women with breast cancer should take into account functional reserve, tolerance to antineoplastic therapies, competing causes of morbidity and death, and patient goals of care.
- Further research investigating the role of geriatric assessment in treatment selection and tolerance, tumor biology, and specific clinical interventions/therapeutics in a clinical trial setting.

INTRODUCTION

In 2015, breast cancer will remain the most common cancer in women with an estimated 232,000 new cases and 40,000 deaths (**Fig. 1**).[1] Despite the fact that most new breast cancer diagnoses occur in women less than 65 years of age (58%), most breast cancer deaths (60%) occur in women aged 65 years and older (37% in women aged 75 years and older). Furthermore, of the approximately 3 million survivors of breast cancer in the United States, most are aged 65 years and older.[2] These alarming demographics coupled with the aging of the US population portend for a tsunami of older women with breast cancer.

[a] Department of Breast Medical Oncology, MD Anderson Cancer Center, 1515 Holcombe Boulevard, Unit 1354, Houston, TX 77030, USA; [b] Department of Radiation Oncology, University of Tennessee West Cancer Center, 1265 Union Avenue, Thomas Basement, Memphis, TN 38104, USA; [c] Lineberger Comprehensive Cancer Center and Department of Medicine, University of North Carolina, Chapel Hill, NC 27514, USA
* Corresponding author.
E-mail address: hyman_muss@med.unc.edu

Clin Geriatr Med 32 (2016) 133–153
http://dx.doi.org/10.1016/j.cger.2015.08.011
0749-0690/16/$ – see front matter © 2016 Elsevier Inc. All rights reserved.

geriatric.theclinics.com

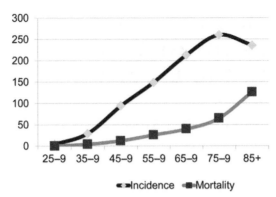

Fig. 1. Surveillance, Epidemiology, and End Results' incidence and mortality rates for breast cancer by age. X-axis is age in years. Y-axis is number of cases × 1000 per year. (*Data from* SEER cancer statistics factsheets: breast cancer. Bethesda (MD): National Cancer Institute; 2015. Available at: http://seer.cancer.gov/statfacts/html/breast.html.)

Although the mortality rates for breast cancer have decreased substantially over the last 2 decades, older patients have not shared as well in these successes when compared with younger ones.[3,4] In one study, the absolute risk of breast cancer death decreased by 15.3% for women aged 50 to 64 years but only 7.5% for women 75 years and older.[3] These major improvements in mortality have likely resulted from the more widespread use of mammographic screening as well as adjuvant therapy: the use of radiation therapy, chemotherapy, endocrine therapy, or a combination of these modalities. Then why do older woman make up most of those who die of breast cancer? Some suggest that poorer survival may be associated with diagnosis at a higher stage; if older woman had the same stage distribution as their younger peers, their survival would be better.[5,6] Additionally, adjuvant therapy has not been as frequently given to older patients as compared with younger patients, mainly because of age bias, concerns of toxicity, and the effects of treatment on quality of life.[7,8] Such underuse, especially of chemotherapy, may be largely responsible for reduced improvement in breast cancer–specific survival in older patients.[8] An increasing amount of data show that older women in good health tolerate state-of-the-art breast cancer treatments as well as younger women and derive the same disease-free and overall survival (OS) benefits.[9] Several excellent reviews addressing the use of adjuvant therapy in older women are available.[10,11]

Older patients tend to have more favorable breast cancers at diagnosis and when compared with younger patients are more likely to have smaller tumors, less lymph node involvement, more tumors that express both estrogen and/or progesterone receptors, more lower-grade tumors, and more tumors that are human epidermal growth factor receptor (HER-2) negative (**Fig. 2**).[12,13] These more favorable phenotypes in older women are reinforced by new studies using molecular genetics to characterize breast cancer subtypes, which show that more favorable subtypes (luminal A and luminal B) increase with increasing age.[14] Nevertheless, older women also present with unfavorable breast cancer subtypes (basal type and HER-2 overexpressed) that are best managed with more aggressive therapy, especially chemotherapy. The small but significant increase in more favorable tumor characteristics and molecular subtypes in older patients, however, has not translated into major improvements in survival. Generally speaking, approach to treatment is determined by the identification of the breast cancer phenotype: (1) hormone receptor positive (estrogen and/or

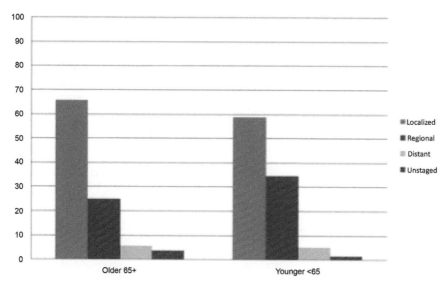

Fig. 2. Surveillance, Epidemiology, and End Results' description of stage distribution by cancer site (65 years of age and older versus less than 65 years of age [all races]), 2002 to 2011.

progesterone receptors are positive) and HER-2 overexpression negative; (2) HER-2 positive (HER-2 is overexpressed irrespective of hormone receptor status); and (3) estrogen, progesterone, and HER-2 overexpression all negative (so-called triple-negative breast cancer). Characteristics of these 3 cancer phenotypes are shown in **Table 1**.

CHALLENGES IN CARING FOR OLDER PATIENTS WITH BREAST CANCER

Oncologists caring for patients with breast cancer are challenged by the great heterogeneity of older women with breast cancer. Chronologic age is a weak surrogate for patient function and comorbidities, yet ageism is still a problem among specialists and may account for substantial undertreatment.[15] Most older women with early stage breast cancer, especially those that present with smaller hormone receptor positive tumors with no or limited nodal involvement, are much more likely to die of non–breast cancer causes. On occasion, medical oncologists partner with physicians experienced in managing older patients, but frequently such collaborators are not available. Geriatric assessment, the cornerstone for detecting functional, social, and other medical problems associated with aging, is an area of limited awareness and use among cancer specialists. An extensive body of data has shown that geriatric assessment can identify major issues, many with proven beneficial interventions (eg, falls). To combat this problem, brief screening instruments and geriatric assessments to detect major geriatric-associated problems are being used more and more to formally evaluate older patients with cancer.[16]

When making treatment decisions in older women, the authors recommend that clinicians first estimate patients' life expectancy due to non–breast cancer causes in order to put the potential benefits of the varying treatment options into perspective. Several calculators that estimate life expectancy of community-dwelling and institutionalized older patients are readily available (see www.eprognosis.ucsf.org). Older women with early stage breast cancer with life expectancies of 5 to 10 years because of other

Table 1 Tumor phenotypes		
Tumor Phenotype (Frequency)	Natural History of Disease	Treatment Considerations
Hormone receptor positive and HER-2 negative (about 75% of older patients)	It is slower growing, with most locoregional and distant recurrences occulting after 5 y.	Systemic adjuvant therapy: endocrine therapy with tamoxifen or aromatase inhibitor for most; chemotherapy and endocrine therapy for some with high risk of recurrence Metastatic disease: endocrine therapy followed by single-agent chemotherapy once refractory to endocrine treatment
Triple negative (About 15% of older patients)	About 95% of recurrences happen within the first 5 y after diagnosis.	Systemic adjuvant therapy: chemotherapy if it improves survival at least 3% Metastatic disease: single-agent chemotherapy for most
HER-2 positive (about 15% of older patients)	Most recurrences occur in first 5 y. Hormone receptor–positive and HER-2–positive tumors have a better natural history and later recurrences than hormone receptor–negative, HER-2–positive tumors.	Systemic adjuvant therapy: chemotherapy and anti-HER2–directed therapy for most and endocrine therapy for hormone receptor–positive tumors Metastatic disease: single-agent and anti-HER2–directed therapy for most; endocrine therapy and anti-HER directed therapy for some

comorbid illnesses are not likely to derive any survival benefit from mammographic screening or treatments that can be associated with major toxicity, such as chemotherapy. However, healthy older women with life expectancies exceeding 10 years should receive state-of-the art breast cancer treatment. Trials have shown that this healthy older age group tolerates treatment as well as younger patients, including breast and axillary surgery, radiation therapy, and chemotherapy. **Table 2** provides a list of helpful Web sites that can help in managing breast and other cancers in older patients.

Another major challenge in managing older women with breast cancer is the lack of information from large clinical trials that can help guide treatment decisions. Historically older patients were excluded from clinical trials based on age alone. Even now, older women remain underrepresented when such upper age limits have been lifted. This is especially concerning for patients who are candidates for chemotherapy or newer biological therapies whereby the bulk of published trials have few older patients limiting the information on acute and long-term toxicity among older patients.[17] This poor representation is frequently due to age bias on the part of the clinician.[15] Studies have shown that when older patients are offered trials, they have a similar rate of

Table 2
Useful Web sites helpful in managing older patients with breast and other cancers

Name	Description	URL/Link
SIOG	An international organization that focuses on geriatric oncology: Web site has useful links to geriatric oncology guidelines and other educational materials	http://www.siog.org/
ePrognosis	A series of calculators based on systematic review of literature that allows for estimation of life expectancy in older adults over a wide range of years and in various settings	http://eprognosis.ucsf.edu/default.php
POGOe	Comprehensive site totally devoted to geriatrics with free collections of expert-contributed materials for educators and learners; includes videos and slideshows	http://www.pogoe.org/about
Lineberger Comprehensive Cancer Center Geriatric Oncology	A collection of free PowerPoint (Microsoft Corporation, Redmond, WA) slide sets of core lectures in geriatrics as well as resources and links developed by the Geriatric Oncology program at the University of North Carolina	http://unclineberger.org/geriatric

Abbreviations: POGOe, Portal of Geriatrics Online Education; SIOG, International Society of Geriatric Oncology.

participation as younger patients.[15,18–21] In addition, a limited number of trials have focused exclusively on frail patients.

STAGING

For older women in good health who have a breast mass on physical examination, or a mammogram highly suspicious for breast cancer, management is similar to younger women. A core biopsy is the preferred method of diagnosis over fine-needle aspiration (FNA). These procedures are well tolerated, usually performed by surgeons or radiologists, and provide information on tumor phenotype.

To assess the appropriate treatment of older patients with breast cancer, an understanding of how to correctly stage and estimate outcomes in this patient population is critical. Another possible explanation for the higher breast cancer death rate in older woman could be that older woman may be inappropriately staged. In other words, there may be many older women who undergo limited staging and are treated as if they have early stage/low-risk breast cancer when in reality they have regional or even distant disease. The current American Joint Committee on Cancer (AJCC) staging edition uses a tumor (T), nodal, metastasis model to stage patients.[22] The T stage can be derived by clinical imaging and ultimately by pathologic size. According to the current National Comprehensive Cancer Network's (NCCN) guidelines,[23] systemic staging using computerized tomographic or PET imaging is only needed for patients with stage IIIA cancer and greater or patients showing clinical signs of systemic disease. The current guidelines from the NCCN recommend clinical and surgical staging of all patients with invasive breast cancer.[23] For those with clinically positive nodes that are biopsy proven with FNA or core biopsies, they recommend patients undergo axillary lymph node dissection. For those without clinically evident abnormal lymph nodes, the guideline recommends at least sentinel lymph node (SLN) mapping and excision.

Before the sentinel lymph node biopsy (SLNB) era, older women were less likely to undergo axillary dissection.[24] The avoidance of axillary dissection was probably in women with small primary tumors and no clinical evidence of axillary lymph nodes, as the risks (including arm pain, paresthesia, lymphedema, infection, and poor quality of life) in women who were not at full health to begin with possibly outweighed the benefits.[25] The omission of axillary lymph node dissection (ALND) has since been supported by the results of a randomized clinical trial, which randomized older woman (65 years of age and older, with clinical T1 N0 hormone receptor, positive tumors, with plans to receive adjuvant breast radiotherapy [RT], and 5 years of tamoxifen) to axillary dissection or not.[26] With 15 years' median follow-up, they found no difference in OS, distant metastases, or breast cancer mortality. Additionally, there was only 6% cumulative incidence of axillary failure over a 15-year period for patients without dissection.[26] There is concern, however, that these data may be extrapolated to patients who do not meet the inclusion criteria of that study, making it likely that patients with higher-risk disease will be mismanaged. Today, in the SLN era, when the risks associated with the SLNB are significantly lower than ALND,[27,28] there should be less risk of older women receiving inappropriate axillary staging. Yet, older woman are still less likely to undergo SLN mapping when compared with their younger peers.[29,30] Avoidance of SLNB in relatively healthy older woman with early stage breast cancer is not recommended, as the results of this low-risk procedure can significantly change treatment recommendations.[31,32] Whether understaging of older women leads to worse survival though is still not clear from the current data. However, a logical deduction can be made that if older women are incorrectly staged, it could lead to mistreatment and, thus, worse survival.

EARLY STAGE BREAST CANCER (STAGE 0–3)
Surgery and Primary Endocrine Therapy

Breast surgery is tolerated as well in older women as in younger women[33] except for frail elders or those with a life expectancy less than a year. Even older patients with substantial comorbidity can tolerate partial mastectomy (lumpectomy) with a minimum of operative risk. Body image is of major importance to many older women, and they should be offered breast conservation when appropriate. For those with larger tumors not amenable to breast conservation, preoperative systemic therapy (see earlier discussion) should be considered. Sentinel node biopsy is the preferred method of nodal evaluation in women without evidence of nodal involvement on imaging or physical examination. However, if these clinically node-negative patients have poor performance status and could not receive systemic therapy, SLNB could potentially be avoided. However, the decision to omit or offer adjuvant radiation becomes harder in patients who have not had some type of surgical evaluation of their axilla.

Some older patients are too frail to tolerate surgery. Those with hormone receptor–positive tumors can be treated with endocrine therapy alone (primary endocrine therapy). Most will have a decrease in tumor size of greater than 50%, with an average duration of response of about 18 to 24 months.[34] For frail patients with hormone receptor–negative tumors who are unable to tolerate surgery and when endocrine therapy is not an option, radiation therapy alone may offer disease control.

Radiation Therapy

Adjuvant RT plays an important role in most women with early stage breast cancer. The National Surgical Adjuvant Breast and Bowel Project (NSABP) B-06 study randomized 1851 patients between mastectomy, lumpectomy, and lumpectomy with radiation. With greater than 20 years of follow-up, NSABP-B06 demonstrated an absolute local control benefit of 24.9% to the addition of radiation to lumpectomy (34.2% vs 14.3%).[35] The Early Breast Cancer Trialists Collaborative Group (EBCTG) meta-analysis demonstrated that the addition of RT to breast conservation surgery decreased breast cancer–related death by 3.8% (25.2% vs 21.4%) at 15 years.[36] For every 4 local recurrences prevented at 10 years by radiation, 1 breast cancer–related death was prevented at 15 years.[36] This meta-analysis nicely supports the theorem that local regional treatment could improve survival in patients with early stage breast cancer given enough time. Yet, in patients with a lower risk of recurrence and a higher likelihood of death from causes other than breast cancer, should RT, with its associated economic, social, and medical costs, be offered as standard therapy for all patients?

Adjuvant radiation has traditionally entailed the delivery of photons in fractionated doses to the effected breast using a linear accelerator. Radiation is thought to cause the death of microscopic tumor cells via both direct (double-stranded DNA breaks) and indirect (generation of oxygen radicals that cause DNA damage) mechanisms.[37,38] The previous standard of care, set by multiple randomized studies,[35,39–43] was to deliver 50 Gy to the ipsilateral breast over 25 fractions of 2 Gy per fraction followed by a 10 to 16 Gy boost to the lumpectomy cavity.[44] Thus, adjuvant RT could often take up to 6.0 to 6.5 weeks to complete. Over the last 10 years, standard-of-care RT for early stage breast cancer has been changing. Thanks to the publication of multiple randomized studies comparing hypofractionated (higher doses per fraction to lower overall doses) treatment courses with standard fractionation, which all demonstrated equal efficacy, noninferiority, and equal if not improved toxicity with shorter (3–4 week) courses of radiation,[45–48] the American Society of Radiation Oncology has made the use of shorter courses of RT for early stage breast cancer part of their Choosing Wisely campaign.[49] In the Canadian study, a dose of 42.56 Gy was given over 16 fractions of 2.66 Gy per fraction.[45] With 10 years of follow-up, they found no difference in local recurrence (6.2% vs 6.7%) or cosmetic outcome.[45] Recently, a large database study demonstrated the use of hypofractionation for breast cancer RT has increased from only 10% of patients in 2008 to greater than 30% of endorsed patients by 2013.[50] Additionally, shorter radiation techniques targeting the lumpectomy cavity alone, including one-time intraoperative RT, and accelerated partial breast irradiation (APBI) in which RT is delivered twice a day over 1 week, have been studied[51,52] or are being studied (https://www.clinicaltrials.gov/ct2/show/NCT00103181) in randomized clinical trials for which we are still awaiting long-term follow-up.

Yet, for older women with early stage low-risk hormone-positive breast cancer, the question for oncologists is not how long to radiate our patients but rather whether it is needed at all. Luckily, this question has been well studied. There are at least 4 large randomized studies of older women with early stage breast cancer that compared adjuvant RT with no adjuvant RT (**Table 3**).[53–56] Arguably, the most important of these studies thus far has been the Cancer and Leukemia Group B (CALGB) 9343. In this study, Hughes and colleagues[55] randomized 636 women aged 70 years and older with hormone-positive or unknown tumors, less than 2 cm in size (T1), with no evidence of nodal disease to adjuvant tamoxifen with or without standard fractionated

Table 3
Overview of pivotal studies on adjuvant radiation approaches in the elderly

Study	Key Eligibility Criteria	Study Arms	Local Recurrence Results	OS Results
Fyles et al (Princess Margaret)	50 y of age and older Breast-conserving surgery Negative margins T1 or T2 (5 cm or less) Negative nodes No adjuvant chemotherapy allowed	Tamoxifen alone (n = 383) vs RT + tamoxifen (n = 386)	5-y rate: 7.7% vs 0.6% (P<.001)	5-y rate: 93.2% vs 92.8% (P = .83)
Pötter et al (ABCSG 8A)	Postmenopausal women Breast-conserving surgery Negative margins T1 or T2 (<3 cm) Hormone positive Negative nodes Grade 1 or 2	Tamoxifen or anastrozole (n = 417) vs RT + tamoxifen or anastrozole (n = 414)	5-y rate: 5.1% vs 0.4% (P<.001)	5-y rate: 94.5% vs 97.9% (P = .18)
Hughes et al (CALGB 9343)	70 y of age and older Breast-conserving surgery Negative margins T1 (2 cm or less) Hormone positive or unknown Negative nodes	Tamoxifen alone (n = 319) vs RT + tamoxifen (n = 317)	Locoregional recurrence: 5-y rate: 4% vs 1% (P<.001) 10-y rate: 9% vs 2% (P<.001)	5-y rate: 86% vs 87% (P = .94) 10-y rate: 66% vs 67% (P = .64)
Kunkler et al (PRIME II)	65 y of age and older Breast-conserving surgery Negative margins T1 or T2 (<3 cm) Negative nodes Hormone positive Grade 3 or LVSI but not both	Endocrine therapy + RT (n = 658) vs endocrine therapy no RT (n = 668)	5-y rate: 4% vs <1% (P<.001)	5-y rate: 94% vs 95% (P = .34)

Abbreviations: ABCSG, Austrian Breast Cancer Study Group; CALGB, Cancer and Leukemia Group B; LVSI, lymphovascular space invasion; PRIME, Post-operative Radiotherapy in Minimum-Risk Elderly.
Data from Refs.[53–56]

radiation. In a recently published 10-year update, the investigators reported a locoregional recurrence rate of 10% in those not receiving radiation and 2% in those who received radiation (P<.001), with no difference in disease-specific or OS. Because of the relatively low risk of locoregional recurrence even without radiation, this study has been used to justify the consideration to omit radiation therapy in older women with T1N0 hormone-positive breast cancer.[23] Patterns-of-care studies suggest that CALGB 9343 has led to a decrease in the use of RT among older women with early stage breast cancer,[57] but its impact has not been as great as expected.[58] It is possible now with the publication of the 10-year follow-up that radiation oncologists will be more comfortable with omitting radiation if they and their patients agree that 10% local recurrence is acceptable. Other concerns with CALGB 9343 include the lack of information regarding the grade of tumor and tamoxifen adherence. Some have suggested that the CALGB results may not apply to women with grade 3 disease.[59] Similarly, for those women who are at higher risk of discontinuing tamoxifen before 5 years, an argument can be made to strongly consider radiation.

The recently published Post-operative Radiation in Minimal-Risk Elderly II study significantly supports and adds to the CALGB study.[56] In this study, Kunkler and colleagues[56] randomized 1326 women aged 65 years and older with T1-T2 (up to 3 cm), hormone-positive cancers with clear margins and grade 3 or lymphovascular invasion (but not both) to adjuvant hormone treatment with or without standard or hypofractionated RT. With a median follow-up of 5 years, there was a 2.9% absolute local control benefit to the addition of radiation (4.1% vs 1.3%, P<.001) but no difference in regional recurrence, distant metastases, or OS. These numbers are very similar to the 5-year results of CALGB 9343.[60] One important difference, however, was the inclusion of women 65 to 69 years of age, which could justify omission of radiation in women of those ages as well.

Yet, many older women, when faced with the option of omission of radiation leading to a 5-year recurrence rate of 4% or a 10-year recurrence rate of 10%, may choose to undergo RT. A big factor in that decision is the expected costs (economic, time, morbidity) of the radiation treatments. In terms of toxicity, breast irradiation is generally well tolerated in the older patient population.[53,60,61] Cardiovascular toxicity, one of the more concerning late toxicities of RT,[62,63] may be improving with newer techniques.[64] Additionally, with the increased use of hypofractionated RT[50,57] or APBI, the time and economic constraint on many women has also decreased in today's environment.

When counseling older patients with early stage hormone-positive breast cancer, it is important to consider each individual patient's priorities and expectations. Although generally this patient population is at low risk of breast cancer–related death,[55,56] local or regional recurrences can be difficult for both patients and their family members. Some women, when presented with the aforementioned data, will choose to omit radiation, whereas others will choose RT. Multidisciplinary consultations with breast surgeons, medical oncologists, and radiation oncologists for all patients (even those in whom radiation may be safely omitted) is recommended.

Systemic Therapy

Treatment considerations

Adjuvant systemic therapy refers to treatment given after curative surgery and/or radiation. The primary goal is to prolong survival by preventing breast cancer recurrence (locally, regionally, or in a distant site). Several factors must be taken into consideration in selecting patients suitable to receive adjuvant systemic therapy. These factors include functional status, social support, physiologic reserve, comorbidity, and life expectancy. As discussed earlier, consideration of estimated life expectancy and competing causes of mortality are of particular importance in determining how likely patents are to succumb to their breast cancer as opposed to another cause.[65] Standard-of-care treatments should be used in those healthy older adults whose life expectancy is equal to or greater than 10 years. The value of adjuvant therapies in patients whose life expectancy is less than 5 years requires greater discretion.[66–68]

Treatment decisions should also be guided by patient specific organ dysfunction, which can lead to certain side effects and toxicities. However, there is much controversy surrounding the extent to which pharmacokinetic and pharmacodynamics interactions of various cancer therapeutic agents differ in the elderly.[69] An instance in which the necessity for dose-modification is more established is renal insufficiency. Decisions regarding the use of specific endocrine or cytotoxic agents may be also be impacted by preexisting comorbidities, such as the use of anthracyclines or trastuzumab in the setting of cardiovascular disease, taxanes in the setting of preexisting neuropathy, tamoxifen in the presence of a history of thromboembolism, and aromatase inhibitors (AIs) in the setting of osteoporosis.[70]

Endocrine therapy

Endocrine therapy is the most commonly used systemic treatment in older patients with breast cancer in both the adjuvant and metastatic settings.[71–73] All women with hormone receptor (estrogen/progesterone)–positive breast cancer should be considered as candidates for adjuvant endocrine therapy with an aromatase inhibitor or tamoxifen. Tamoxifen belongs to a class of drugs recognized as selective estrogen receptor (ER) modulators. It acts as an antagonist of the ER in breast tissue but an agonist in others, which accounts for its adverse effect profile. AIs are another important class of drugs that decrease levels of circulating estrogen by inhibiting aromatase, the enzyme that converts androgens to estrogen in several tissues, such as adipose and the adrenal glands. Although AIs have similar survival benefits as compared with tamoxifen, they are associated with a lower overall risk of relapse.[74]

The EBCTCG published an overview showing that women aged 70 years and older with early stage hormone receptor–positive breast cancer treated with tamoxifen for 5 years benefit from a similar reduction in risk of breast cancer recurrence and death as compared with their younger counterparts.[75,76] Furthermore, a recent prospective cohort study showed a 4% absolute increase in breast cancer–specific survival and 11% absolute increase in OS at a 5-year follow-up in older women treated with adjuvant tamoxifen.[73]

Studies have also shown that AI-based therapy for a duration of 5 years is more effective than tamoxifen for the same duration, resulting in fewer recurrences in women older than 60 years.[74] Alternatively, as compared with their younger counterparts, women aged 70 years and older who receive an additional 5 years of treatment with letrozole after taking tamoxifen for 5 years experience fewer recurrences with no decrement in quality of life.[77] AIs only work in women who are postmenopausal; the median age of women enrolled in clinical trials of AIs as the treatment of both early stage, locally advanced and metastatic breast cancer has often been older than 60 years.

With regard to toxicities, tamoxifen is known to have a 1% to 3% risk of thromboembolism (including stroke), in addition to a 1% to 2% risk of endometrial cancer after 5 years of therapy.[78] AIs are known for an increase risk of bone loss and/or osteoporosis with a corresponding increase in risk of factures, a 10% to 40% incidence of potentially functionally limiting arthralgias and myalgias, and a possible increased risk of cardiovascular events. A final consideration in treatment with adjuvant endo-crine therapy is that studies have demonstrated poorer adherence in older compared with younger women, which may impact clinical outcomes.[79]

Chemotherapy

Generally speaking, adjuvant chemotherapy is recommended for women with ER-negative or Her-2/neu–amplified tumors that are larger than 1 cm or any subtype in which lymph node involvement is found. A retrospective review of 4 randomized studies has also shown that the administration of intensive chemotherapy regimens in older patients results in a reduction in breast cancer recurrence and morality, regardless of age.[9] A consensus expert panel, a part of the NCCN's published recom-mendations in 2008, suggested that recommendations for the use of adjuvant chemo-therapy in older patients should be guided by a well-balanced consideration of benefit-fit risk ratio. Oncologists should carefully consider factors, such as life expec-tancy, impact of comorbidities, specific toxicity profile of various agents, and patient-specific goals of care. Risk-prediction models, such as Adjuvant Online (www.adjuvantonline.org) and PREDICT (http://www.predict.nhs.uk/predict.html), are useful in providing the added value of chemotherapy in addition to other treatments, although their validity in patients older than 70 years has not been clearly documented. When used in the appropriate setting and patient population, validated molecular testing, such as mammaprint and oncotype Dx, provides estimates on the predictive benefit of chemotherapy based on molecular and genetic features of a patient's spe-cific tumor.[80,81] No one specific adjuvant chemotherapy regimen is preferable in the treatment of elderly patients, aside from caution that should be exercised in the use of anthracyclines. General treatment recommendations include consideration of he-patic and renal function, attention to dosing schedules (such as weekly administra-tion), and early use of growth factors to minimize the risk of neutropenic fever.[70] Another area of interest that is underevaluated in the older population is the potential interactions of chemotherapeutic drugs with other medications.

The risk of recurrence for ER-negative breast cancer is known to be higher in the first 5 years as compared with ER-positive breast cancer, whereby a small risk of recur-rence extends to more than 15 years. However, in both settings, the benefit of chemo-therapy is most pronounced in the first 5 years.[75,82] A meta-analysis of randomized trials published by the EBCTCG demonstrated that adjuvant polychemotherapy pro-vides a significant impact on recurrence rate and breast cancer–specific mortality in women with ER-negative disease regardless of age. Women younger than 50 years were shown to have a 12% reduction in 10-year recurrence risk and 8% reduction in breast cancer mortality, as compared with 10% and 6%, respectively, in patients aged 50 to 69 years. For older women with ER-negative breast cancer, several retro-spective analyses also support the use of adjuvant chemotherapy. Two recent ana-lyses using the Surveillance, Epidemiology, and End Results database have demonstrated that adjuvant chemotherapy in the treatment of node-positive, ER-negative breast cancer is associated with a reduction in mortality.[82,83]

Analysis by the EBCTCG have also shown that patients with ER-positive disease derive less benefit from adjuvant chemotherapy than ER-negative disease, particularly in an older group of patients aged 50 to 69 years as compared with those younger than 50 years.[75] The benefit of adjuvant chemotherapy with cyclophosphamide, metho-trexate, and fluorouracil in addition to tamoxifen was also found to be less pronounced in a subset of women older than 60 years with ER-positive disease enrolled in 2 large coop-erative group trials, NSABP B14 and B20.[84] One randomized study published by the French adjuvant group specifically evaluated the role of adjuvant-epicurubicin-based chemotherapy in addition to tamoxifen in women 65 years or older with predominantly ER-positive breast cancer that was operable and node positive. Although adjuvant chemotherapy followed by tamoxifen demonstrated a significant increase in disease-free survival, no impact on survival was seen at 6 years.[85]

With regard to toxicity, an analysis of 3 randomized cooperative group trials that included 6642 patients showed that the reduction in disease-free and breast cancer related mortality in older patients occurred at the risk of greater toxicity.[86] This increased toxicity translated to a higher rate of treatment-related death. However, it is likely that the increase risk of chemotherapy-related toxicity may be due more to the type of regimen than the patient's age. Specific treatment-related complications that older patients are at increased risk for include cardiac toxicity and secondary malignancies that include acute myelogenous leukemia/myelodysplastic syndromes.[86,87]

Biological agents

Another consideration in older women is the use of trastuzumab in the setting of Her-2–positive breast cancer. Although the use of trastuzumab in the adjuvant setting is associated with significant improvement in clinical outcomes that include disease-free survival and OS, the magnitude of benefit in older patients is difficult to estimate given that few elderly patients were enrolled in the randomized trials.[88,89] In a joint analysis of 2 large cooperative group trials (NSABP B-31 and North Central Cancer Treatment Group 9831), only 16% of patients were aged 60 years and older, with 6% of patients older than 65 years. Older age is a recognized risk factor for trastuzumab-related cardiotoxicity.[90–92] Additionally, at a follow-up period of 5 years, older age was found to be a risk factor for congestive heart failure (CHF), with an incidence of 2.3% for patients less than 50 years as compared with 5.1% for patients aged 50 to 59 years and 5.4% for patients 60 years old or older ($P = .03$). In this analysis, significant associations with CHF and trastuzumab exposure included use of hypertensive medications, lower baseline left ventricular ejection fraction (LVEF), and lower LVEF following treatment with doxorubicin/cyclophosphamide. Rates of CHF following trastuzumab-based adjuvant therapy were found to be 6.8% and 3.0%, respectively, in patients treated with and without concurrent antihypertensive therapy. Taking all evidence into consideration, expert consensus opinion issued by the NCCN is that the small numbers of cardiac-related deaths and added valued and therapeutic index of adjuvant trastuzumab should not preclude its use in the treatment of most fit elderly women.[70] Given that adjuvant trastuzumab is always given to patients with chemotherapy, a similar decision process taking into account competing risk and functional reserve should occur in selecting patients for treatment.

A final consideration regarding chemotherapy-induced cardiotoxicity is prevention. Both beta-blockers and angiotensin-converting enzyme inhibitors have been shown to have a potential benefit.[93] Treatment with beta-blockers was found to preserve ejection-fraction before anthracycline-based chemotherapy in a randomized study of 50 patients assigned to receive carvedilol versus placebo, with similar findings in a study using nebivolol.[94,95] A larger randomized study involving 473 patients treated with enalapril showed a benefit in the prevention of cardiotoxicity. However, the mean age in this study was 45 years. Currently, ongoing randomized phase II trials are evaluating the role of treatment of the aforementioned agents in comparison with placebo following trastuzumab-based treatment.[96]

METASTATIC DISEASE

Although metastatic beast cancer is incurable, currently available treatments have led to modest improvement in survival with improvement in quality of life. As is encouraged for all patients, older patients should be enrolled into studies evaluating novel agents and therapeutic approaches when possible and appropriate. As in the adjuvant setting, selection of treatment in the metastatic setting is guided by tumor phenotype and other negative prognostic factors related to tumor biology and patient-specific clinical characteristics. Identified factors include ER-negative tumors, presence of visceral dominant disease, and a short disease-free survival interval (time from diagnosis until detection of metastases) for those who received adjuvant treatment. However, older age alone has not been found to impact clinical outcomes.[97]

Endocrine therapy is preferred as the first-line therapy for patients with HR-positive disease. Chemotherapy should be reserved for those with HR-negative breast cancer, patients in which a rapid response is needed (patients that are particularly symptomatic or with a high burden of disease), or patients who develop disease that is refractory to endocrine therapy. On progression, sequential endocrine therapies can be used in patients with HR-positive breast cancer. A unique disease subtype in which targeted therapies should be used is Her-2/neu–positive breast cancer. The use of Her-2–targeted agents (eg, trastuzumab, pertuzumab, TDM-1, lapatinib) in older women with or without chemotherapy and endocrine therapy is beneficial. Single-agent use may be considered to avoid certain treatment-related side effects. As is the case with the adjuvant setting, the evaluation of trastuzumab in elderly patients in the metastatic setting is limited given the underrepresentation of older patients in randomized trials. In the pivotal trials of trastuzumab plus chemotherapy and single-agent trastuzumab, the mean age of enrolled patients was 54 years.[98,99]

A case-control study of women receiving chemotherapy for metastatic breast cancer identified no significant difference in time to disease progression and survival for women younger than 50 years, aged 50 to 69 years, and 70 years and older.[100] Despite similar clinical outcomes, the study found that women aged 70 years and older were more likely to receive lower doses of chemotherapy. Given increased toxicity with combination chemotherapy, single-agent cytotoxic therapy is generally preferred. Supporting this is a randomized study for first-line combination chemotherapy (doxorubicin/paclitaxel) compared with sequential single-agent chemotherapy in women with metastatic breast cancer with a median age of 56 to 58 years. Although no difference was seen in OS or quality of life between the treatment arms, those who received combination therapy experienced greater treatment-related toxicity.

Choice of specific agents and regimens should be determined by therapeutic efficacy and toxicity profile. Specific trials evaluating the role of various agents in older women are small in size. Taxanes are a class of drugs that are highly efficacious and well-tolerated when administered weekly.[101] The main dose-limiting side effect is neurotoxicity. A small trial evaluating single-agent taxanes in elderly or frail women revealed that response rates were higher with weekly paclitaxel as compared with docetaxel (48% vs 38%), with a different side effect accompanying each drug.[102,103] Vinorelbine as a single agent is another good option in elderly patients with cancer, given its relatively favorable side-effect profile with less alopecia and neuropathy.[79] Despite being an anthracycline, pegylated liposomal doxorubicin has been found to be effective with convenient dosing on a monthly schedule.[104] Another good cytotoxic option in elderly women is capecitabine, a fluorouracil prodrug, with benefits including a favorable toxicity profile and availability in an oral formulation.[28] A recent analysis of capecitabine from 2 single-arm phase II studies and one open-label randomized phase II study showed improved clinical outcomes (OS, progression-free survival, response rate, and clinical benefit rate) comparable with younger counterparts in selected elderly patients with a good baseline performance status. Furthermore, incidence of adverse effects was not associated with older age.[105]

| Table 4 | |
| ASCO and NCCN follow-up guidelines | |
Recommended Test	Frequency
History and examination (update family history)	Every 3–6 mo × 3 y Every 6 mo × 2 y Yearly after 5 y (NCCN 1-4 × per year × 5 y)
Mammography	Yearly[a]
Breast self-examination	Monthly[b]
Not recommended for routine screening in asymptomatic patients	CBCs, chemistry panels, bone scans, chest radiographs, liver ultrasounds, computed tomography scans, PET scan, MRI, or tumor markers (CEA, CA 15–3, and CA 27.29).

Abbreviations: CBCs, complete blood counts; CEA, carcinoembryonic antigen.
[a] For older patients with life expectancies less than 5 years, the authors suggest mammography be discontinued.
[b] Level of evidence for this low and can be omitted for many.

Perhaps mention a line or two of some of the newer agents just approved by the Food and Drug Administration, for example, Ibrance, Palbociclib with letrozole, and also pertuzumab in combination with trastuzumab (Herceptin) and chemotherapy.

FOLLOW-UP AND SURVIVORSHIP

Older women with early stage breast cancer should have follow-up evaluations similar to younger women that adhere to the guidelines of the American Society of Clinical Oncology (ASCO) or NCCN (**Table 4**). These guidelines are prudent, effective, and minimize the costs of care. Although the risk of ipsilateral breast cancer (in women who have breast conservation) and contralateral breast cancer is higher in women who have a history of prior breast cancer, it is reasonable to consider eliminating screening mammography in these patients it they have a life expectancy of less than 5 years. It is essential in these patients that breast examination be done yearly to detect recurrence.

Most breast cancer survivors are greater than 65 years of age. Although oncologists are likely to remain involved in the care of many of these women, most are likely to die of non–breast cancer causes. Nevertheless, oncologists are likely to see these patients at least yearly for the first 5 years after diagnosis, especially those on endocrine therapy. In addition to making sure patients are compliant with their endocrine therapy, oncologists can best serve these patients by becoming aware and questioning such patients about falls, loss of function, social support, and other geriatric issues. Oncologists should make sure that primary care practitioners, experienced in geriatrics, are part of the patients' care team to maximize the quality of care for all older patients with cancer.

SUMMARY

The complexities of treatment decision making in older women with cancer are attributable to changes in functional reserve, an increase in competing causes of morbidity and death, and differing tolerance to certain various interventions and cancer therapies. Individualized treatment decisions in the geriatric patient population require careful consideration of tumor biology, a comprehensive geriatric assessment, clinical trial results, and patient preferences. As the population of older women with breast cancer continues to increase, there is an urgent need to bolster evidence-based guidelines.

REFERENCES

1. Siegel RL, Miller KD, Jemal A. Cancer statistics, 2015. CA Cancer J Clin 2015; 65(1):5–29.
2. SEER cancer statistics factsheets: breast cancer. Bethesda (MD): National Cancer Institute; 2015. Available at: http://seer.cancer.gov/statfacts/html/breast.html.
3. Smith BD, Jiang J, McLaughlin SS, et al. Improvement in breast cancer outcomes over time: are older women missing out? J Clin Oncol 2011; 29(1527–7755 (Electronic)):4647–53.
4. Early Breast Cancer Trialists' Collaborative Group (EBCTCG), Clarke M, Coates AS, et al. Adjuvant chemotherapy in oestrogen-receptor-poor breast cancer: patient-level meta-analysis of randomised trials. Lancet 2008; 371(9606):29–40.
5. Lyratzopoulos G, Abel GA, Brown CH, et al. Socio-demographic inequalities in stage of cancer diagnosis: evidence from patients with female breast, lung, colon, rectal, prostate, renal, bladder, melanoma, ovarian and endometrial cancer. Ann Oncol 2013;24(3):843–50.
6. Rutherford MJ, Abel GA, Greenberg DC, et al. The impact of eliminating age inequalities in stage at diagnosis on breast cancer survival for older women. Br J Cancer 2015;112(Suppl 1):S124–8.
7. Owusu C, Lash TL, Silliman RA. Effect of undertreatment on the disparity in age-related breast cancer-specific survival among older women. Breast Cancer Res Treat 2007;102(2):227–36.
8. van de Water W, Markopoulos C, van de Velde CJ, et al. Association between age at diagnosis and disease-specific mortality among postmenopausal women with hormone receptor-positive breast cancer. JAMA 2012;307(6):590–7.
9. Muss HB, Woolf S, Berry D, et al. Adjuvant chemotherapy in older and younger women with lymph node-positive breast cancer. JAMA 2005;293(9):1073–81.
10. Williams GR, Jones E, Muss HB. Challenges in the treatment of older breast cancer patients. Hematol Oncol Clin North Am 2013;27(4):785–804.
11. Biganzoli L, Wildiers H, Oakman C, et al. Management of elderly patients with breast cancer: updated recommendations of the International Society of Geriatric Oncology (SIOG) and European Society of Breast Cancer Specialists (EU-SOMA). Lancet Oncol 2012;13(4):e148–60.
12. Diab SG, Elledge RM, Clark GM. Tumor characteristics and clinical outcome of elderly women with breast cancer. J Natl Cancer Inst 2000;92(7):550–6.
13. Daidone MG, Coradini D, Martelli G, et al. Primary breast cancer in elderly women: biological profile and relation with clinical outcome. Crit Rev Oncol Hematol 2003;45(3):313–25.
14. Jenkins EO, Deal AM, Anders CK, et al. Age-specific changes in intrinsic breast cancer subtypes: a focus on older women. Oncologist 2014;19(10):1076–83.
15. Kemeny MM, Peterson BL, Kornblith AB, et al. Barriers to clinical trial participation by older women with breast cancer. J Clin Oncol 2003;21(12):2268–75.
16. Sattar S, Alibhai SM, Wildiers H, et al. How to implement a geriatric assessment in your clinical practice. Oncologist 2014;19(10):1056–68.
17. Talarico L, Chen G, Pazdur R. Enrollment of elderly patients in clinical trials for cancer drug registration: a 7-year experience by the US Food and Drug Administration. J Clin Oncol 2004;22(22):4626–31.

18. Javid SH, Unger JM, Gralow JR, et al. A prospective analysis of the influence of older age on physician and patient decision-making when considering enrollment in breast cancer clinical trials (SWOG S0316). Oncologist 2012;17(9): 1180–90.

19. Dixon JM, Renshaw L, Macaskill EJ, et al. Increase in response rate by prolonged treatment with neoadjuvant letrozole. Breast Cancer Res Treat 2009; 113(1):145–51.

20. Brandt J, Garne JP, Tengrup I, et al. Age at diagnosis in relation to survival following breast cancer: a cohort study. World J Surg Oncol 2015;13(1):33.

21. Vestal RE. Aging and pharmacology. Cancer 1997;80(7):1302–10.

22. Edge SB. AJCC cancer staging manual. 7th edition. Chicago: Springer; 2010.

23. National Comprehensive Cancer Network clinical practice guidelines in oncology: breast cancer. 2014; Version 3.2014. Available at: http://www.nccn.org/. Accessed May 20, 2015.

24. Merchant TE, McCormick B, Yahalom J, et al. The influence of older age on breast cancer treatment decisions and outcome. Int J Radiat Oncol Biol Phys 1996;34(3):565–70.

25. Mandelblatt JS, Edge SB, Meropol NJ, et al. Predictors of long-term outcomes in older breast cancer survivors: perceptions versus patterns of care. J Clin Oncol 2003;21(5):855–63.

26. Martelli G, Boracchi P, Ardoino I, et al. Axillary dissection versus no axillary dissection in older patients with T1N0 breast cancer: 15-year results of a randomized controlled trial. Ann Surg 2012;256(6):920–4.

27. Giuliano AE, Hunt KK, Ballman KV, et al. Axillary dissection vs no axillary dissection in women with invasive breast cancer and sentinel node metastasis: a randomized clinical trial. JAMA 2011;305(6):569–75.

28. Bajetta E, Procopio G, Celio L, et al. Safety and efficacy of two different doses of capecitabine in the treatment of advanced breast cancer in older women. J Clin Oncol 2005;23(10):2155–61.

29. Chen AY, Halpern MT, Schrag NM, et al. Disparities and trends in sentinel lymph node biopsy among early-stage breast cancer patients (1998-2005). J Natl Cancer Inst 2008;100(7):462–74.

30. Rescigno J, Zampell JC, Axelrod D. Patterns of axillary surgical care for breast cancer in the era of sentinel lymph node biopsy. Ann Surg Oncol 2009;16(3): 687–96.

31. Lyman GH, Temin S, Edge SB, et al. Sentinel lymph node biopsy for patients with early-stage breast cancer: American Society of Clinical Oncology clinical practice guideline update. J Clin Oncol 2014;32(13):1365–83.

32. Utada M, Ohno Y, Shimizu S, et al. Comparison between overall, cause-specific, and relative survival rates based on data from a population-based cancer registry. Asian Pac J Cancer Prev 2012;13(11):5681–5.

33. Kemeny MM, Busch-Devereaux E, Merriam LT, et al. Cancer surgery in the elderly. Hematol Oncol Clin North Am 2000;14(1):169–92.

34. Hind D, Wyld L, Beverley CB, et al. Surgery versus primary endocrine therapy for operable primary breast cancer in elderly women (70 years plus). Cochrane Database Syst Rev 2006;(1):CD004272.

35. Fisher B, Anderson S, Bryant J, et al. Twenty-year follow-up of a randomized trial comparing total mastectomy, lumpectomy, and lumpectomy plus irradiation for the treatment of invasive breast cancer. N Engl J Med 2002;347(16):1233–41.

36. Early Breast Cancer Trialists' Collaborative Group (EBCTCG), Darby S, McGale P, et al. Effect of radiotherapy after breast-conserving surgery on

10-year recurrence and 15-year breast cancer death: meta-analysis of individual patient data for 10,801 women in 17 randomised trials. Lancet 2011; 378(9804):1707–16.

37. Hall EJ, Giaccia AJ. Radiobiology for the radiologist. 6th edition. Philadelphia: Lippincott Williams & Wilkins; 2006.

38. Regaud C, Blanc J. générations de la lignée spermatique: extreme sensibilité des spermatogonies à ces rayons. Comptes Rendus Des Seances De La Societe De Biologie Et De Ses Filiales 1906;61:163–5.

39. van Dongen JA, Voogd AC, Fentiman IS, et al. Long-term results of a randomized trial comparing breast-conserving therapy with mastectomy: European Organization for Research and Treatment of Cancer 10801 trial. J Natl Cancer Inst 2000;92(14):1143–50.

40. Liljegren G, Holmberg L, Bergh J, et al. 10-Year results after sector resection with or without postoperative radiotherapy for stage I breast cancer: a randomized trial. J Clin Oncol 1999;17(8):2326–33.

41. Forrest AP, Stewart HJ, Everington D, et al. Randomised controlled trial of conservation therapy for breast cancer: 6-year analysis of the Scottish trial. Scottish Cancer Trials Breast Group. Lancet 1996;348(9029):708–13.

42. Holli K, Hietanen P, Saaristo R, et al. Radiotherapy after segmental resection of breast cancer with favorable prognostic features: 12-year follow-up results of a randomized trial. J Clin Oncol 2009;27(6):927–32.

43. Fisher B, Bryant J, Dignam JJ, et al. Tamoxifen, radiation therapy, or both for prevention of ipsilateral breast tumor recurrence after lumpectomy in women with invasive breast cancers of one centimeter or less. J Clin Oncol 2002; 20(20):4141–9.

44. Bartelink H, Horiot JC, Poortmans P, et al. Recurrence rates after treatment of breast cancer with standard radiotherapy with or without additional radiation. N Engl J Med 2001;345(19):1378–87.

45. Whelan TJ, Pignol JP, Levine MN, et al. Long-term results of hypofractionated radiation therapy for breast cancer. N Engl J Med 2010;362(6):513–20.

46. START Trialists' Group, Bentzen SM, Agrawal RK, et al. The UK Standardisation of Breast Radiotherapy (START) Trial A of radiotherapy hypofractionation for treatment of early breast cancer: a randomised trial. Lancet Oncol 2008;9(4):331–41.

47. START Trialists' Group, Bentzen SM, Agrawal RK, et al. The UK Standardisation of Breast Radiotherapy (START) Trial B of radiotherapy hypofractionation for treatment of early breast cancer: a randomised trial. Lancet 2008;371(9618): 1098–107.

48. Haviland JS, Owen JR, Dewar JA, et al. The UK Standardisation of breast radiotherapy (START) trials of radiotherapy hypofractionation for treatment of early breast cancer: 10-year follow-up results of two randomised controlled trials. Lancet Oncol 2013;14(11):1086–94.

49. ASTRO releases list of five radiation oncology treatments to question as part of national Choosing Wisely® campaign. September 23, 2013.

50. Bekelman JE, Sylwestrzak G, Barron J, et al. Uptake and costs of hypofractionated vs conventional whole breast irradiation after breast conserving surgery in the United States, 2008-2013. JAMA 2014;312(23):2542–50.

51. Veronesi U, Orecchia R, Maisonneuve P, et al. Intraoperative radiotherapy versus external radiotherapy for early breast cancer (ELIOT): a randomised controlled equivalence trial. Lancet Oncol 2013;14(13):1269–77.

52. Vaidya JS, Wenz F, Bulsara M, et al. Risk-adapted targeted intraoperative radiotherapy versus whole-breast radiotherapy for breast cancer: 5-year results for

local control and overall survival from the TARGIT-A randomised trial. Lancet 2014;383(9917):603–13.

53. Fyles AW, McCready DR, Manchul LA, et al. Tamoxifen with or without breast irradiation in women 50 years of age or older with early breast cancer. N Engl J Med 2004;351(10):963–70.

54. Potter R, Gnant M, Kwasny W, et al. Lumpectomy plus tamoxifen or anastrozole with or without whole breast irradiation in women with favorable early breast cancer. Int J Radiat Oncol Biol Phys 2007;68(2):334–40.

55. Hughes KS, Schnaper LA, Bellon JR, et al. Lumpectomy plus tamoxifen with or without irradiation in women age 70 years or older with early breast cancer: long-term follow-up of CALGB 9343. J Clin Oncol 2013;31(19):2382–7.

56. Kunkler IH, Williams LJ, Jack WJ, et al. Breast-conserving surgery with or without irradiation in women aged 65 years or older with early breast cancer (PRIME II): a randomised controlled trial. Lancet Oncol 2015;16(3):266–73.

57. Rutter CE, Lester-Coll NH, Mancini BR, et al. The evolving role of adjuvant radiotherapy for elderly women with early-stage breast cancer. Cancer 2015;121(14): 2331–40.

58. Soulos PR, Yu JB, Roberts KB, et al. Assessing the impact of a cooperative group trial on breast cancer care in the Medicare population. J Clin Oncol 2012;30(14):1601–7.

59. VanderWalde N, Hebert B, Jones E, et al. The role of adjuvant radiation treatment in older women with early breast cancer. J Geriatr Oncol 2013;4(4): 402–12.

60. Hughes KS, Schnaper LA, Berry D, et al. Lumpectomy plus tamoxifen with or without irradiation in women 70 years of age or older with early breast cancer. N Engl J Med 2004;351(10):971–7.

61. Rayan G, Dawson LA, Bezjak A, et al. Prospective comparison of breast pain in patients participating in a randomized trial of breast-conserving surgery and tamoxifen with or without radiotherapy. Int J Radiat Oncol Biol Phys 2003; 55(1):154–61.

62. Darby SC, Ewertz M, McGale P, et al. Risk of ischemic heart disease in women after radiotherapy for breast cancer. N Engl J Med 2013;368(11):987–98.

63. Darby S, McGale P, Peto R, et al. Mortality from cardiovascular disease more than 10 years after radiotherapy for breast cancer: nationwide cohort study of 90 000 Swedish women. BMJ 2003;326(7383):256–7.

64. Eldredge-Hindy HB, Duffy D, Yamoah K, et al. Modeled risk of ischemic heart disease following left breast irradiation with deep inspiration breath hold. Pract Radiat Oncol 2015;5(3):162–8.

65. Balducci L, Extermann M. Management of cancer in the older person: a practical approach. Oncologist 2000;5(3):224–37.

66. Punglia RS, Hughes KS, Muss HB. Management of older women with early-stage breast cancer. Am Soc Clin Oncol Educ Book 2015;35:48–55.

67. Balducci L. Aging, frailty, and chemotherapy. Cancer Control 2007;14(1):7–12.

68. Koroukian SM, Murray P, Madigan E. Comorbidity, disability, and geriatric syndromes in elderly cancer patients receiving home health care. J Clin Oncol 2006;24(15):2304–10.

69. Hurria A, Lichtman SM. Pharmacokinetics of chemotherapy in the older patient. Cancer Control 2007;14(1):32–43.

70. Carlson RW, Moench S, Hurria A, et al. NCCN task force report: breast cancer in the older woman. J Natl Compr Canc Netw 2008;6(Suppl 4):S1–25 [quiz: S26–7].

71. Mustacchi G, Ceccherini R, Milani S, et al. Tamoxifen alone versus adjuvant tamoxifen for operable breast cancer of the elderly: long-term results of the phase III randomized controlled multicenter GRETA trial. Ann Oncol 2003; 14(3):414–20.
72. Crivellari D, Aapro M, Leonard R, et al. Breast cancer in the elderly. J Clin Oncol 2007;25(14):1882–90.
73. Owusu C, Lash TL, Silliman RA. Effectiveness of adjuvant tamoxifen therapy among older women with early stage breast cancer. Breast J 2007;13(4): 374–82.
74. Dowsett M, Cuzick J, Ingle J, et al. Meta-analysis of breast cancer outcomes in adjuvant trials of aromatase inhibitors versus tamoxifen. J Clin Oncol 2010;28(3): 509–18.
75. Early Breast Cancer Trialists' Collaborative Group (EBCTCG). Effects of chemotherapy and hormonal therapy for early breast cancer on recurrence and 15-year survival: an overview of the randomised trials. Lancet 2005;365(9472): 1687–717.
76. Clarke M, Collins R, Darby S, et al. Effects of radiotherapy and of differences in the extent of surgery for early breast cancer on local recurrence and 15-year survival: an overview of the randomised trials. Lancet 2005;366(9503): 2087–106.
77. Muss HB, Tu D, Ingle JN, et al. Efficacy, toxicity, and quality of life in older women with early-stage breast cancer treated with letrozole or placebo after 5 years of tamoxifen: NCIC CTG intergroup trial MA.17. J Clin Oncol 2008; 26(12):1956–64.
78. Amir E, Seruga B, Niraula S, et al. Toxicity of adjuvant endocrine therapy in postmenopausal breast cancer patients: a systematic review and meta-analysis. J Natl Cancer Inst 2011;103(17):1299–309.
79. Tew WP, Muss HB, Kimmick GG, et al. Breast and ovarian cancer in the older woman. J Clin Oncol 2014;32(24):2553–61.
80. Paik S, Shak S, Tang G, et al. A multigene assay to predict recurrence of tamoxifen-treated, node-negative breast cancer. N Engl J Med 2004;351(27): 2817–26.
81. Fan C, Oh DS, Wessels L, et al. Concordance among gene-expression-based predictors for breast cancer. N Engl J Med 2006;355(6):560–9.
82. Giordano SH, Duan Z, Kuo YF, et al. Use and outcomes of adjuvant chemotherapy in older women with breast cancer. J Clin Oncol 2006;24(18):2750–6.
83. Elkin EB, Hurria A, Mitra N, et al. Adjuvant chemotherapy and survival in older women with hormone receptor-negative breast cancer: assessing outcome in a population-based, observational cohort. J Clin Oncol 2006; 24(18):2757–64.
84. Fisher B, Jeong JH, Bryant J, et al. Treatment of lymph-node-negative, oestrogen-receptor-positive breast cancer: long-term findings from National Surgical Adjuvant Breast and Bowel Project randomised clinical trials. Lancet 2004; 364(9437):858–68.
85. Fargeot P, Bonneterre J, Roché H, et al. Disease-free survival advantage of weekly epirubicin plus tamoxifen versus tamoxifen alone as adjuvant treatment of operable, node-positive, elderly breast cancer patients: 6-year follow-up results of the French adjuvant study group 08 trial. J Clin Oncol 2004;22(23): 4622–30.
86. Muss HB, Biganzoli L, Sargent DJ, et al. Adjuvant therapy in the elderly: making the right decision. J Clin Oncol 2007;25(14):1870–5.

87. Pinder MC, Duan Z, Goodwin JS, et al. Congestive heart failure in older women treated with adjuvant anthracycline chemotherapy for breast cancer. J Clin Oncol 2007;25(25):3808–15.

88. Piccart-Gebhart MJ, Procter M, Leyland-Jones B, et al. Trastuzumab after adjuvant chemotherapy in HER2-positive breast cancer. N Engl J Med 2005;353(16): 1659–72.

89. Smith I, Procter M, Gelber RD, et al. 2-year follow-up of trastuzumab after adjuvant chemotherapy in HER2-positive breast cancer: a randomised controlled trial. Lancet 2007;369(9555):29–36.

90. al, R.e. Five year update of cardiac dysfunction on NSABP B-31, a randomized trial of sequential AC/paclitaxel vs. AC/paclitaxel/trastuzumab. J Clin Oncol 2007;25(Suppl 1) [abstract: LBA 513].

91. al, G.C.e. Update of cardiac dysfunction on NSABP B-31, a randomized trial of sequential AC vs. ACT with trastuzumab [abstract]. J Clin Oncol 2006;24(Suppl 1) [abstract: 581].

92. Tan-Chiu E, Yothers G, Romond E, et al. Assessment of cardiac dysfunction in a randomized trial comparing doxorubicin and cyclophosphamide followed by paclitaxel, with or without trastuzumab as adjuvant therapy in node-positive, human epidermal growth factor receptor 2-overexpressing breast cancer: NSABP B-31. J Clin Oncol 2005;23(31):7811–9.

93. Colombo A, Meroni CA, Cipolla CM, et al. Managing cardiotoxicity of chemotherapy. Curr Treat Options Cardiovasc Med 2013;15(4):410–24.

94. Kalay N, Basar E, Ozdogru I, et al. Protective effects of carvedilol against anthracycline-induced cardiomyopathy. J Am Coll Cardiol 2006;48(11): 2258–62.

95. Kaya MG, Ozkan M, Gunebakmaz O, et al. Protective effects of nebivolol against anthracycline-induced cardiomyopathy: a randomized control study. Int J Cardiol 2013;167(5):2306–10.

96. Lisinopril and Coreg CR in reducing side effects in women with breast cancer receiving trastuzumab.

97. Sledge GW, Neuberg D, Bernardo P, et al. Phase III trial of doxorubicin, paclitaxel, and the combination of doxorubicin and paclitaxel as front-line chemotherapy for metastatic breast cancer: an intergroup trial (E1193). J Clin Oncol 2003;21(4):588–92.

98. Slamon DJ, Leyland-Jones B, Shak S, et al. Use of chemotherapy plus a monoclonal antibody against HER2 for metastatic breast cancer that overexpresses HER2. N Engl J Med 2001;344(11):783–92.

99. Vogel VG. Why do we still use hormone replacement therapy? Why don't we use it more? J Clin Oncol 2002;20(3):616–9.

100. Christman K, Muss HB, Case LD, et al. Chemotherapy of metastatic breast cancer in the elderly. The Piedmont Oncology Association experience. JAMA 1992; 268(1):57–62 [see comment].

101. Lichtman SM, Hurria A, Cirrincione CT, et al. Paclitaxel efficacy and toxicity in older women with metastatic breast cancer: combined analysis of CALGB 9342 and 9840. Ann Oncol 2012;23(3):632–8.

102. Beuselinck B, Wildiers H, Wynendaele W, et al. Weekly paclitaxel versus weekly docetaxel in elderly or frail patients with metastatic breast carcinoma: a randomized phase-II study of the Belgian Society of Medical Oncology. Crit Rev Oncol Hematol 2010;75(1):70–7.

103. Hurria A, Fleming MT, Baker SD, et al. Pharmacokinetics and toxicity of weekly docetaxel in older patients. Clin Cancer Res 2006;12(20 Pt 1):6100–5.

104. Biganzoli L, Coleman R, Minisini A, et al. A joined analysis of two European Organization for the Research and Treatment of Cancer (EORTC) studies to evaluate the role of pegylated liposomal doxorubicin (Caelyx) in the treatment of
elderly patients with metastatic breast cancer. Crit Rev Oncol Hematol 2007;
61(1):84–9.
105. Ershler WB. Capecitabine monotherapy: safe and effective treatment for metastatic breast cancer. Oncologist 2006;11(4):325–35.

Myelodysplastic Syndromes and Acute Myeloid Leukemia in the Elderly

CrossMark

Heidi D. Klepin, MD, MS

KEYWORDS

- Myelodysplasia • Acute myeloid leukemia • Older • Treatment • Management
- Elderly

KEY POINTS

- Myelodysplastic syndromes (MDS) are a heterogeneous group of hematologic disorders with variable natural history.
- Treatment recommendations for MDS are risk adapted and range from supportive care to high-intensity therapy.
- Optimal therapy for older patients with acute myeloid leukemia (AML) is unclear.
- Management of older adults with MDS and AML needs to be individualized, accounting for both the heterogeneity of disease biology and patient characteristics, which can influence life expectancy and treatment tolerance.

MYELODYSPLASTIC SYNDROMES

Myelodysplastic syndromes (MDS) constitute a heterogenous group of clonal hematopoietic disorders characterized by ineffective hematopoiesis and peripheral blood cytopenias. MDS can be indolent or rapidly progressive with complications secondary to profound cytopenias and the risk of evolution into acute myeloid leukemia (AML). MDS also impair quality of life, and are associated with high symptom burden[1] and high rates of health care use. Estimated 3-year survival rates are less than 50% in aggregate,[2] although survival can vary widely based on risk stratification. MDS are most commonly diagnosed among older adults (80% among adults ≥70 years of age) with approximately 15,000 to 20,000 new cases per year in the United States.[3]

Disclosure: Dr H.D. Klepin is supported by a Paul Beeson Career Development Award in Aging Research (K23AG038361; supported by NIA, AFAR, The John A. Hartford Foundation, and The Atlantic Philanthropies), The Gabrielle's Angel Foundation for Cancer Research, and NCI Cancer Center Support Grant (CCSG) P30CA012197. Dr H.D. Klepin has no other disclosures.
Section on Hematology and Oncology, Department of Internal Medicine, Wake Forest School of Medicine, Medical Center Boulevard, Winston-Salem, NC 27157, USA
E-mail address: hklepin@wakehealth.edu

Given population aging, these are diseases that will frequently be encountered in geriatric practices.

Diagnosis and Work-up

Diagnosis of MDS relies mainly on peripheral blood and bone marrow findings. The diagnosis should be suspected in individuals presenting with cytopenia. A common presentation is progressive macrocytic anemia followed by pancytopenia in older adults. Classic peripheral blood findings associated with MDS include macrocytosis and hypogranular, hypolobated (dysplastic) neutrophils. A bone marrow biopsy with cytogenetic analysis is required to confirm the diagnosis. Cytogenetic abnormalities (often involving chromosomes 5, 7, 8, 17, or 20) play a critical role in the diagnosis and natural history of MDS.

Risk Stratification: Disease Characteristics

Because of the heterogeneity inherent in diseases classified as MDS, several risk stratification schemes have been proposed to inform trial design and treatment decisions. The International Prognostic Scoring System (IPSS) is the most commonly referenced risk stratification schema and was developed to assess risk at the time of diagnosis.[4] The IPSS incorporates specific cytogenetic abnormalities, the percentage of marrow blasts, and the number of hematopoietic lineages involved in the cytopenia. A 5-category revised IPSS (IPSS-R) was developed, which further subdivides cytogenetic abnormalities and increases the weight of higher blast percentages.[5,6] The IPSS-R highlights differences in the natural history of the disease by contrasting survival and time to AML progression (**Table 1**). In the development cohort, age was a prognostic factor for survival but not for progression to AML, having more impact in lower versus higher risk disease. The IPSS does not account for severity of cytopenia or for transfusion dependence.

Risk Stratification: Patient Characteristics

Selection of treatment of patients with MDS depends not only on disease characteristics but on assessment of the patient's overall fitness and competing comorbid conditions. Patient characteristics that influence life expectancy and treatment tolerance (eg, comorbidity, functional status, cognition) vary widely among similarly aged patients. Although measurement of these characteristics is not routine in most clinical trials, there is evidence regarding the prevalence and prognostic importance of comorbidity.[7–9] Studies suggest that more than half of older adults diagnosed with MDS have competing comorbid conditions and that comorbidity is associated with

Table 1 Overall survival (OS) and risk of AML evolution by revised IPSS score			
Risk Group	**IPSS-R Score**	**Median OS (y)**	**Median Time to 25% AML Evolution (y)**
Very low	<1.5	8.8	>14.5
Low	<1.5–3.0	5.3	10.8
Intermediate	>3–4.5	3.0	3.2
High	>4.5–6	1.6	1.4
Very high	>6	0.8	0.7

Abbreviation: IPSS-R, Revised International Prognostic Scoring System.
   Data from Greenberg PL, Tuechler H, Schanz J, et al. Revised International Prognostic Scoring System (IPSS-R) for myelodysplastic syndromes. Blood 2012;120(12):2454–65.

shorter survival independent of age or disease risk.[7–10] A study using questions from a baseline quality of life (QOL) questionnaire to predict survival indicated that self-reported physical function (eg, ease of taking a long walk) was predictive of survival.[11] A prospective study investigating the predictive utility of a geriatric assessment (GA) among older adults treated nonintensively for MDS (N = 51) and AML (N = 69) found that requiring assistance with activities of daily living (ADL) and high fatigue rating were independently associated with survival.[12] These characteristics and others detected by GA may help identify patients who are vulnerable to the toxicities of therapies and can inform decisions related to the intensity and chronicity of treatment. Larger prospective studies validating these findings are needed to optimally predict treatment benefit and individualize management.

Treatment

Treatment strategies have been evolving to target patients with higher risk MDS and subgroups defined by specific cytogenetic abnormalities. Current treatment recommendations are based on a risk-adapted therapeutic approach and are further refined by addition of patient-specific characteristics (**Tables 2** and **3**). In general, treatment goals for lower risk patients are to minimize the morbidity of disease (maximize QOL, and minimize symptoms and transfusion dependence); goals for higher risk patients include altering the natural history of the disease.

Supportive care, designed to control symptoms related to cytopenias, is indicated for all patients and remains the primary treatment of lower risk patients with MDS or those who are frail. Key components of supportive care are transfusion support and antibiotics for infection. Hematopoietic growth factors (eg, erythropoietin) are used to minimize transfusion requirements for patients with symptomatic anemia and can improve QOL.[13,14] Over time, most patients become transfusion dependent, increasing the risk of iron overload; iron chelation therapy should be started for those with lower risk MDS, ongoing transfusion dependence, and expected survival greater than 1 year.

Patients in the higher risk IPSS categories are more likely to experience complications from cytopenias and to progress to acute leukemia more quickly after diagnosis. Hypomethylating agents that inhibit DNA methyltransferases (azacitidine and decitabine) are the primary treatment of most patients. Randomized studies with azacitidine compared with placebo have shown improvements in survival and QOL, and a longer time to progression to acute leukemia.[15–18] The survival advantage associated with azacitidine has been shown for adults more than 75 years of age.[19] Registry data comparing differing treatment schedules among patients greater than or equal to 75 years of age provide additional real-world information on the benefits (40% transfusion independence) and complications (29% cycles delayed, 47% hospitalized for infection) of treatment in this age group.[19] The US Food and Drug Administration also approved decitabine for the treatment of higher risk MDS based on data showing decreased transfusion requirements and symptoms.[20]

Challenges for older adults using hypomethylating agents include long-term management of myelosuppression, which often worsens for several months before response is detectable. The duration of treatment can be challenging both physically and psychologically; the median duration of treatment on clinical trials is at least 6 months and often more than 12 months for responders.[15,18]

Additional treatment options exist for patients with the 5q minus (5q−) syndrome, defined by a deletion of the long arm of chromosome 5 as the sole abnormality. The 5q− syndrome often presents as refractory, severe anemia with a preserved platelet count. It is considered a more favorable subtype of MDS with lower risk

Table 2
Treatment options for older adults with MDS based on disease and patient characteristics

Disease Characteristics (IPSS-R)	Goal of Therapy	Patient Characteristics	Treatment Considerations (Comments)
Very low risk, low risk. Asymptomatic	Improve QOL	Any	Observation (evidence is lacking to support QOL or survival advantage with early therapy)
Very low/low/intermediate. Symptomatic			
5q deletion	Improve QOL	Any	Lenalidomide (understudied in vulnerable/frail patients. Dose adjust for impaired creatinine clearance)
Absence of 5q− with erythropoietin level <500 uM/mL	Improve QOL	Any	Erythropoietin ± GCSF (discontinue if no response in 8 wk)
	Improve QOL	Good PS/minimal comorbidity	Consider lenalidomide (especially if isolated anemia)
			Consider hypomethylating agents (observational data suggest benefit in lower risk MDS)
Intermediate/high/very high	Delay progression, extend life	Any age, good PS, absence of major comorbidity	Hypomethylating agents (strongest evidence supports use of 7-d azacitidine regimen)
	Cure	Age 60–75 y, excellent PS, absence of major comorbidity	Consider referral for RIC HSCT vs hypomethylating agents (comprehensive GA may help inform fitness, randomized data to support benefits of HCST are lacking)
	Delay progression, extend life	Poor PS and/or major comorbidity	Consider hypomethylating agents vs supportive care (absence of data in frail patients; however, given potential to improve survival and QOL, would discuss with patient)

Abbreviations: GCSF, granulocyte colony-stimulating factor; HSCT, hematopoietic stem cell transplantation; PS, performance status; RIC, reduced-intensity conditioning.

Adapted from Klepin HD, Rao AV, Pardee TS. Acute myeloid leukemia and myelodysplastic syndromes in older adults. J Clin Oncol 2014;32(24):2541–52.

Table 3
Selected randomized treatment trials for MDS

Treatment	N	Disease Risk Category	Positive Outcomes	Toxicity
Azacitidine[16] 75 mg/m² SQ × 7 d Q 4 wk vs supportive care	191	IPSS Int-1/Int-2/high	Improved response rate (23% vs 5%) Improved time to AML or death (21 vs 13 mo) Decreased AML transformation (15% vs 38%) Improved QOL (physical function, symptoms, psychological state)	Grade 3–4 myelosuppression (43%–58%) Infection (20%)
Azacitidine[15] 75 mg/m² SQ × 7 d Q 4 wk vs conventional care (supportive, low-dose cytarabine, intensive chemotherapy)	358	IPSS Int-2 or high	OS (median 24.5 vs 15 mo)	Myelosuppression
Decitabine 15 mg/m² IV Q 8 h for 3 d Q 6 wk vs supportive care[20]	170	IPSS Int or high	Response rate (17% vs 0%) Improved QOL (global health, fatigue, dyspnea)	Dose reductions/delays (35%) Grade 4 myelosuppression (>50%)
Lenalidomide 10 mg/d days 1–21 vs 5 mg/ d days 1–28 vs placebo on 28-d cycle[21]	205	MDS with del5q31 IPSS low or Int-1 RBC transfusion dependence	RBC transfusion independence for ≥26 wk (56.1% vs 42.6% vs 5.9%) RBC transfusion independence >8 wk associated with decreased risk of death and AML progression	Myelosuppression in first 2 cycles DVT (5.8%) in 10-mg group

Abbreviations: DVT, deep venous thrombosis; ECOG, Eastern Cooperative Oncology Group; Int, intermediate; IV, intravenous; Q, every; RBC, red blood cell; SQ, subcutaneous.

of AML progression. Lenalidomide, an oral immunomodulatory drug, decreases transfusion requirements and reverses cytogenetic abnormalities in patients with 5q− syndrome.[21,22] Myelosuppression is the primary toxicity of lenalidomide, often requiring dose reduction or dose delay. Studies suggest that treatment with lenalidomide may also benefit patients with low-risk MDS without 5q deletion and it can be considered an option for these patients as well if they are transfusion dependent.[23]

To date the only curative therapy for MDS is allogeneic hematopoietic stem cell transplantation (HSCT), which is generally restricted to younger adults with acceptable donors because of treatment-associated morbidity and mortality risk. However, HSCT is increasingly considered for selected adults between the ages of 60 and 80 years with good functional status and minimal comorbidity with the use of reduced-intensity conditioning (RIC) regimens. HSCT can result in appreciable survival rates among patients with high-risk disease,[24] although most older adults in this context are aged less than 70 years. At present, HSCT is reserved for fit patients (good performance status [PS], minimal comorbidity) with higher risk disease. Specifically, among patients 60 to 70 years of age, evidence suggests that survival may be improved by RIC HSCT for patients who are int-2/high IPSS (36 vs 28 months) but not for patients who are low/int-1 IPSS (38 vs 77 months).[24] Balancing the risk of disease versus treatment is critical and remains an active area of research. Because the criteria for fitness in the context of stem cell transplantation are further refined with the use of standardized strategies such as GA,[25] the real-world applicability of transplantation will increase.

Unresolved Questions for Older Adults with Myelodysplastic Syndromes

Trials targeting vulnerable and frail patients are needed, as are consistent definitions of fit, vulnerable, and frail in each treatment setting. In the noncurative setting, the duration and timing of treatment to optimally balance disease control and QOL are unclear. The role of HSCT for older adults needs to be defined; evidence remains confounded by the lack of randomized controlled trials, inadequate characterization of fitness, and inconsistent collection of additional patient-centered outcomes (functional independence, health care use, QOL, treatment satisfaction).

ACUTE MYELOID LEUKEMIA

AML refers to a group of clonal hematopoietic disorders characterized by proliferation of immature myeloid cells in the bone marrow. Accumulation of leukemic cells impairs the normal hematopoietic function, resulting in cytopenias with or without leukocytosis. AML is most commonly diagnosed among older adults (median age, 68–72 years).[3] In 2014, the American Cancer Society estimated that 18,860 patients would be diagnosed with AML, with most (10,460) anticipated to die from the disease.[26]

Diagnosis

The diagnosis of AML depends primarily on detection of leukemic blasts of myeloid lineage ($\geq$20%) in the bone marrow. The World Health Organization classifies AML into 4 major categories (each with 2 or more subtypes) using morphologic, immunophenotypic, genetic, and clinical features. The main categories are (1) AML with recurrent genetic abnormalities, (2) AML with myelodysplasia-related features, (3) therapy-related AML and MDS, and (4) AML not otherwise specified. Genetic and molecular abnormalities highlight the heterogeneity of AML and identify subsets associated with better or worse prognosis. For example, the core binding factor leukemias [inv16, t(8;21), t(16;16)], and acute promyelocytic leukemia [t(15;17)] are associated with better prognosis. The presence of mutations in *FLT-3* in the setting of a normal karyotype is associated with worse outcomes.

Treatment

If untreated or unresponsive to chemotherapy, AML is rapidly fatal (median survival <2 months). The major causes of death are infection and hemorrhage related to the disease-associated cytopenias. Increased age is associated with poor outcomes[27] (**Fig. 1**). There is no consensus regarding optimal therapy for older adults (often defined by age ≥60 years) with AML[28,29] in part because of the higher morbidity and mortality seen in clinical trials. In the United States, less than 40% of older adults receive any therapy for newly diagnosed AML.[30] However, it is clear from both clinical trial and population-based data that chemotherapy can provide a survival benefit compared with supportive care for selected older adults, even among octagenarians.[28,30–33] Age is a surrogate measure representing both age-related changes in tumor biology (contributing to treatment resistance) and patient characteristics (contributing to decreased treatment tolerance). Individualized decision making based on evolving stratification of both tumor biology and patient characteristics will help inform the tailoring of treatment and supportive care.

Tumor Biology

Age-related differences in tumor biology are a major factor contributing to poor outcomes among older adults. Cytogenetic abnormalities are the most important prognostic factors in AML. Older adults are more likely to have poor-risk karyotypes (−7, 7q−, −5, 5q−; abnormalities of 11q, 17p, Inv3; or complex karyotypes involving

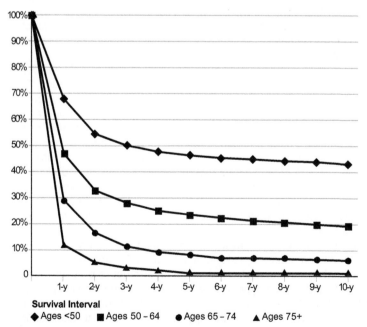

Fig. 1. Relative survival by time and age for AML. (*Adapted from* Surveillance Epidemiology End Results (SEER). Available at: www.Seer.cancer.gov. Accessed April 3, 2014.)

$\geq$3 chromosomes) and fewer good-risk karyotypes [i16, t(16;16), t(8;21), or t(15;17)] compared with younger patients.[34,35] In an analysis of more than 1000 older adults treated on clinical trials, the proportions with favorable, intermediate, and adverse cytogenetics were 7.3%, 79.1%, and 13.6% respectively associated with 5-year overall survival (OS) rates of 34%, 13%, and 2% respectively.[35] Molecular mutations and gene deregulation also contribute to prognosis.[36,37] Older adults also have higher expression of the multidrug resistance gene MDR1.[38] MDR1 encodes a membrane transporter protein responsible for drug efflux and chemotherapy resistance. In addition, older patients are more likely to have a secondary AML arising from underlying MDS, which is less responsive to standard therapy. The biology of AML in the elderly is complex and contributes directly to poor outcomes with conventional therapies.

Review of Elderly-specific Clinical Trial Data

Most clinical trials in AML have enrolled patients aged 60 to 80 years with good oncology PS (**Table 4**). Median survival in AML has historically been less than 1 year, with improvements seen in more recent trials.[27,39] In general, older adults are less likely to achieve remission (although rates are 30%–80%), are more likely to relapse, and experience higher 30-day treatment mortalities (10%–30%).[27,39,40]

Standard induction therapy for AML is combination chemotherapy that includes cytosine arabinoside (Ara-C) and an anthracycline administered in the inpatient setting. These drugs yield complete remissions (CRs) in ~50% of patients. The poorer prognosis associated with increased age is related to both a higher frequency of induction deaths (treatment-related mortality) and to chemotherapy failure caused by residual or resistant leukemia. Evidence suggests that selected older adults can benefit from standard intensive therapy, although survival improvement is often measured in months.[28,32] Attempts to improve durable response rates in older patients with AML have included dose attenuation, anthracycline substitution, use of growth factors, modulation of multidrug resistance, and targeting of molecular subsets.[39,41–48] Improvements have been incremental, without a clear practice-changing regimen identified.[39,42]

The role of lower intensity therapies, including the DNA hypomethylating agents (eg, azacitidine and decitabine), is an area of active investigation.[18,49,50] These agents have shown some efficacy for older adults with AML and are increasingly used in clinical practice, particularly among patients with comorbidity or poor functional status. In many cases, the goal of therapy is disease control or palliation. A recent randomized trial among adults 65 years of age or older with newly diagnosed AML showed a survival advantage for azacitidine compared with conventional care.[51] Conventional care included a wide variety of treatment options, from intensive induction to supportive care alone. The role of lower intensity regimens remains an active area of investigation. To date, none have been shown to be superior to intensive induction as a single comparator in randomized trials; cross-study comparisons are challenging.

For patients who achieve remission, the median duration of CR is approximately 1 year; a small percentage ($\leq$15%) may be cured. Patients who achieve remission are considered for postremission therapy in an attempt to prevent or delay relapse. The exact role and optimal type of postremission therapy remains poorly defined for older adults. On clinical trials, up to 20% of older adults who achieve remission never receive any postremission therapy, possibly related to declines in functional status or acquired comorbid conditions.[52] Strategies that are routinely used for younger patients, including high-dose Ara-C[53] and stem cell transplantation, are

Table 4
Selected randomized trials of induction chemotherapy for older adults with AML

Chemotherapy Regimens[a]	Age Range (y)	N	CR (%)	Median OS (mo)	P Value for OS	Induction Death Rate (%)	Comments
Intensive vs Supportive Care							
Ara-C, daunorubicin, vincristine	65–85	31	58	5.3	<.05	9.7	No difference in days hospitalized
Supportive care[32]		29	0	2.8		NA	
Type and Dose of Anthracycline							
Ara-C, daunorubicin 80 mg/m²	50–70	156	70	No difference	.16	8	Median OS 17 mo for entire study cohort
Ara-C, idarubicin 12 mg/m² × 3 d		155	83			3	
Ara-C, idarubicin 12 mg/m² × 4 d[47]		157	78			6	
Ara-C, daunorubicin 45 mg/m²[43]	60–83	411	54		.16	11	Benefits suggested among patients aged 60–65 y
Ara-C, daunorubicin 90 mg/m²		402	64			12	
Dose-attenuated Induction							
Rubidazone, Ara-C	65–83	46	52	12.8	.12	31	
Low-dose Ara-C[46]		41	32	8.8		10	
Growth Factor Support							
Ara-C, daunorubicin[45]	60–80[b]	195	54	9.4	.10	16	
Ara-C, daunorubicin + GM-CSF		193	51	9.4		20	
MDR1 Modulation							
Ara-C, daunorubicin, etoposide	60–84	61	46	No difference	.48	20	
Ara-C, daunorubicin, etoposide, +PSC-833[41]		59	39			44	
Addition of Gemtuzumab Ozogamicin							
Ara-C, daunorubicin[39]	50–70	139	75[c]	11	<.05	4	
Ara-C, daunorubicin + gemtuzumab		139	81[c]	28		6	
Daunorubicin, Ara-C, or clofarabine	51–84	556	58	Improved	.05	9	Improved 3-y survival (25% vs 20%)
Daunorubicin, Ara-C, or clofarabine + gemtuzumab[42]		559	65			8	

(continued on next page)

Table 4
(continued)

Chemotherapy Regimens[a]	Age Range (y)	N	CR (%)	Median OS (mo)	P Value for OS	Induction Death Rate (%)	Comments
Lower Intensity Therapy							
Supportive care or low-dose Ara-C	64–91	243	8	5	.2	8	Poor-risk/intermediate-risk cytogenetics only
Decitabine[50]		242	18	8		9	ECOG PS 0–2 with minimal comorbid conditions
Low-dose Ara-C ± ATRA[49]	51–90	103	18	Improved	<.05	26	No specific fitness criteria except comorbidity if <70 y old
Hydroxyurea ± ATRA		99	1			26	
Azacitidine[51]	64–91	241	20	10.4	.1	7	In adjusted analyses, survival benefit or azacitidine (*P* = .03)
Conventional care (supportive, low-dose cytarabine, intensive chemotherapy)		247	22	6.5		10	

Abbreviations: Ara-C, cytarabine; ATRA, all-*trans* retinoic acid; CR, complete remission; GM-CSF, granulocyte macrophage colony-stimulating growth factor; N, number of patients enrolled; NA, not applicable.
[a] One limitation in translating clinical trial data into best practices is the lack of consistency in patient populations recruited and in drug doses used, making comparisons of results between trials challenging.
[b] Four percent greater than or equal to 80 years old.
[c] Rates represent CR with incomplete platelet count recovery.

associated with increased toxicity among older adults. However, with RIC HSCT regimens, an increasing number of older adults who achieve remission are being referred for allogeneic transplantation in an effort to improve longer-term disease-free survival and cure rates.[54] Although feasible in selected older adults,[55] it remains unclear whether this strategy is superior to nontransplant approaches with respect to survival and QOL.

Treatment recommendations differ for patients with acute promyelocytic leukemia (APL). APL is characterized by a translocation between chromosomes 15 and 17 leading to the fusion of the promyelocytic leukemia (*PML*) gene with the retinoic acid receptor alpha (*RARα*) gene, resulting in disruption of normal cell differentiation. Although uncommon among older adults, this disease has a high response and cure rate with current therapies that include use of all-*trans* retinoic acid (ATRA), which overcomes the differentiation block. Remission and disease-free survival rates approximate 90% and thus patients with APL should be treated aggressively with ATRA and arsenic trioxide.[56]

Risk Stratification

Improving outcomes for older adults with AML requires more accurate discrimination between those older patients who are more or less likely to benefit from therapies regardless of chronologic age. There are several prognostic models developed from clinical trial or registry data that can be used to predict outcomes for older adults treated with induction chemotherapy[29,57–59] (**Table 5**). Application of these models highlights the heterogeneity of expected treatment outcomes for older adults; estimates of early mortality (16%–71%),[29] remission (12%–91%),[57] and 3-year survival (3%–40%[58]) vary widely. Each model provides useful information to help individualize treatment choices for older patients. However, these models are weighted toward characterization of tumor biology and primarily rely on chronologic age to predict treatment tolerance. Disease characteristics alone do not fully explain age-related outcome disparity in AML. Even among older adults with favorable disease biology, outcomes are worse than for younger patients.[27] Patient characteristics that are more common with aging, such as increased comorbidity, and functional and cognitive impairment complicate therapy and contribute to decreased treatment tolerance and benefit. Systematic measurement of patient-specific characteristics can help discriminate between fit, vulnerable, and frail patients for a given treatment.

In studies of older adults, comorbidity burden, typically measured with a modified Charlson Comorbidity Index (CCI) or the Hematopoietic Cell Transplantation Comorbidity Index (HCT-CI) is associated with lower remission rates, increased treatment-related mortality, and decreased survival.[60–62] For example, among 177 patients aged 60 years or older who received induction, HCT-CI score was 0 (no major comorbidity) in 22%, 1 to 2 in 30%, and greater than or equal to 3 in 48%, corresponding with early death rates (3%, 11%, and 29%, respectively) and OS (45, 31, and 19 weeks, respectively).[61] Current evidence supports pretreatment comorbidity assessment using the CCI or HCT-CI. The prognostic implications of individual comorbid conditions are not well studied.

Evidence is strong that functional status also influences treatment tolerance. In oncology practice, functional status is frequently assessed using the Eastern Cooperative Oncology Group (ECOG) Performance Score (0–4 scale, higher scores indicating impaired function) and the Karnofsky Performance Scale (scale 10%–100%, higher scores indicating better function). The relationship between ECOG PS at diagnosis, age, and 30-day mortality during intensive induction is dramatic. Data from

Table 5
Factors associated with survival among older adults receiving chemotherapy for AML

Study	Treatment	Tumor Characteristics	Clinical Variables	Patient Characteristics	Outcomes
Predictive Models Developed from Treatment Trials					
Kantarjian et al,[29] 2010 (N = 446)	Intensive	Complex karyotype	Creatinine >1.3 mg/dL	Age >80 y, ECOG PS >1	Early mortality (8 wk)
Krug et al,[57] 2010 (N = 1406)	Intensive	Secondary AML or prior hematologic disease, Molecular/cytogenetic risk	Body temperature, Hemoglobin, Platelets, LDH, Fibrinogen	Age	Early mortality (60 d), CR
Rollig et al,[58] 2010 (N = 909)	Intensive	Karyotype, NPM1 mutation, CD34 expression >10%	White cell count >20/μL, LDH >700 U/L	Age >65 y	Survival
Wheatley et al,[59] 2009 (N = 2208)	Intensive	Cytogenetic risk group, Secondary AML	White cell count	Age, ECOG PS	Survival
Predictors Derived from GA Studies					
Deschler et al,[12] 2013 (N = 107)	Nonintensive (prospective)	Bone marrow blast %, Cytogenetic risk group	—	Impaired ADLs, KPS <80, High fatigue score, HCT-CI ≥3	Survival
Klepin et al,[63] 2013 (N = 74)	Intensive (prospective)	Cytogenetic risk group, Prior MDS	Hemoglobin	Cognitive impairment (3MS <77), Impaired physical performance (SPPB <9)	Survival
Sherman et al,[66] 2013 (N = 101)	Mixed (retrospective)	Adverse cytogenetics, Secondary AML	—	HCT-CI >1, Difficulty with strenuous activity, Pain (more often vs less), ECOG PS >1	Survival

Abbreviations: 3MS, Modified Mini Mental State Examination; HCT-CI, Hematopoietic Cell Transplantation Comorbidity Index; KPS, Karnofsky Performance Scale; LDH, lactate dehydrogenase level; SPPB, Short Physical Performance Battery.
Adapted from Klepin HD, Rao AV, Pardee TS. Acute myeloid leukemia and myelodysplastic syndromes in older adults. J Clin Oncol 2014;32(24):2541–52.

older adults enrolled on induction trials showed similar 30-day mortality (11%–15%) for patients aged 56 to 65 years, 66 to 75 years, and greater than 75 years with excellent PS (ECOG 0), contrasted with rates of 29%, 47%, and 82%, respectively, for poor baseline PS (ECOG 3).[27] Fit older adults, even those greater than 75 years old, may tolerate induction chemotherapy similarly to those in middle age but the negative prognostic implications of poor PS increase with chronologic age. Although ECOG PS is useful in identifying frail patients (ECOG>2), it is an insensitive and subjective measure of physical function. Further refinement is needed to identify vulnerable older adults. Studies have shown that assessment of self-reported ADL and objectively measured physical performance (testing consisted of walking speed, chair stands, and balance) are predictive of survival after accounting for PS.[12,63,64]

Pretreatment assessment of older adults needs to take into account the complexity of variables that may differ from patient to patient. GA is an approach to measure the complexity of patient characteristics present in older populations. Pretreatment GA is feasible in the context of AML and suggests that chronologic age may not be a robust predictor of outcome after accounting for function, comorbidity, and symptoms (see **Table 5**).[12,65] In a prospective study of adults 60 years of age or older treated intensively, pretreatment GA detected significant impairments even among those with good oncology PS (ECOG 0–1): cognitive impairment, 24%; depression, 26%; distress, 50%; ADL impairment, 34%; impaired physical performance, 31%; and comorbidity, 40%.[65] Importantly, most patients (63%) were impaired in more than 1 measured characteristic. Overall, studies using a GA approach have identified impaired cognition, impaired physical performance, ADL impairment, and symptoms (eg, fatigue, pain) as independent predictors of worse survival.[12,63,66] The utility of GA is currently under investigation in multisite trials.

Treatment recommendations for older adults with AML should be individualized based on tumor biology and patient characteristics. Although validation is needed, available evidence can inform practical strategies to differentiate fit, vulnerable, and frail patients when considering therapy (**Table 6**). In general, patients categorized as frail are at high risk for treatment toxicity; risks may outweigh benefits. Clinical trials are needed to test novel therapies in this subgroup. Fit patients are most likely to benefit from curative therapy and strong consideration should be given to offering standard therapies similar to those used for middle-aged patients. For fit patients, older age is associated with similar QOL and physical function to younger age during and after intensive induction therapy.[67,68] Optimal therapy for the large proportion of older adults who are between these two extremes is unclear. In practice, consideration should be given to enhanced supportive care for vulnerable patients by targeting modifiable risk factors (ie, early physical therapy for patients with impaired physical performance).

Unanswered Questions for Older Adults with Acute Myeloid Leukemia

There are many unanswered questions regarding best practices for older adults with AML. Many questions concern improved characterization of fitness to optimally predict treatment tolerance in a given setting. The interactions between patient characteristics and tumor biology require further study. Ideally, trials targeting biologically defined subtypes of AML within the context of defined patient subgroups (fit, vulnerable, frail) are needed. In addition, patient-centered outcomes capturing QOL, symptoms, functional independence, patient preference, and health care use are needed to fully inform treatment decisions.

Table 6
Considerations for risk stratification and treatments for older adults with AML

Patient Risk Category	Characteristics	Treatment Considerations (Clinical Trials Preferred)
Frail	Poor oncology PS (ECOG PS score ≥3) Major comorbidity (ie, HCT-CI >2) Impairment in ADLs	High treatment-related mortality (particularly for adults >75 y old) Favorable tumor biology[a]: consider lower intensity therapy (HMAs, low-dose Ara-C). Patients with poor PS (particularly aged 60–75 y) but without end-stage comorbidity may consider intensive treatment if risks/benefits are consistent with goals of care Intermediate/unfavorable: consider best supportive care, including palliative care consultation if available vs lower intensity therapy (HMAs, low-dose Ara-C) Clinical trials targeting frail patients are needed; randomized evidence is lacking
Vulnerable	ECOG PS score 0–2 Absence of major comorbidity (HCT-CI ≤2) Presence of: Impairment in IADLs/self-reported mobility Impaired physical performance (SPPB <9) Impaired cognition (3MS score <77) High symptom burden (fatigue, pain)	Outcomes for this subgroup are poorly defined in clinical trials because of lack of characterization. In nonrandomized studies this group is at risk for shorter survival compared with fit patients Favorable tumor biology: consider intensive therapy Intermediate/unfavorable: consider intensive therapy if risks and benefits are consistent with goals of care vs lower intensity therapies (HMAs, low-dose Ara-C) Consider enhanced supportive care targeting vulnerabilities such as early physical therapy for impaired mobility Clinical trials are needed to validate definitions of vulnerability and to test treatment and supportive care strategies to improve outcomes in this group
Fit	ECOG PS score 0–1 Minimal comorbidity (ie, HCT-CI <1) Absence of any risk factors mentioned earlier	Best evidence suggests fit older adults derive benefit from aggressive therapy Favorable tumor biology: intensive therapy should be offered Intermediate/unfavorable: consider intensive treatment with possible RIC allogeneic HSCT if risks/benefits consistent with goals of care vs lower intensity therapies (HMAs, low-dose Ara-C) Future clinical trials should compare investigational therapies with standard intensive treatment among fit older adults

Abbreviations: Ara-C, cytarabine; HMA, hypomethylating agent; IADLs, instrumental ADL; TRM, treatment-related mortality.

[a] Favorable tumor biology: inv(16), t(16;16), t(8;21), t(15;17). Intermediate risk: normal cytogenetics, +8 alone, t(9;11), other nondefined. Unfavorable: complex (≥3 clonal abnormalities), −5, 5q−, −7, 7q−, abnormalities of 11q, inv(3), t(3;3), t(6;9). In the normal cytogenetic category, NPM1 mutation in the absence of FLT3-ITD or isolated biallelic CEBPA mutation confers better risk than the presence of FLT3-ITD, which confers worse risk.

Adapted from Klepin HD, Rao AV, Pardee TS. Acute myeloid leukemia and myelodysplastic syndromes in older adults. J Clin Oncol 2014;32(24):2541–52.

SUMMARY

MDS and AML are heterogeneous diseases affecting older adults. Significant advances are being made in understanding the complexity of both tumor biology and the patient characteristics that influence outcomes. Optimal treatment decision making requires a frank discussion regarding risks and benefits of therapy interpreted in the context of individualized assessment and each patient's values and goals of care.

REFERENCES

1. Efficace F, Gaidano G, Breccia M, et al. Prevalence, severity and correlates of fatigue in newly diagnosed patients with myelodysplastic syndromes. Br J Haematol 2015;168:361–70.
2. Rollison DE, Howlader N, Smith MT, et al. Epidemiology of myelodysplastic syndromes and chronic myeloproliferative disorders in the United States, 2001-2004, using data from the NAACCR and SEER programs. Blood 2008;112:45–52.
3. SEER cancer statistics review 1975-2009. 2012. Available at: www.seer.cancer.gov. Accessed July 21, 2015.
4. Greenberg P, Cox C, LeBeau MM, et al. International scoring system for evaluating prognosis in myelodysplastic syndromes. Blood 1997;89:2079–88.
5. Greenberg PL, Tuechler H, Schanz J, et al. Revised International Prognostic Scoring System for myelodysplastic syndromes. Blood 2012;120:2454–65.
6. Voso MT, Fenu S, Latagliata R, et al. Revised International Prognostic Scoring System (IPSS) predicts survival and leukemic evolution of myelodysplastic syndromes significantly better than IPSS and WHO Prognostic Scoring System: validation by the Gruppo Romano Mielodisplasie Italian Regional Database. J Clin Oncol 2013; 31:2671–7.
7. Della Porta MG, Malcovati L, Strupp C, et al. Risk stratification based on both disease status and extra-hematologic comorbidities in patients with myelodysplastic syndrome. Haematologica 2011;96:441–9.
8. Daver N, Naqvi K, Jabbour E, et al. Impact of comorbidities by ACE-27 in the revised-IPSS for patients with myelodysplastic syndromes. Am J Hematol 2014; 89:509–16.
9. Naqvi K, Garcia-Manero G, Sardesai S, et al. Association of comorbidities with overall survival in myelodysplastic syndrome: development of a prognostic model. J Clin Oncol 2011;29:2240–6.
10. Balleari E, Salvetti C, Del Corso L, et al. Age and comorbidities deeply impact on clinical outcome of patients with myelodysplastic syndromes. Leuk Res 2015; 39(8):846–52.
11. Fega KR, Abel GA, Motyckova G, et al. Non-hematologic predictors of mortality improve the prognostic value of the international prognostic scoring system for MDS in older adults. J Geriatr Oncol 2015;6(4):288–98.
12. Deschler B, Ihorst G, Platzbecker U, et al. Parameters detected by geriatric and quality of life assessment in 195 older patients with myelodysplastic syndromes and acute myeloid leukemia are highly predictive for outcome. Haematologica 2013;98:208–16.
13. Jadersten M, Malcovati L, Dybedal I, et al. Erythropoietin and granulocyte-colony stimulating factor treatment associated with improved survival in myelodysplastic syndrome. J Clin Oncol 2008;26:3607–13.
14. Moyo V, Lefebvre P, Duh MS, et al. Erythropoiesis-stimulating agents in the treatment of anemia in myelodysplastic syndromes: a meta-analysis. Ann Hematol 2008;87:527–36.

15. Fenaux P, Mufti GJ, Hellstrom-Lindberg E, et al. Efficacy of azacitidine compared with that of conventional care regimens in the treatment of higher-risk myelodysplastic syndromes: a randomised, open-label, phase III study. Lancet Oncol 2009;10:223–32.

16. Silverman LR, Demakos EP, Peterson BL, et al. Randomized controlled trial of azacitidine in patients with the myelodysplastic syndrome: a study of the cancer and leukemia group B. J Clin Oncol 2002;20:2429–40.

17. Kornblith AB, Herndon JE, Silverman LR, et al. Impact of azacytidine on the quality of life of patients with myelodysplastic syndrome treated in a randomized phase III trial: a Cancer and Leukemia Group B study. J Clin Oncol 2002;20: 2441–52.

18. Fenaux P, Mufti GJ, Hellstrom-Lindberg E, et al. Azacitidine prolongs overall survival compared with conventional care regimens in elderly patients with low bone marrow blast count acute myeloid leukemia. J Clin Oncol 2010;28: 562–9.

19. Xicoy B, Jimenez MJ, Garcia O, et al. Results of treatment with azacitidine in patients aged $\geq$ 75 years included in the Spanish Registry of Myelodysplastic Syndromes. Leuk Lymphoma 2014;55:1300–3.

20. Kantarjian H, Issa JP, Rosenfeld CS, et al. Decitabine improves patient outcomes in myelodysplastic syndromes: results of a phase III randomized study. Cancer 2006;106:1794–803.

21. Fenaux P, Giagounidis A, Selleslag D, et al. A randomized phase 3 study of lenalidomide versus placebo in RBC transfusion-dependent patients with Low-/Intermediate-1-risk myelodysplastic syndromes with del5q. Blood 2011; 118:3765–76.

22. List A, Dewald G, Bennett J, et al. Lenalidomide in the myelodysplastic syndrome with chromosome 5q deletion. N Engl J Med 2006;355:1456–65.

23. Sibon D, Cannas G, Baracco F, et al. Lenalidomide in lower-risk myelodysplastic syndromes with karyotypes other than deletion 5q and refractory to erythropoiesis-stimulating agents. Br J Haematol 2012;156:619–25.

24. Koreth J, Pidala J, Perez WS, et al. Role of reduced-intensity conditioning allogeneic hematopoietic stem-cell transplantation in older patients with de novo myelodysplastic syndromes: an international collaborative decision analysis. J Clin Oncol 2013;31:2662–70.

25. Muffly LS, Kocherginsky M, Stock W, et al. Geriatric assessment to predict survival in older allogeneic hematopoietic cell transplantation recipients. Haematologica 2014;99(8):1373–9.

26. American Cancer Society. 2009. Available at: http://www.cancer.org/docroot/ home/index.asp. Accessed July 21, 2015.

27. Appelbaum FR, Gundacker H, Head DR, et al. Age and acute myeloid leukemia. Blood 2006;107:3481–5.

28. Juliusson G. Most 70- to 79-year-old patients with acute myeloid leukemia do benefit from intensive treatment. Blood 2011;117:3473–4.

29. Kantarjian H, Ravandi F, O'Brien S, et al. Intensive chemotherapy does not benefit most older patients (age 70 years or older) with acute myeloid leukemia. Blood 2010;116:4422–9.

30. Oran B, Weisdorf DJ. Survival for older patients with acute myeloid leukemia: a population-based study. Haematologica 2012;97:1916–24.

31. Juliusson G, Antunovic P, Derolf A, et al. Age and acute myeloid leukemia: real world data on decision to treat and outcomes from the Swedish Acute Leukemia Registry. Blood 2009;113:4179–87.

32. Lowenberg B, Zittoun R, Kerkhofs H, et al. On the value of intensive remission-induction chemotherapy in elderly patients of 65+ years with acute myeloid leukemia: a randomized phase III study of the European Organization for Research and Treatment of Cancer Leukemia Group. J Clin Oncol 1989;7:1268–74.
33. Wetzler M, Mrozek K, Kohlschmidt J, et al. Intensive induction is effective in selected octogenarian acute myeloid leukemia patients: prognostic significance of karyotype and selected molecular markers used in the European LeukemiaNet classification. Haematologica 2014;99:308–13.
34. Farag SS, Archer KJ, Mrozek K, et al. Pretreatment cytogenetics add to other prognostic factors predicting complete remission and long-term outcome in patients 60 years of age or older with acute myeloid leukemia: results from Cancer and Leukemia Group B 8461. Blood 2006;108:63–73.
35. Grimwade D, Walker H, Harrison G, et al. The predictive value of hierarchical cytogenetic classification in older adults with acute myeloid leukemia (AML): analysis of 1065 patients entered into the United Kingdom Medical Research Council AML11 trial. Blood 2001;98:1312–20.
36. Rao AV, Valk PJ, Metzeler KH, et al. Age-specific differences in oncogenic pathway dysregulation and anthracycline sensitivity in patients with acute myeloid leukemia. J Clin Oncol 2009;27:5580–6.
37. Scholl S, Theuer C, Scheble V, et al. Clinical impact of nucleophosmin mutations and Flt3 internal tandem duplications in patients older than 60 yr with acute myeloid leukaemia. Eur J Haematol 2008;80:208–15.
38. Leith CP, Kopecky KJ, Godwin J, et al. Acute myeloid leukemia in the elderly: assessment of multidrug resistance (MDR1) and cytogenetics distinguishes biologic subgroups with remarkably distinct responses to standard chemotherapy. A Southwest Oncology Group study. Blood 1997;89:3323–9.
39. Castaigne S, Pautas C, Terre C, et al. Effect of gemtuzumab ozogamicin on survival of adult patients with de-novo acute myeloid leukaemia (ALFA-0701): a randomised, open-label, phase 3 study. Lancet 2012;379:1508–16.
40. Kantarjian H, O'Brien S, Cortes J, et al. Results of intensive chemotherapy in 998 patients age 65 years or older with acute myeloid leukemia or high-risk myelodysplastic syndrome: predictive prognostic models for outcome. Cancer 2006;106:1090–8.
41. Baer MR, George SL, Dodge RK, et al. Phase 3 study of the multidrug resistance modulator PSC-833 in previously untreated patients 60 years of age and older with acute myeloid leukemia: Cancer and Leukemia Group B Study 9720. Blood 2002;100:1224–32.
42. Burnett AK, Russell NH, Hills RK, et al. Addition of gemtuzumab ozogamicin to induction chemotherapy improves survival in older patients with acute myeloid leukemia. J Clin Oncol 2012;30:3924–31.
43. Lowenberg B, Ossenkoppele GJ, van Putten W, et al. High-dose daunorubicin in older patients with acute myeloid leukemia. N Engl J Med 2009;361:1235–48.
44. Lowenberg B, Suciu S, Archimbaud E, et al. Mitoxantrone versus daunorubicin in induction-consolidation chemotherapy–the value of low-dose cytarabine for maintenance of remission, and an assessment of prognostic factors in acute myeloid leukemia in the elderly: final report. European Organization for the Research and Treatment of Cancer and the Dutch-Belgian Hemato-Oncology Cooperative Hovon Group. J Clin Oncol 1998;16:872–81.
45. Stone RM, Berg DT, George SL, et al. Granulocyte-macrophage colony-stimulating factor after initial chemotherapy for elderly patients with primary acute myelogenous leukemia. Cancer and Leukemia Group B. N Engl J Med 1995;332:1671–7.

46. Tilly H, Castaigne S, Bordessoule D, et al. Low-dose cytarabine versus intensive chemotherapy in the treatment of acute nonlymphocytic leukemia in the elderly. J Clin Oncol 1990;8:272–9.

47. Pautas C, Merabet F, Thomas X, et al. Randomized study of intensified anthracycline doses for induction and recombinant interleukin-2 for maintenance in patients with acute myeloid leukemia age 50 to 70 years: results of the ALFA-9801 study. J Clin Oncol 2010;28:808–14.

48. Serve H, Krug U, Wagner R, et al. Sorafenib in combination with intensive chemotherapy in elderly patients with acute myeloid leukemia: results from a randomized, placebo-controlled trial. J Clin Oncol 2013;31:3110–8.

49. Burnett AK, Milligan D, Prentice AG, et al. A comparison of low-dose cytarabine and hydroxyurea with or without all-trans retinoic acid for acute myeloid leukemia and high-risk myelodysplastic syndrome in patients not considered fit for intensive treatment. Cancer 2007;109:1114–24.

50. Kantarjian HM, Thomas XG, Dmoszynska A, et al. Multicenter, randomized, open-label, phase III trial of decitabine versus patient choice, with physician advice, of either supportive care or low-dose cytarabine for the treatment of older patients with newly diagnosed acute myeloid leukemia. J Clin Oncol 2012;30:2670–7.

51. Dombret H, Seymour JF, Butrym A, et al. International phase 3 study of azacitidine vs conventional care regimens in older patients with newly diagnosed AML with >30% blasts. Blood 2015;126:291–9.

52. Stone RM, Berg DT, George SL, et al. Postremission therapy in older patients with de novo acute myeloid leukemia: a randomized trial comparing mitoxantrone and intermediate-dose cytarabine with standard-dose cytarabine. Blood 2001;98:548–53.

53. Mayer RJ, Davis RB, Schiffer CA, et al. Intensive postremission chemotherapy in adults with acute myeloid leukemia. Cancer and Leukemia Group B. N Engl J Med 1994;331:896–903.

54. Hahn T, McCarthy PL Jr, Hassebroek A, et al. Significant improvement in survival after allogeneic hematopoietic cell transplantation during a period of significantly increased use, older recipient age, and use of unrelated donors. J Clin Oncol 2013;31:2437–49.

55. McClune BL, Weisdorf DJ, Pedersen TL, et al. Effect of age on outcome of reduced-intensity hematopoietic cell transplantation for older patients with acute myeloid leukemia in first complete remission or with myelodysplastic syndrome. J Clin Oncol 2010;28:1878–87.

56. Lo-Coco F, Avvisati G, Vignetti M, et al. Retinoic acid and arsenic trioxide for acute promyelocytic leukemia. N Engl J Med 2013;369:111–21.

57. Krug U, Rollig C, Koschmieder A, et al. Complete remission and early death after intensive chemotherapy in patients aged 60 years or older with acute myeloid leukaemia: a web-based application for prediction of outcomes. Lancet 2010;376:2000–8.

58. Rollig C, Thiede C, Gramatzki M, et al. A novel prognostic model in elderly patients with acute myeloid leukemia: results of 909 patients entered into the prospective AML96 trial. Blood 2010;116:971–8.

59. Wheatley K, Brookes CL, Howman AJ, et al. Prognostic factor analysis of the survival of elderly patients with AML in the MRC AML11 and LRF AML14 trials. Br J Haematol 2009;145:598–605.

60. Etienne A, Esterni B, Charbonnier A, et al. Comorbidity is an independent predictor of complete remission in elderly patients receiving induction chemotherapy for acute myeloid leukemia. Cancer 2007;109:1376–83.

61. Giles FJ, Borthakur G, Ravandi F, et al. The haematopoietic cell transplantation comorbidity index score is predictive of early death and survival in patients over 60 years of age receiving induction therapy for acute myeloid leukaemia. Br J Haematol 2007;136:624–7.
62. Malfuson JV, Etienne A, Turlure P, et al. Risk factors and decision criteria for intensive chemotherapy in older patients with acute myeloid leukemia. Haematologica 2008;93:1806–13.
63. Klepin HD, Geiger AM, Tooze JA, et al. Geriatric assessment predicts survival for older adults receiving induction chemotherapy for acute myelogenous leukemia. Blood 2013;121:4287–94.
64. Wedding U, Rohrig B, Klippstein A, et al. Impairment in functional status and survival in patients with acute myeloid leukaemia. J Cancer Res Clin Oncol 2006; 132:665–71.
65. Klepin HD, Geiger AM, Tooze JA, et al. The feasibility of inpatient geriatric assessment for older adults receiving induction chemotherapy for acute myelogenous leukemia. J Am Geriatr Soc 2011;59:1837–46.
66. Sherman AE, Motyckova G, Fega KR, et al. Geriatric assessment in older patients with acute myeloid leukemia: a retrospective study of associated treatment and outcomes. Leuk Res 2013;37:998–1003.
67. Alibhai SM, Breunis H, Timilshina N, et al. Quality of life and physical function in adults treated with intensive chemotherapy for acute myeloid leukemia improve over time independent of age. J Geriatr Oncol 2015;6(4):262–71.
68. Mohamedali H, Breunis H, Timilshina N, et al. Older age is associated with similar quality of life and physical function compared to younger age during intensive chemotherapy for acute myeloid leukemia. Leuk Res 2012;36:1241–8.

Chronic Lymphocytic Leukemia and Other Lymphoproliferative Disorders

Sarah Wall, MD, Jennifer A. Woyach, MD*

KEYWORDS

- Chronic lymphocytic leukemia • Non-Hodgkin lymphoma • Elderly

KEY POINTS

- Chronic lymphocytic leukemia and other non-Hodgkin lymphomas primarily affect older patients.
- When making treatment decisions for older patients, it is important to consider not only chronologic age but also fitness level and comorbid conditions.
- Clinical trials that recruit and enroll older and/or less fit patients will improve the treatment options available to this important and growing population.
- Therapies targeting the B-cell receptor signaling pathway are changing the treatment paradigms of many B-cell lymphoproliferative disorders.

CHRONIC LYMPHOCYTIC LEUKEMIA
Epidemiology

Chronic lymphocytic leukemia (CLL) is a disease mainly of the elderly, with a median age at diagnosis of 71 years. Although it accounts for less than 1% of all new cancers diagnosed each year, the prevalence has grown because of improvements in therapy and overall survival, and at this time it is the most common adult leukemia. In 2007, the 5-year overall survival had increased to 87.9% from 69% in 1980, and, with the advent of newer targeted therapies, survival is likely even better for patients diagnosed with CLL in 2015. CLL is more common in men than in women by approximately 2:1, more common in white people than in African Americans, and far less common in any other race.[1]

CLL is a chronic and incurable disease outside of allogeneic stem cell transplantation (AlloSCT). Because of the high treatment-related morbidity and mortality of

Disclosures: The authors have no disclosures related to this work.
Division of Hematology, Department of Internal Medicine, The Ohio State University Comprehensive Cancer Center, 445A Wiseman Hall, 410 West 12th Avenue, Columbus, OH 43210, USA
* Corresponding author.
E-mail address: Jennifer.Woyach@osumc.edu

Clin Geriatr Med 32 (2016) 175–189
http://dx.doi.org/10.1016/j.cger.2015.08.006
0749-0690/16/$ – see front matter © 2016 Elsevier Inc. All rights reserved.

geriatric.theclinics.com

AlloSCT, especially in older patients, this is rarely an option for most patients with CLL. Despite the chronicity of disease and indolent nature experienced by many, patients with CLL have a shorter survival than age-matched controls. Importantly, although many patients with CLL have impaired organ function and reduced performance status, these patients are treated at the same frequency as those with adequate organ function and intact performance status, but they have a shorter overall survival.[2] Thus, management strategies focused on older adults and those with impaired organ function and performance status are needed.

Spectrum of Disease and Prognosis

CLL presents as a spectrum of disease that encompasses monoclonal B lymphocytosis (MBL), small lymphocytic lymphoma (SLL), and the more common CLL. CLL is often found incidentally by the presence of lymphocytosis on routine blood work, with most patients asymptomatic at diagnosis. Unexplained lymphocytosis on a complete blood count differential should prompt peripheral blood immunophenotyping to differentiate a reactive lymphocytosis from one that is malignancy associated. The diagnosis of CLL is established by detecting a clonal population of B cells in the peripheral blood and does not require bone marrow biopsy. On immunophenotyping, this B-cell population typically expresses the surface markers CD5, CD19, CD20(dim), and CD23, with dim expression of surface kappa or lambda immunoglobulin.[3] Patients with greater than 5000 of these monoclonal cells per microliter are classified as having CLL. Those with less than this threshold but with enlarged lymph nodes or spleen are classified as having SLL, and those with less than this threshold and no other signs of disease are best categorized as having MBL. SLL and CLL are managed identically, and are referred to as CLL throughout this article.

Recent studies suggest that approximately 4% of the general population more than 40 years of age harbor a population of clonal B cells with the phenotype of either CLL or another low-grade non-Hodgkin lymphoma (NHL).[4] Three subcategories of MBL have been identified according to the immunophenotypic features: CLL-like, CD5+ atypical, and CD5− MBL. CLL-like MBL is the most frequent and best studied and can be further divided into low-count (LC) and high-count (HC) MBL, based on a cutoff value of 500/μL clonal B cells. LC-MBL typically remains stable and likely represents an age-related immune senescence rather than a premalignant state. HC-MBL is associated with an annual risk of progression requiring therapy at a rate of 1.1%.[5] Patients with MBL share a similar risk of infection and development of nonhematologic cancer to those patients with CLL, highlighting the similarity in disease biology and need for aggressive surveillance.[6,7]

CLL follows a very heterogeneous course, ranging from indolent disease that never requires therapy to short time to initial therapy and an aggressive disease course with multiple relapses. Because of this heterogeneity, prognostic factors are of great importance in counseling newly diagnosed patients. The earliest prognostic tools were the 2 widely used staging schema described by Binet and colleagues[8] and Rai and colleagues[9] (Table 1). Increasing stage is related to shortened survival; however, the exact survival statistics have improved since the development of the staging systems.

In addition to clinical staging, cytogenetic and molecular markers can add to prognostication. All newly diagnosed patients with CLL should undergo fluorescence in situ hybridization (FISH) testing for common CLL abnormalities as well as stimulated cytogenetics to determine whether the karyotype is complex (≥3 cytogenetic abnormalities). Complex karyotype is associated with an aggressive disease course, and specific cytogenetic abnormalities on FISH are also strong predictors of disease

Table 1	
Rai and Binet staging systems in CLL	
Rai 0: Lymphocytosis alone	Binet A: <3 groups of enlarged lymph nodes
Rai I: Stage 0 with enlarged lymph nodes	Binet B: ≥3 groups of enlarged lymph nodes
Rai II: Stage 0–I with palpable organomegaly	Binet C: Hemoglobin <10 g/dL and/or platelets
Rai III: Stage 0–II with hemoglobin <11 g/dL	counts <100 × 10³/μL
Rai IV: Stage 0–III with platelet counts <100 × 10³/μL	

Adapted from Binet JL, Auquier A, Dighiero G, et al. A new prognostic classification of chronic lymphocytic leukemia derived from a multivariate survival analysis. Cancer 1981;48:198–206; and Rai KR, Sawitsky A, Cronkite EP, et al. Clinical staging of chronic lymphocytic leukemia. Blood 1975;46:219–34.

biology.[10,11] The presence of *del13q* imparts favorable prognosis, trisomy 12 confers standard or intermediate risk, and *del11q* and *del17p* are associated with poor prognosis.[12,13] Karyotypes can change over time and become more complex, known as clonal evolution, and specific cytogenetic abnormalities can be acquired, especially after cytotoxic chemotherapy, so reassessment of cytogenetics and FISH at the time of each treatment is recommended. Another strong predictor of disease course is the degree of somatic hypermutation of immunoglobulin heavy chain variable region gene (IGHV), which does not change over time. Somatic hypermutation (>2% difference from germline) indicates a postgerminal center–derived cell, and is associated with a much more indolent course than unmutated CLL cells. Patients with mutated CLL are less likely to require therapy, respond better to most standard therapies, and have prolonged survival compared with those with unmutated IGHV.[14,15] Zap70 expression, CD38 expression, and TP53 sequencing can be helpful in some circumstances but are not always required.

Monitoring and Therapy

At diagnosis, patients with CLL should be followed every 3 months with complete history, physical examination, and complete blood count with differential. There is no role for routine computed tomography (CT) scanning in asymptomatic patients. If the disease follows an indolent course through the first few visits, then assessments can be spread out to every 6 months.[16] Patients with CLL are at increased risk of infection[17] and nonhematologic cancers[18] and so should be monitored for these regardless of disease status. Patients should receive pneumococcal vaccination every 5 years and influenza vaccination annually. Zoster vaccine and other live vaccines should be avoided in patients with CLL because of risk of disseminated infection.[3] Patients should be encouraged to stay up to date on their age-appropriate cancer screening tests, including at least annual skin examinations, but there is no indication for more stringent screening based on the presence of CLL alone. There is also an increased incidence of autoimmune hemolytic anemia and immune thrombocytopenia in patients with CLL. In the event of an acute or disproportionate reduction in hemoglobin or platelet levels, these diagnoses should be considered and appropriate work-up undertaken.[19] Another potential complication of CLL is transformation of CLL to a more aggressive lymphoma, either Richter or prolymphocytic transformation.[20] This transformation should be suspected if a patient presents with rapidly progressive B symptoms or node enlargement. Work-up should include a PET scan to help direct biopsy to the most fluorodeoxyglucose (FDG)-avid area.

At present, CLL is managed expectantly, with therapy deferred until the onset of symptoms. The role for early treatment has been explored with no significant difference in overall survival found between early and deferred treatment with intensive chemoimmunotherapy (fludarabine/cyclophosphamide/ rituximab) in high-risk patients. There was a significant benefit in event-free survival (EFS) in the early treatment group but at the cost of significant toxicity (73.2% with grade 3 or 4 hematologic toxicity, 19.5% with grade 3 or 4 infections, and 3.7% with fatal infectious complications).[21] Indications for treatment at this time include progressive marrow failure manifested by anemia and/or thrombocytopenia, massive organomegaly or nodes that are symptomatic, autoimmune anemia or thrombocytopenia poorly responsive to standard treatment, or the presence of moderate to severe B symptoms (weight loss, fatigue, fever, night sweats). Lymphocyte doubling time and absolute lymphocyte count are parameters that are often monitored but neither of them alone is an indication for treatment.[3,22]

When an indication for treatment is present in an elderly patient, the patient's fitness level should be assessed. There are a variety of tools available to assess patient fitness and the impact of comorbid illnesses, but at this time there are no formal guidelines as to which should be used in individual patients. Ideally, fitness assessment should involve multiple tools to assess various domains. Karnofsky[23] and Eastern Cooperative Oncology Group (ECOG)[24] performance statuses are widely used methods to evaluate patient activity level. A measure of comorbidity such as the Cumulative Illness Rating Score[25] can be helpful in assessing baseline comorbidities as well as helping to predict treatment-related toxicity for specific agents. In addition, functional status assessments such as the Timed Up and Go test can be extremely useful to quickly and objectively assess function.[26] A comprehensive geriatric assessment (CGA) consists of evaluation of functional status, comorbid medical conditions, cognition, psychological state, social support, nutritional status, and a review of the patient's medications. This assessment would be the gold standard for fitness assessment; however, the CGA is often impractical because of time constraints, and may be best used in patients in whom shorter screening tests indicate functional deficits.[27]

Using these tools, patients can be stratified into 3 distinct groups: Go-Go, Slow-Go, and No-Go. The Go-Go group is made up of fit patients with few to no comorbidities and normal life expectancy. Patients in the Go-Go group should be treated with aggressive chemoimmunotherapy and ideally on a clinical trial. It should be noted that this treatment recommendation is made regardless of chronologic age, although it is unlikely that many elderly patients are in this category. The Slow-Go group consists of less medically fit patients with multiple or severe comorbidities and unknown life expectancy. Treatment should be offered on clinical trial whenever possible, and, outside of clinical trial, careful consideration for potential toxicities of treatment is important. In addition, the No-Go group consists of medically frail patients with fatal comorbidities and very short life expectancy, and these patients are unlikely to tolerate or benefit from CLL-directed therapy. Hospice referral should be considered.[28]

For Go-Go patients younger than 65 years, 2 pivotal studies have established fludarabine, cyclophosphamide, and rituximab (FCR) as the standard initial therapy.[29,30] In patients older than 65 years, there does not seem to be a difference in efficacy between FCR and the less toxic bendamustine plus rituximab (BR) regimen, so BR should be considered as one standard for this age group. Clinical trials should be considered for all patients.

Slow-Go patients tolerate intensive chemoimmunotherapy with FCR or BR poorly. A better tolerated therapy is chlorambucil, either alone or in combination with monoclonal CD20 antibody, such as obinutuzumab, ofatumumab, or rituximab. The noninferiority of chlorambucil compared with fludarabine in older patients has been shown in both the prospective German CLL5 study[31] and a retrospective analysis of frontline

US Cancer and Leukemia Group B (CALGB) studies.[32] In the CLL5 trial, patients more than 65 years of age were randomized to receive either fludarabine or chlorambucil monotherapy. There was no difference in overall survival (OS) between groups, although a trend toward prolonged OS in the chlorambucil group was noted (64 vs 46 months). The CALGB data reinforced that fludarabine was not superior to chlorambucil in the subgroup of patients older than 70 years, but showed that the addition of rituximab prolonged survival in all patients, regardless of age.

There have been 2 phase III trials investigating chlorambucil in combination with CD20 antibodies, primarily in older patients with significant comorbidities. The German CLL11 study compared single-agent chlorambucil with rituximab-chlorambucil and obinutuzumab-chlorambucil and showed a survival advantage to both obinutuzumab-chlorambucil and rituximab-chlorambucil compared with chlorambucil alone.[33,34] Follow-up is ongoing, with the most recent assessment showing a significant benefit in OS with obinutuzumab-chlorambucil versus chlorambucil monotherapy (hazard ratio [HR], 0.47; 95% confidence interval [CI], 0.29–0.76; $P = .0014$) as well as rituximab-chlorambucil versus chlorambucil (HR, 0.60; 95% CI, 0.38–0.94; $P = .0242$). Progression-free survival (PFS) with obinutuzumab-chlorambucil is significantly longer than with rituximab-chlorambucil, but at this time there is no survival advantage.

The COMPLEMENT1 study compared single-agent chlorambucil with ofatumumab-chlorambucil. The ofatumumab-chlorambucil group experienced prolonged PFS compared with the chlorambucil monotherapy group (22.4 vs 13.1 months; HR, 0.57; 95% CI, 0.45–0.72; $P<.0001$). With a median follow-up time of 28.9 months, median OS was not reached in either treatment group and no survival advantage has been shown (3-year survival 85% chlorambucil plus ofatumumab vs 83% chlorambucil alone).[35]

For relapsed or refractory disease, there are many options, so this article is limited to the 2 US Food and Drug Administration (FDA)–approved small molecule kinase inhibitors that have changed the standard of care for patients with relapsed disease. These agents, which target the B-cell receptor (BCR) signaling pathway, are excellent options, especially for older patients. By virtue of specificity for their target, these therapies avoid many of the cytotoxic effects of traditional chemotherapy. Another ideal feature of new targeted therapies is that many are administered orally, limiting the need for frequent clinic visits and infusions, which can be important in an older population that may have limited means to travel to clinic frequently. The first-in-class Bruton tyrosine kinase inhibitor, ibrutinib, is a targeted agent that is administered orally. It has garnered FDA approval for treatment of relapsed/refractory CLL or frontline treatment of patients with del17p. This approval in large part resulted from the phase III RESONATE trial comparing ibrutinib with ofatumumab monotherapy, which showed an OS benefit for ibrutinib with short follow-up.[36] Longer follow-up data come from a phase Ib/II trial, which was recently updated to reflect the first 3 years of follow-up. Estimated 30-month PFS for patients with relapsed disease was 69% (95% CI, 58–78%). This trial also included a group of 31 patients who were all age 65 or older and previously untreated, and in this group, estimated 30-month PFS was 96% (95% CI, 76.5–99.5%). In the same group, the most commonly experienced grade 3 toxicities were diarrhea (16%) and hypertension (23%).[37]

Another drug active in BCR signaling inhibition is idelalisib, a first-in-class phosphatidylinositol 3 kinase (PI3K) delta inhibitor. Idelalisib was FDA approved in 2014 for use in combination with rituximab for relapsed/refractory CLL. This approval was largely based on a phase III trial comparing idelalisib-rituximab with placebo-rituximab. All responses were partial but overall response rate (ORR) was 81% in the idelalisib group compared with 13% in the placebo group (odds ratio, 29.92; P<.001). The 12-month OS in the idelalisib group was superior to that in the placebo group (92% vs 80% respectively).[38]

The outcomes thus far with the oral kinase inhibitors have been outstanding. Current research is focusing on moving these agents, especially ibrutinib, to the frontline setting and determining the best combination strategies for these therapies. However, we expect that these drugs, and those like them currently in clinical development, will continue to improve outcomes for patients with CLL.

OTHER COMMON NON-HODGKIN LYMPHOMAS
Epidemiology

NHLs are a heterogeneous group of diseases ranging from indolent to very aggressive. NHL is the seventh most common cancer in the United States by incidence, with an estimated 71,850 new cases predicted in 2015, and they are the fifth leading cause of cancer death in the United States in 2015. The median age at diagnosis is 66 years.[39] Approximately 85% of NHLs are of B-cell origin, with the remainder mostly T-cell origin. Diffuse large B-cell lymphoma (DLBCL) is the most common NHL, making up 31% of new NHL cases, followed by follicular lymphoma (FL), an indolent B-cell lymphoma that accounts for 22% of NHLs.

DLBCL is a disease of the elderly, with a median age at diagnosis of 70 years and an incidence that increases with increasing age.[40] In a recent French population study, the 5-year net survival decreased significantly in men older than 75 years (45% for those aged 65–74 years vs 23% for those older than 75 years).[41] The immunoblastic morphologic variant, activated B cell–like (ABC) variant, and EBV-positive DLBCL subtypes confer poorer prognosis and are more prevalent in elderly patients.[42,43] Mantle cell lymphoma (MCL) is also an important disease of the elderly, although it only accounts for about 6% of NHL as of 2004.[44] Through 2009, there was a linear rate of increase in incidence rate for each decade beyond age 50 years, up to a 429.24% increase in the group of white men more than 80 years old. There was also an increase of 192.73% in incidence rate in women more than 80 years old.[45] Identification of trends like these seen in DLBCL and MCL has contributed to an increase in clinical trials for elderly and unfit patients. FL is the most common indolent NHL, with a median age at diagnosis of 60 to 65 years and no gender predilection.[46]

Diagnosis and Staging

If lymphoma is suspected, the general approach to diagnosis includes complete physical examination; complete blood count; lactate dehydrogenase level; imaging of chest, abdomen, and pelvis; and an excisional biopsy of an enlarged lymph node or other involved tissue. Pathologic diagnosis is the most important component of the work-up and should be supplemented by immunophenotyping and cytogenetics (**Table 2**).

Complete staging varies by type of lymphoma. Recently, the Lugano Classification was established with a goal of modernizing the initial evaluation, staging, and assessment of response for both NHL and Hodgkin lymphoma.[47] Per these updated guidelines, bone marrow biopsy is no longer required for staging of DLBCL, but there were insufficient data to make a recommendation about biopsy in other NHLs. Imaging at baseline and follow-up should be performed using PET-CT in cases of FDG-avid nodal lymphomas, including essentially all diseases except CLL/SLL, Waldenstrom macroglobulinemia, and the indolent marginal zone lymphomas.[48,49] In addition to staging studies, a transthoracic echocardiogram and hepatitis B serologies should also be obtained if anthracycline chemotherapy or rituximab are being considered.

Table 2
Typical immunophenotype and chromosomal abnormalities for select NHL

Disease	Typical Immunophenotype	Chromosomal Abnormalities
DLBCL	CD20+, CD45+; notably negative for CD3	None diagnostic
MCL	CD5+, CD19+, CD20+, CD43+, CyclinD1+	t(11;14)
FL	CD10+, CD20+, BCL-2+, BCL-6+; notably negative for CD5 and CyclinD1	t(14;18)
Marginal zone lymphoma	CD20+; notably negative for CD5, CD10, and CyclinD1	None diagnostic
Burkitt lymphoma	CD10+, CD20+, BCL-6+, sIg+, Ki-67+; notably negative for TdT	t(8;14) or others involving myc (chromosome 8)

One of the most commonly used tools in lymphoma prognostication is the International Prognostication Index (IPI), which was first described in 1993. The IPI has been modified for use in other NHLs, including MCL (MIPI) and FL (FLIPI). Although both the IPI and FLIPI were developed in the prerituximab era, they remain good predictive tools in the age of rituximab.[50,51] **Table 3** summarizes the risk factors, risk groups, and associated OS for each of the IPI tools. The FLIPI has also been used as a prognostic tool for other indolent lymphomas.[52,53] An Elderly IPI has been proposed using an age cutoff of 70 years but has not yet been validated. The National LymphoCare Study group has also very recently validated an elderly FL prognostic score with poor risk features consisting of male gender, presence of B symptoms, and hemoglobin level less than 12 g/dL.[54]

Beyond the IPI, there are many additional prognostic factors used in NHL. In DLBCL, the combination of MYC and BCL2 gene rearrangement is termed double-hit lymphoma and responds poorly to standard of care treatment with rituximab, cyclophosphamide, adriamycin, vincristine, and prednisone (R-CHOP), so clinical trials are investigating alternative regimens. Also in DLBCL, ABC and germinal B-cell (GBC) subtypes of DLBCL represent different prognostic groups with the ABC subtype associated with a much poorer prognosis compared with GBC (5-year OS 16% vs 76%) when treated with anthracycline-based therapy.[55–57] There are 4 subtypes of MCL distinguished by cytology: small cell, marginal zone, diffuse or pleomorphic, and blastic or blastoid, with pleomorphic and blastoid subtypes associated with a poorer prognosis.[58] Complex karyotype has been associated with shortened PFS in MCL.[59] Mutated IGHV genes and the absence of the transcription factor SOX11 have been associated with more indolent disease in MCL.[60,61]

Monitoring and Therapy

Treatment of DLBCL, MCL, and FL is discussed here, in both the first-line and relapsed or refractory settings. The standard of care for each of these processes remains chemoimmunotherapy, and is discussed later; however, as in CLL, the role for targeted therapies is likely to change the treatment landscape of these diseases. Some targeted therapies have already been approved in the relapsed and refractory settings and are outlined later.

Diffuse large B-cell lymphoma

For limited stage DLBCL (I or II), low risk by IPI, and no bulky disease, the standard of care in North America is to give 3 cycles of cyclophosphamide, adriamycin, vincristine, and prednisone (CHOP) and 4 doses of rituximab followed by involved field radiation

Table 3
Prognostic indices for select NHL with associated OS

Prognostic Index	Adverse Risk Factors	Risk Stratification	5-y OS (%)
IPI (DLBCL)[90]	1 point for each risk factor • Age >60 y • LDH >1 × ULN • ECOG >2 • Extensive stage (III or IV) • >1 extranodal site	LR: 0–1 point LIR: 2 points HIR: 3 points HR: 4–5 points	LR: 73 LIR: 51 HIR: 43 HR: 26
MIPI (MCL)[91]	Age • 50–59 y: 1 point • 60–69 y: 2 points • 70+ y: 3 points LDH • 2/3–1 × ULN: 1 point • 1–1.5 × ULN: 2 points • >1.5 × ULN: 3 points ECOG • >2: 2 points WBC • 6.7–9.9 × 10³/uL: 1 point • 10–14.9 × 10³/uL: 2 points • 15+ × 10³/uL: 3 points	LR: 0–3 points IR: 4–5 points HR: 6–11 points	LR: 60 IR: 40 HR: 15
FLIPI (FL)[92]	1 point for each risk factor • Age >60 y • LDH >1 × ULN • Extensive stage (III or IV) • Hemoglobin <12 g/dL • >4 nodal areas	LR: 0–1 point IR: 2 points HR: 3–5 points	LR: 90.6 (70.7 10-y) IR: 77.6 (50.9 10-y) HR: 52.5 (35.5 10-y)

Abbreviations: HIR, high intermediate risk; HR, high risk; IR, intermediate risk; LDH, lactate dehydrogenase level; LIR, low intermediate risk; LR, low risk; ULN, upper limit of normal; WBC, white blood cell count.
Data from Refs.[90–92]

treatment (IFRT). This regimen is associated with a 4-year OS of 92% and a 4-year PFS of 88%.[62]

In extensive stage DLBCL disease (III or IV), R-CHOP therapy is the standard of care. The RICOVER-60 trial was crucial to establishing the superiority of R-CHOP compared with CHOP in terms of OS, PFS, and EFS. The noninferiority of 6 cycles compared with 8 was also established in this trial.[63] Following RICOVER-60, the GELA trial studied the benefit of 14-day versus 21-day cycles. There was no significant difference in outcome between the 2 groups with nearly one-quarter of dose-dense patients receiving less than 80% of planned treatment and most requiring hematopoietic support.[64] These two trials have established the standard dosing of R-CHOP, which is every 21 days for 6 cycles.

In relapsed or refractory disease, the first step in evaluation is to determine fitness for autologous stem cell transplant. Data from 2 different registries revealed treatment-related mortality to be higher in those greater than or equal to 60 years old compared with younger patients.[65,66] For unfit or frail patients, clinical trial options should be investigated. Outside of clinical trials, multiple options exist, including single-agent options such as etoposide and lenalidomide, bendamustine-containing or gemcitabine-containing combination regimens, and metronomic regimens with low-dose oral chemotherapy agents.[67–71]

Mantle cell lymphoma

Almost all patients with MCL have advanced stage disease (bulky II or III/IV) at diagnosis. Because of this limitation, the treatment guidelines for limited stage disease are based on retrospective data and include involved field radiation therapy plus or minus chemotherapy. Although ORR is excellent (95%) with combination therapy, the 5-year OS was only 62%, with most recurrence occurring at distant sites.[72] Chemotherapy with IFRT achieves local control but has less impact on prevention of distant recurrence, so there may be a role for a watch-and-wait strategy in frail elderly patients who are asymptomatic.

There is no clearly superior regimen for first-line treatment of MCL so enrollment on a clinical trial should be offered to all eligible patients. In an elderly population, most patients are unlikely to be fit for transplant; however, for the rare fit patients younger than 70 years, an aggressive regimen should be considered in first-line treatment with the goal of inducing a complete response (CR). There are many aggressive regimens with dose-intensified chemoimmunotherapy that have proved to be very active in MCL.[73] These cytarabine-containing regimens are associated with significant toxicity, including severe infections, high rate of grade 3 or higher hematologic toxicity, and toxicity-associated death rate of 2% to 8%, and as such should only be offered to very fit patients.

Less aggressive regimens have been studied in elderly and unfit patients, with 2 frontrunner regimens emerging: R-CHOP and BR. Both of these regimens were evaluated in clinical trials that included patients with MCL and indolent NHL. BR has proved to be an effective regimen in noninferiority trials with R-CHOP. BR was associated with a longer PFS (35.4 months BR vs 22.1 months R-CHOP; $P = .0044$) and with a better tolerated side effect profile with less paresthesia, fewer infectious episodes, and less sepsis than R-CHOP and no alopecia, compared with 100% with R-CHOP.[74] The noninferiority of BR compared with R-CHOP was confirmed by the BRIGHT trial.[75] There is also a role for maintenance rituximab after R-CHOP induction, which was established in a second randomization in the trial of R-FC versus R-CHOP. Rituximab maintenance was associated with significantly longer PFS and OS compared with interferon-alfa maintenance.[76]

As in the treatment of CLL, there is an emerging role for targeted therapies in the treatment of MCL. Ibrutinib has already gained FDA approval for treatment of relapsed or refractory MCL. This approval was based on phase II data that showed an ORR of 68% with 21% achieving CR. With a median follow-up of 15.3 months, the estimated median PFS was 13.9 months (95% CI, 7.0 to not reached) and the median OS was not reached.[77] Ibrutinib and idelalisib are also currently under investigation in combination with other agents such as BR or lenalidomide. In phase I data from combination BR with ibrutinib in relapsed/refractory MCL, the ORR was 94% with a 76% CR rate.[78] Other treatment options include single-agent rituximab, chlorambucil alone or in combination with rituximab, and the well-tolerated oral metronomic regimen of PEP-C (prednisone, etoposide, procarbazine, and cyclophosphamide).[79–81]

Follicular lymphoma

FL is typically managed with a watch-and-wait strategy, with treatment reserved for symptomatic patients with a goal of inducing a durable remission. Trials investigating early treatment compared with watch and wait did not show a survival advantage in the prerituximab and postrituximab eras.[82–85] There are multiple criteria for treatment of FL, but consensus recommends treatment in cases of marrow compromise and B symptoms. Patients with limited stage disease are rare, making prospective study difficult. A large retrospective meta-analysis showed no significant difference in OS between watchful waiting and a variety of treatment regimens, including chemotherapy, radiation, and immunotherapy.[85] The National Comprehensive Cancer Network guidelines recommend IFRT in these circumstances.[3]

Low-bulk, extensive stage FL that requires therapy does not have 1 clear standard of care for frontline therapy, so all eligible patients should be offered enrollment in a clinical trial. Outside of clinical trials, treatment with BR or R-CHOP represents standards of care based on the previously reviewed data.[74,75] For unfit or frail elderly patients, single-agent rituximab is often used as both induction and maintenance therapy and has shown improved response rates and EFS without benefit in OS.[86,87] More recently, maintenance rituximab has been compared with retreatment at relapse with no significant difference in OS or time to treatment failure, representing a more cost-effective approach to treatment.[88] Given the likelihood of relapse regardless of response to initial therapy, inducing even a partial response may be adequate to prolong the need for future treatment. In the setting of relapsed or refractory FL, idelalisib has gained FDA approval based on the results of a phase II study in indolent NHL, in which the median PFS was 11 months.[89]

SUMMARY

Lymphoproliferative disorders are common in the elderly population, frequently presenting at age 65 years or beyond. Clinical trials traditionally select for a younger, fitter patient population and the resulting data may not be applicable to an elderly, less fit population. When considering treatment options for an elderly patient, fitness level is an important consideration and these patients often need to be treated differently than their younger counterparts. There has been a recent interest in enrolling elderly and less fit patients on clinical trials for treatment of CLL, MCL, and DLBCL and these have yielded important new data that have changed the way these patients are treated. Future clinical trials should continue to focus on this important patient population and eligible patients should be offered enrollment whenever possible.

The role of novel targeted therapies is expected to continue to grow in the future. These agents are ideal for elderly and unfit patients given their favorable side effect profiles and ease of administration because most are available orally. Although many targeted therapies are available only in relapsed or refractory disease and/or on clinical trials, this is expected to change as more data become available from phase III trials, especially those conducted in the up-front setting. The introduction of these therapies seems to herald a paradigm shift in the B-cell lymphoproliferative disorders, and may bring well-tolerated targeted therapies a step closer for patients with CLL and NHL.

REFERENCES

1. Chronic lymphocytic leukemia - SEER stat fact sheets. 2015. Available at: http://seer.cancer.gov/statfacts/html/clyl.html. Accessed May 20, 2015.
2. Thurmes P, Call T, Slager S, et al. Comorbid conditions and survival in unselected, newly diagnosed patients with chronic lymphocytic leukemia. Leuk Lymphoma 2008;49:49–56.
3. Non-Hodgkin's lymphomas [Version 2.2015]. 2015. Available at: http://www.nccn.org/professionals/physician_gls/pdf/nhl.pdf. Accessed May 20, 2015.
4. Shanafelt TD, Ghia P, Lanasa MC, et al. Monoclonal B-cell lymphocytosis (MBL): biology, natural history and clinical management. Leukemia 2010;24:512–20.
5. Kalpadakis C, Pangalis GA, Sachanas S, et al. New insights into monoclonal B-cell lymphocytosis. Biomed Res Int 2014;2014:258917.

6. Moreira J, Rabe KG, Cerhan JR, et al. Infectious complications among individuals with clinical monoclonal B-cell lymphocytosis (MBL): a cohort study of newly diagnosed cases compared to controls. Leukemia 2012;27:136–41.

7. Solomon BM, Rabe KG, Moreira J, et al. Risk of cancer in patients with clinical monoclonal B-cell lymphocytosis (MBL): A cohort study of newly diagnosed patients compared to controls. Poster presented at the 54th Annual Meeting of the American Society of Hematology. Atlanta, GA, December 8-11, 2012.

8. Binet JL, Auquier A, Dighiero G, et al. A new prognostic classification of chronic lymphocytic leukemia derived from a multivariate survival analysis. Cancer 1981; 48:198–206.

9. Rai KR, Sawitsky A, Cronkite EP, et al. Clinical staging of chronic lymphocytic leukemia. Blood 1975;46:219–34.

10. Juliusson G, Oscier DG, Fitchett M, et al. Prognostic subgroups in B-cell chronic lymphocytic leukemia defined by specific chromosomal abnormalities. N Engl J Med 1990;323:720–4.

11. Mayr C, Speicher MR, Kofler DM, et al. Chromosomal translocations are associated with poor prognosis in chronic lymphocytic leukemia. Blood 2005;107:742–51.

12. Dohner H, Stilgenbauer S, Fischer K, et al. Cytogenetic and molecular cytogenetic analysis of B cell chronic lymphocytic leukemia: specific chromosome aberrations identify prognostic subgroups of patients and point to loci of candidate genes. Leukemia 1997;11(Suppl 2):S19–24.

13. Dohner H, Stilgenbauer S, Benner A, et al. Genomic aberrations and survival in chronic lymphocytic leukemia. N Engl J Med 2001;343:1910–6.

14. Damle RN, Wasil T, Fais F, et al. Ig V gene mutation status and CD38 expression as novel prognostic indicators in chronic lymphocytic leukemia. Blood 1999;94: 1840–7.

15. Hamblin TJ, Davis Z, Gardiner A, et al. Unmutated Ig V(H) genes are associated with a more aggressive form of chronic lymphocytic leukemia. Blood 1999;94: 1848–54.

16. Gribben JG. How I treat CLL up front. Blood 2009;115:187–97.

17. Molica S. Infections in chronic lymphocytic leukemia: risk factors, and impact on survival, and treatment. Leuk Lymphoma 1994;13:203–14.

18. Manusow D, Weinerman BH. Subsequent neoplasia in chronic lymphocytic leukemia. JAMA 1975;232:267–9.

19. Hodgson K, Ferrer G, Pereira A, et al. Autoimmune cytopenia in chronic lymphocytic leukaemia: diagnosis and treatment. Br J Haematol 2011;154:14–22.

20. Kjeldsberg CR, Marty J. Prolymphocytic transformation of chronic lymphocytic leukemia. Cancer 1981;48:2447–57.

21. Schweighofer CD, Cymbalista F, Muller C, et al. Early versus deferred treatment with combined fludarabine, cyclophosphamide and rituximab (FCR) improves event-free survival in patients with high-risk Binet stage A chronic lymphocytic leukemia – first results of a randomized German-French cooperative phase III trial. Paper presented at the 55th Annual Meeting of the American Society of Hematology. New Orleans, LA, December 7-10, 2013.

22. Hallek M, Cheson BD, Catovsky D, et al. Guidelines for the diagnosis and treatment of chronic lymphocytic leukemia: a report from the International Workshop on Chronic Lymphocytic Leukemia updating the National Cancer Institute-Working Group 1996 guidelines. Blood 2008;111:5446–56.

23. Karnofsky D, Burchenal J. The clinical evaluation of chemotherapeutic agents in cancer. In: MacCleod C, editor. Evaluation of chemotherapeutic agents. New York: Columbia University Press; 1949. p. 191–205.

24. Oken MM, Creech RH, Tormey DC, et al. Toxicity and response criteria of the Eastern Cooperative Oncology Group. Am J Clin Oncol 1982;5:649–55.
25. Linn BS, Linn MW, Gurel L. Cumulative illness rating scale. J Am Geriatr Soc 1968;16:622–6.
26. Hurria A, Wildes T, Blair SL, et al. Senior adult oncology, version 2.2014: clinical practice guidelines in oncology. J Natl Compr Canc Net 2014;12:82–126.
27. Extermann M, Hurria A. Comprehensive geriatric assessment for older patients with cancer. J Clin Oncol 2007;25:1824–31.
28. Eichhorst B, Goede V, Hallek M. Treatment of elderly patients with chronic lymphocytic leukemia. Leuk Lymphoma 2009;50:171–8.
29. Eichhorst B, Fink A-M, Busch R, et al. Frontline chemoimmunotherapy with fludarabine (F), cyclophosphamide (C), and rituximab (R) (FCR) shows superior efficacy in comparison to bendamustine (B) and Rituximab (BR) in previously untreated and physically fit patients (pts) with advanced chronic lymphocytic leukemia (CLL): final analysis of an international, randomized study of the German CLL Study Group (GCLLSG) (CLL10 study). Paper presented at the 56th Annual Meeting of the American Society of Hematology. San Francisco, CA, December 6-9, 2014.
30. Hallek M, Fischer K, Fingerle-Rowson G, et al. Addition of rituximab to fludarabine and cyclophosphamide in patients with chronic lymphocytic leukaemia: a randomised, open-label, phase 3 trial. Lancet 2010;376:1164–74.
31. Eichhorst BF, Busch R, Stilgenbauer S, et al. First-line therapy with fludarabine compared with chlorambucil does not result in a major benefit for elderly patients with advanced chronic lymphocytic leukemia. Blood 2009;114:3382–91.
32. Woyach JA, Ruppert AS, Rai K, et al. Impact of age on outcomes after initial therapy with chemotherapy and different chemoimmunotherapy regimens in patients with chronic lymphocytic leukemia: results of sequential cancer and leukemia group B studies. J Clin Oncol 2012;31:440–7.
33. Goede V, Fischer K, Busch R, et al. Obinutuzumab plus chlorambucil in patients with CLL and coexisting conditions. N Engl J Med 2014;370:1101–10.
34. Goede V, Fischer K, Engelke A, et al. Obinutuzumab as frontline treatment of chronic lymphocytic leukemia: updated results of the CLL11 study. Leukemia 2015;29:1602–4.
35. Hillmen P, Robak T, Janssens A, et al. Chlorambucil plus ofatumumab versus chlorambucil alone in previously untreated patients with chronic lymphocytic leukaemia (COMPLEMENT 1): a randomised, multicentre, open-label phase 3 trial. Lancet 2015;385:1873–83.
36. Byrd JC, Brown JR, O'Brien S, et al. Ibrutinib versus ofatumumab in previously treated chronic lymphoid leukemia. N Engl J Med 2014;371:213–23.
37. Byrd JC, Furman RR, Coutre SE, et al. Three-year follow-up of treatment-naive and previously treated patients with CLL and SLL receiving single-agent ibrutinib. Blood 2015;125:2497–506.
38. Furman RR, Sharman JP, Coutre SE, et al. Idelalisib and rituximab in relapsed chronic lymphocytic leukemia. N Engl J Med 2014;370:997–1007.
39. Non-Hodgkin lymphoma - SEER stat fact sheets. 2015. Available at: http://seer.cancer.gov/statfacts/html/nhl.html. Accessed May 20, 2015.
40. Williams JN, Rai A, Lipscomb J, et al. Disease characteristics, patterns of care, and survival in very elderly patients with diffuse large B-cell lymphoma. Cancer 2015;121:1800–8.
41. Monnereau A, Troussard X, Belot A, et al. Unbiased estimates of long-term net survival of hematological malignancy patients detailed by major subtypes in France. Int J Cancer 2012;132:2378–87.

42. Morrison VA, Hamlin P, Soubeyran P, et al. Diffuse large B-cell lymphoma in the elderly: impact of prognosis, comorbidities, geriatric assessment, and supportive care on clinical practice. An International Society of Geriatric Oncology (SIOG) expert position paper. J Geriatr Oncol 2014;6:141–52.

43. Pfreundschuh M. How I treat elderly patients with diffuse large B-cell lymphoma. Blood 2010;116:5103–10.

44. Zhou Y, Wang H, Fang W, et al. Incidence trends of mantle cell lymphoma in the United States between 1992 and 2004. Cancer 2008;113:791–8.

45. Aschebrook-Kilfoy B, Caces DB, Ollberding NJ, et al. An upward trend in the age-specific incidence patterns for mantle cell lymphoma in the USA. Leuk Lymphoma 2013;54:1677–83.

46. Nabhan C, Aschebrook-Kilfoy B, Chiu BC, et al. The impact of race, age, and sex in follicular lymphoma: a comprehensive SEER analysis across consecutive treatment eras. Am J Hematol 2014;89:633–8.

47. Cheson BD, Fisher RI, Barrington SF, et al. Recommendations for initial evaluation, staging, and response assessment of Hodgkin and non-Hodgkin lymphoma: the Lugano classification. J Clin Oncol 2014;32:3059–68.

48. Barrington SF, Mikhaeel NG, Kostakoglu L, et al. Role of imaging in the staging and response assessment of lymphoma: consensus of the International Conference on Malignant Lymphomas Imaging Working Group. J Clin Oncol 2014;32:3048–58.

49. Seam P, Juweid ME, Cheson BD. The role of FDG-PET scans in patients with lymphoma. Blood 2007;110:3507–16.

50. Ziepert M, Hasenclever D, Kuhnt E, et al. Standard International Prognostic Index remains a valid predictor of outcome for patients with aggressive CD20+ B-cell lymphoma in the rituximab era. J Clin Oncol 2010;28:2373–80.

51. Nooka AK, Nabhan C, Zhou X, et al. Examination of the Follicular Lymphoma International Prognostic Index (FLIPI) in the National LymphoCare study (NLCS): a prospective US patient cohort treated predominantly in community practices. Ann Oncol 2012;24:441–8.

52. Troch M, Wohrer S, Raderer M. Assessment of the prognostic indices IPI and FLIPI in patients with mucosa-associated lymphoid tissue lymphoma. Anticancer Res 2010;30:635–9.

53. Heilgeist A, McClanahan F, Ho AD, et al. Prognostic value of the Follicular Lymphoma International Prognostic Index score in marginal zone lymphoma: an analysis of clinical presentation and outcome in 144 patients. Cancer 2012;119:99–106.

54. Nabhan C, Byrtek M, Rai A, et al. Disease characteristics, treatment patterns, prognosis, outcomes and lymphoma-related mortality in elderly follicular lymphoma in the United States. Br J Haematol 2015;170:85–95.

55. Alizadeh AA, Eisen MB, Davis RE, et al. Distinct types of diffuse large B-cell lymphoma identified by gene expression profiling. Nature 2000;403:503–11.

56. Choi WW, Weisenburger DD, Greiner TC, et al. A new immunostain algorithm classifies diffuse large B-cell lymphoma into molecular subtypes with high accuracy. Clin Cancer Res 2009;15:5494–502.

57. Hans CP, Weisenburger DD, Greiner TC, et al. Confirmation of the molecular classification of diffuse large B-cell lymphoma by immunohistochemistry using a tissue microarray. Blood 2003;103:275–82.

58. Bertoni F, Ponzoni M. The cellular origin of mantle cell lymphoma. Int J Biochem Cell Biol 2007;39:1747–53.

59. Cohen JB, Ruppert AS, Heerema NA, et al. Complex karyotype is associated with aggressive disease and shortened progression-free survival in patients with

newly diagnosed mantle cell lymphoma. Clin Lymphoma Myeloma Leuk 2015;15: 278–85.e1.

60. Nodit L, Bahler DW, Jacobs SA, et al. Indolent mantle cell lymphoma with nodal involvement and mutated immunoglobulin heavy chain genes. Hum Pathol 2003; 34:1030–4.

61. Navarro A, Clot G, Royo C, et al. Molecular subsets of mantle cell lymphoma defined by the IGHV mutational status and SOX11 expression have distinct biologic and clinical features. Cancer Res 2012;72:5307–16.

62. Persky DO, Unger JM, Spier CM, et al. Phase II study of rituximab plus three cycles of CHOP and involved-field radiotherapy for patients with limited-stage aggressive B-cell lymphoma: Southwest Oncology Group study 0014. J Clin Oncol 2008;26:2258–63.

63. Pfreundschuh M, Schubert J, Ziepert M, et al. Six versus eight cycles of bi-weekly CHOP-14 with or without rituximab in elderly patients with aggressive CD20+ B-cell lymphomas: a randomised controlled trial (RICOVER-60). Lancet Oncol 2008;9:105–16.

64. Delarue R, Tilly H, Mounier N, et al. Dose-dense rituximab-CHOP compared with standard rituximab-CHOP in elderly patients with diffuse large B-cell lymphoma (the LNH03-6B study): a randomised phase 3 trial. Lancet Oncol 2013;14:525–33.

65. Jantunen E, Canals C, Rambaldi A, et al. Autologous stem cell transplantation in elderly patients (> or =60 years) with diffuse large B-cell lymphoma: an analysis based on data in the European Blood and Marrow Transplantation registry. Haematologica 2008;93:1837–42.

66. Lazarus HM, Carreras J, Boudreau C, et al. Influence of age and histology on outcome in adult non-Hodgkin lymphoma patients undergoing autologous hematopoietic cell transplantation (HCT): a report from the Center for International Blood & Marrow Transplant Research (CIBMTR). Biol Blood Marrow Transplant 2008;14:1323–33.

67. Niitsu N, Umeda M. Evaluation of long-term daily administration of oral low-dose etoposide in elderly patients with relapsing or refractory non-Hodgkin's lymphoma. Am J Clin Oncol 1997;20:311–4.

68. Ohmachi K, Niitsu N, Uchida T, et al. Multicenter phase II study of bendamustine plus rituximab in patients with relapsed or refractory diffuse large B-cell lymphoma. J Clin Oncol 2013;31:2103–9.

69. Coleman M, Martin P, Ruan J, et al. Prednisone, etoposide, procarbazine, and cyclophosphamide (PEP-C) oral combination chemotherapy regimen for recurring/refractory lymphoma: low-dose metronomic, multidrug therapy. Cancer 2008;112:2228–32.

70. Corazzelli G, Capobianco G, Arcamone M, et al. Long-term results of gemcitabine plus oxaliplatin with and without rituximab as salvage treatment for transplant-ineligible patients with refractory/relapsing B-cell lymphoma. Cancer Chemother Pharmacol 2009;64:907–16.

71. Witzig TE, Vose JM, Zinzani PL, et al. An international phase II trial of single-agent lenalidomide for relapsed or refractory aggressive B-cell non-Hodgkin's lymphoma. Ann Oncol 2011;22:1622–7.

72. Bernard M, Tsang RW, Le LW, et al. Limited-stage mantle cell lymphoma: treatment outcomes at the Princess Margaret Hospital. Leuk Lymphoma 2012;54:261–7.

73. Ghielmini M, Zucca E. How I treat mantle cell lymphoma. Blood 2009;114: 1469–76.

74. Rummel MJ, Niederle N, Maschmeyer G, et al. Bendamustine plus rituximab versus CHOP plus rituximab as first-line treatment for patients with indolent

and mantle-cell lymphomas: an open-label, multicentre, randomised, phase 3 non-inferiority trial. Lancet 2013;381:1203–10.

75. Flinn IW, van der Jagt R, Kahl BS, et al. Randomized trial of bendamustine-rituximab or R-CHOP/R-CVP in first-line treatment of indolent NHL or MCL: the BRIGHT study. Blood 2014;123:2944–52.

76. Kluin-Nelemans HC, Hoster E, Hermine O, et al. Treatment of older patients with mantle-cell lymphoma. N Engl J Med 2012;367:520–31.

77. Wang ML, Rule S, Martin P, et al. Targeting BTK with ibrutinib in relapsed or refractory mantle-cell lymphoma. N Engl J Med 2013;369:507–16.

78. Maddocks K, Christian B, Jaglowski S, et al. A phase 1/1b study of rituximab, bendamustine, and ibrutinib in patients with untreated and relapsed/refractory non-Hodgkin lymphoma. Blood 2014;125:242–8.

79. Coleman M, Martin P, Ruan J, et al. Low-dose metronomic, multidrug therapy with the PEP-C oral combination chemotherapy regimen for mantle cell lymphoma. Leuk Lymphoma 2008;49:447–50.

80. Ghielmini M, Schmitz SF, Cogliatti S, et al. Effect of single-agent rituximab given at the standard schedule or as prolonged treatment in patients with mantle cell lymphoma: a study of the Swiss Group for Clinical Cancer Research (SAKK). J Clin Oncol 2004;23:705–11.

81. Bauwens D, Maerevoet M, Michaux L, et al. Activity and safety of combined rituximab with chlorambucil in patients with mantle cell lymphoma. Br J Haematol 2005;131:338–40.

82. Brice P, Bastion Y, Lepage E, et al. Comparison in low-tumor-burden follicular lymphomas between an initial no-treatment policy, prednimustine, or interferon alfa: a randomized study from the Groupe d'Etude des Lymphomes Folliculaires. Groupe d'Etude des Lymphomes de l'Adulte. J Clin Oncol 1997;15:1110–7.

83. Ardeshna KM, Smith P, Norton A, et al. Long-term effect of a watch and wait policy versus immediate systemic treatment for asymptomatic advanced-stage non-Hodgkin lymphoma: a randomised controlled trial. Lancet 2003;362:516–22.

84. Ardeshna KM, Qian W, Smith P, et al. Rituximab versus a watch-and-wait approach in patients with advanced-stage, asymptomatic, non-bulky follicular lymphoma: an open-label randomised phase 3 trial. Lancet Oncol 2014;15:424–35.

85. Michallet AS, Lebras LL, Bauwens DD, et al. Early stage follicular lymphoma: what is the clinical impact of the first-line treatment strategy? J Hematol Oncol 2013;6:45.

86. Hainsworth JD, Litchy S, Burris HA 3rd, et al. Rituximab as first-line and maintenance therapy for patients with indolent non-Hodgkin's lymphoma. J Clin Oncol 2002;20:4261–7.

87. Martinelli G, Schmitz SF, Utiger U, et al. Long-term follow-up of patients with follicular lymphoma receiving single-agent rituximab at two different schedules in trial SAKK 35/98. J Clin Oncol 2010;28:4480–4.

88. Kahl BS, Hong F, Williams ME, et al. Rituximab extended schedule or re-treatment trial for low-tumor burden follicular lymphoma: Eastern Cooperative Oncology Group protocol e4402. J Clin Oncol 2014;32:3096–102.

89. Gopal AK, Kahl BS, de Vos S, et al. PI3Kdelta inhibition by idelalisib in patients with relapsed indolent lymphoma. N Engl J Med 2014;370:1008–18.

90. A predictive model for aggressive non-Hodgkin's lymphoma. The International Non-Hodgkin's Lymphoma Prognostic Factors Project. N Engl J Med 1993;329:987–94.

91. Hoster E, Dreyling M, Klapper W, et al. A new prognostic index (MIPI) for patients with advanced-stage mantle cell lymphoma. Blood 2007;111:558–65.

92. Solal-Celigny P, Roy P, Colombat P, et al. Follicular lymphoma International Prognostic Index. Blood 2004;104:1258–65.

Monoclonal Gammopathy of Undetermined Significance and Multiple Myeloma in Older Adults

Emily J. Guerard, MD[a], Sascha A. Tuchman, MD[b],*

KEYWORDS

- MGUS • Multiple myeloma • Older adult • Elderly • Geriatric • Cancer • Neoplasm

KEY POINTS

- Monoclonal gammopathy of undetermined significance and multiple myeloma (MM) are plasma cell disorders of advanced age.
- Unexplained anemia, hypercalcemia, renal insufficiency, or bone pain, among other symptoms, should prompt a work-up for a plasma cell disorder.
- Chemotherapy is standard of care for MM and, although incurable, survival in MM is progressively improving thanks to new drugs.
- Treating MM in older adults requires careful monitoring, dosing, and management of toxicity to attain good outcomes.
- Geriatric assessment and other novel instruments may soon enable personalization of MM therapy for older adults.

INTRODUCTION AND EPIDEMIOLOGY

Monoclonal gammopathy of undetermined significance (MGUS) and multiple myeloma (MM) are disorders on the spectrum of plasma cell dyscrasias that are diseases of aging. In multiple population-based studies, the prevalence of MGUS increases with age; 5.3% of people greater than or equal to 70 years old and 7.5% of people greater than or equal to 85 years old.[1] The median age at diagnosis of MM

Disclosures: Dr E.J. Guerard has no disclosures. Dr S.A. Tuchman has performed consulting for Celgene and Takeda, and participated in speakers' bureau for Celgene and Takeda.
[a] Division of Hematology & Oncology, Department of Medicine, University of North Carolina at Chapel Hill, 170 Manning Drive, Campus Box 7305, Chapel Hill, NC 27599, USA; [b] Division of Cellular Therapy and Hematologic Malignancies, Duke Cancer Institute, DUMC 3961, Durham, NC 27710, USA
* Corresponding author.
E-mail address: sat6@duke.edu

Clin Geriatr Med 32 (2016) 191–205
http://dx.doi.org/10.1016/j.cger.2015.08.012
0749-0690/16/$ – see front matter © 2016 Elsevier Inc. All rights reserved.

is 69 years, with half of deaths from MM occurring in patients aged 75 years and older (**Fig. 1**).[2] MM accounts for about 10% of all hematologic malignancies and 1.6% of all new cancer cases in the United States.[2,3] It is estimated that there will be 26,850 new cases of MM in 2015. MGUS and MM are more common in men than in women, and in African Americans than in white people.[1,2,4,5]

Five-year overall survival in MM has increased from 29.7% in 1990 to 45.1% in 2007,[2] largely attributable to novel therapies.[6]

Given the anticipated growth in the older adult population and presumably static prevalence rates as a function of age, the raw numbers of older adults with plasma cell disorders will increase over time. Therefore, a familiarity with MM and MGUS is, and will remain, important for geriatricians.

BIOLOGY AND CAUSE

MM is a malignancy of plasma cells, terminally differentiated B lymphocytes that secrete antibodies when exposed to specific antigens. The exact pathogenesis of MM and MGUS is not well understood. Virtually all cases of MM are thought to arise from MGUS, a premalignant, asymptomatic proliferation of plasma cells.[7,8] The initiation of MGUS is likely an abnormal plasma cell response to antigenic stimulation that leads to primary cytogenetic abnormalities and other genomic changes; the resultant derangement of plasma cell biology ultimately causes plasma cell clonal expansion and in some cases clinically significant disease. The expanded plasma cells usually overproduce a complete monoclonal immunoglobulin or some part thereof (eg, light chain only).[9,10] The transition in some cases from MGUS to MM is thought to be caused by additional biological abnormalities (eg, genomic, bone marrow microenvironmental) that lead to further clonal proliferation.[9] Once MGUS has progressed to MM, end organ damage begins because of infiltration of the neoplastic plasma cells into the bones and organ systems, damage mediated by circulating monoclonal

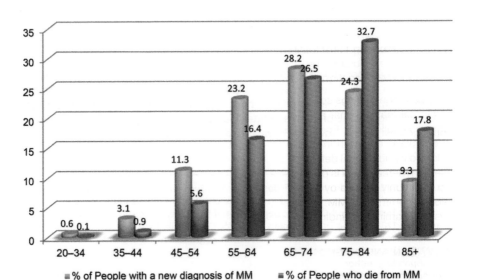

Fig. 1. Age distribution of patients with MM and deaths from MM. (*Data from* Institute NC. SEER stat fact sheets: myeloma. 2015. Available at: http://seer.cancer.gov/statfacts/html/mulmy.html. Accessed May 18, 2015.)

proteins (eg, cast nephropathy), or both. Between MGUS and MM there is an intermediate phase, termed smoldering MM (SMM), which is not always identified before an MM diagnosis. SMM constitutes a higher-burden disease state than MGUS, but one in which end organ damage is similarly absent.

Risk factors such as radiation or pesticide exposure,[11,12] or history of autoimmune or chronic infectious disease,[13] have been described as risk factors for MM or MGUS, but most patients with MM and MGUS have no identifiable risk factors. Perhaps the most important risk factor for these diseases is advanced age. A growing body of research supports the link between aging and MM; as an example, serum levels of the proinflammatory cytokine interleukin 6 (IL-6) increase as a function of age,[14] and, in MM, plasma cells secrete IL-6 and overexpress the IL-6 receptor.[15] In the future, insights such as this are likely to elucidate deeper links between MM and aging and potentially yield beneficial interventions for both conditions.

CLINICAL PRESENTATION OF MULTIPLE MYELOMA

The clinical presentation of patients with MM is variable and can be subtle. The 2 case presentations discussed here highlight this variability.

- Case 1. A 75-year-old woman with osteoporosis presented to the emergency department after experiencing a fall followed by right hip pain. She reported fatigue, poor appetite, and mild weight loss for the past 6 months. Radiographs showed a pathologic fracture involving the distal femur. Intraoperative biopsy showed clonal plasma cells, and complete skeletal radiographs showed diffuse lytic bone lesions. Bone marrow biopsy also revealed clonal plasma cells, indicating a diagnosis of MM.
- Case 2. An 80-year-old man with hypertension and mild cognitive impairment presented to his geriatrician's office for routine follow-up. His only complaint was increased fatigue. Physical examination was nondiagnostic. Routine laboratory evaluation revealed normocytic anemia (hemoglobin level, 9.5 g/dL), increased total protein level, and a mild increase in his creatinine level to 1.35 mg/dL. Serum protein electrophoresis (SPEP) and immunofixation revealed a monoclonal spike of 2.5 g/dL immunoglobulin (Ig) G-kappa, and a bone marrow aspirate and biopsy by a consulting hematologist showed 20% monoclonal plasma cells, confirming MM.

The common findings seen in MM at diagnosis are shown in **Table 1**.[16] The lack of any clinical features that are frequently and uniquely present in MM can make this diagnosis challenging. For example, anemia is present in 73% of patients with MM but anemia is common in community-dwelling older adults and is more commonly explained by nutritional deficiencies, anemia of chronic disease, or chronic kidney disease.[17] Hypercalcemia is present in 28% of patients with a new diagnosis of MM but is also commonly caused by thiazide diuretics or primary hyperparathyroidism. Fatigue, which is common in MM, is seen in innumerable other medical conditions too. No physical examination findings are reliably sensitive and specific for diagnosing MM.[16]

EVALUATION AND DIAGNOSIS

Screening for MGUS and MM is not recommended for older adults.[18] MGUS is highly prevalent, progresses to MM in only a small percentage of patients,[19] and there is no known strategy to prevent that progression.[18] Geriatricians should consider a diagnostic work-up for plasma cell disorders only when a reason to suspect one exists.

Table 1 Clinical features of MM	
Clinical Feature	Frequency (%)
History	
Bone pain	58
Family history of cancer	42
Fatigue	32
Weight loss	24
Known history of MGUS	20
Physical Examination	
Hepatomegaly	4
Splenomegaly	1
Lymphadenopathy	1
Laboratory	
Anemia	73
Increased creatinine level	48
Increased calcium level	28
Leukopenia	20
Thrombocytopenia	5
Radiology	
Lytic lesions	66
Pathologic fractures	26
Osteoporosis	23

Data from Kyle RA, Gertz MA, Witzig TE, et al. Review of 1027 patients with newly diagnosed multiple myeloma. Mayo Clin Proc 2003;78(1):21–33.

The following list represents a sample of clinical findings that could trigger a diagnostic work-up:

- Age-disproportionate osteoporosis or osteopenia
- Increased serum total protein level without increased serum albumin level
- Bone pain, lytic bone lesions, pathologic and/or compression fractures
- Unexplained peripheral neuropathy, hypercalcemia, anemia, proteinuria, or renal insufficiency

The initial diagnostic work-up should include the following laboratory tests:

- SPEP and 24-hour urine protein electrophoresis (UPEP) with immunofixation
- Serum free light chains
- Complete blood count (CBC)
- Serum creatinine and calcium levels
- Quantitative immunoglobulins

The diagnostic criteria for MM, SMM, and MGUS were recently updated (**Box 1**).[20] If a monoclonal protein is not detected on serum or urine studies, then MM is extremely unlikely and most plasma cell diseases can usually be confidently excluded from consideration; nonsecretory myeloma (ie, MM that does not secrete monoclonal protein) does exist but is rare.[21] If a monoclonal protein is detected, then the patient needs additional work-up to clarify the diagnosis. The first step is to determine

---

Box 1
2014 Revision of International Myeloma Working Group diagnostic criteria

MM

Clonal bone marrow plasma cells greater than or equal to 10%, or biopsy-proven bone, or extramedullary plasmacytoma

Plus at least 1 myeloma-defining event.

Myeloma-defining events:
- Hypercalcemia

  ○ Serum calcium level greater than 1 mg/dL higher than upper limit of normal or greater than 11 mg/dL
- Renal insufficiency

  ○ Creatinine clearance less than 40 mL/min or serum creatinine level greater than 2 mg/dL
- Anemia

  ○ Hemoglobin level less than 10 g/dL or greater than 2 g/dL less than the lower limit of normal
- Bone lesions

  ○ One or more osteolytic lesions on skeletal survey, computed tomography (CT), or PET/CT
- Biomarkers of malignancy

  ○ Clonal bone marrow plasma cells greater than or equal to 60%

  ○ Involved/uninvolved serum free light chain ratio greater than 100 with involved light chain greater than 10 g/dL

  ○ Greater than 1 focal lesion on MRI

Smoldering MM

Both criteria must be present:
- Serum monoclonal protein (IgG or IgA) level greater than 3 g/dL, or urinary monoclonal protein level greater than 500 mg per 24 hours, and/or clonal bone marrow plasma cells 10% to 60%
- No myeloma-defining events or evidence of amyloidosis

MGUS

All 3 criteria must be present:
- Serum monoclonal protein level less than 3 g/dL
- Bone marrow plasma cells less than 10%
- No myeloma-defining events or evidence of amyloidosis

Adapted from Rajkumar SV, Dimopoulos MA, Palumbo A, et al. International Myeloma Working Group updated criteria for the diagnosis of multiple myeloma. Lancet Oncol 2014;15(12):e538–48.

---

whether the patient has at least 1 myeloma-defining event: hypercalcemia, renal insufficiency, anemia, bone lesions, or biomarkers of malignancy (see **Box 1**). Next, bone marrow aspiration and biopsy are indicated in patients with a myeloma-defining event, a monoclonal protein level greater than 1.5 g/dL, a non-IgG monoclonal protein level of any amount, or abnormal free light chain ratio. In certain patients, further studies, including complete skeletal radiographs, lactate dehydrogenase, albumin, and β2-microglobulin, should be considered. More sensitive imaging, such as computed tomography (CT) or MRI, should be used as warranted by clinical symptoms (eg, unexplained bone pain) to evaluate for lesions not detected by skeletal radiographs.

If a patient is diagnosed with MGUS, the rate of progression to a true plasma cell cancer, usually MM, is approximately 1% per year.[19] There is no single prognostic marker to determine which patients will progress, but a serum monoclonal protein level of greater than 1.5 g/dL, a non-IgG monoclonal immunoglobulin, and abnormal serum free light chain ratio are known risk factors for progression (**Table 2**).[22,23] Because the risk of progression does not decrease over time, patients with MGUS require lifelong monitoring. It has been suggested that patients with low-risk disease can be monitored by history and physical (HP) only for signs or symptoms of disease progression and do not necessarily need routine laboratory monitoring.[24] All other risk groups should be monitored with an HP and laboratory evaluation with an SPEP, UPEP, CBC, creatinine level, and calcium level every 3 to 12 months, depending on the individual and the characteristics of the plasma cell disease. Older patients with a limited life expectancy (<5 years) do not need routine follow-up given that these patients are likely to die of other causes before MGUS progresses to MM. Older adults with MGUS can be effectively monitored by their primary care physicians.

Unlike in MGUS, approximately half of patients with SMM progress to MM within 5 years and roughly 80% progress over 20 years.[25] Risk factors for progression include an abnormal serum free light chain ratio or both a serum monoclonal protein level of greater than 3 g/dL and clonal bone marrow plasma cells of greater than 10% (only 1 is required to diagnose SMM).[25] Patients with SMM should be monitored at 2 to 3 months after the diagnosis and then every 4 to 6 months with an HP and laboratory testing.[25] There are several therapies currently under investigation to prevent or delay progression to symptomatic MM,[26] but standard of care in the United States arguably remains observation. Medical oncologists and hematologists are often involved in monitoring these higher-risk patients.

STAGING AND PROGNOSIS

The Durie-Salmon system was developed 40 years ago[27] and incorporates multiple known independent markers of prognosis (**Box 2**). Durie-Salmon still retains prognostic capacity. In one comparative study of patients after transplantation for MM, patients who were Durie-Salmon stage 1 versus stage 3 had a median overall survival of 82 versus 50 months, respectively.[28] More recently, the simpler International Staging System (ISS) was developed (see **Box 2**).[29] In the same study as described earlier, patients at ISS stage 1 versus 3 had overall survival of 64 and 45 months respectively. Notably, no study has definitively shown either system to be superior to the other, although ISS is used more commonly because of its simplicity. No large trial has

Table 2	
Mayo Clinic risk stratification for progression of MGUS to MM	
Risk Stratification	**Risk of Progression at 20 y (%)**
High risk (3 risk factors)	58
High to intermediate risk (2 risk factors)	37
Low to intermediate risk (1 risk factor)	21
Low risk (0 risk factors)	5

Risk factors: serum monoclonal (M) protein level greater than 1.5 g/dL, non-IgG M-protein, abnormal serum free light chain ratio.

Adapted from Rajkumar SV, Kyle RA, Therneau TM, et al. Serum free light chain ratio is an independent risk factor for progression in monoclonal gammopathy of undetermined significance. Blood 2005;106(3):812–7.

Box 2
Prognostic systems in MM

Durie-Salmon staging system[27]

Stage 1
   All of:

   Hemoglobin level greater than 10 g/dL

   Normal serum calcium level

   Radiograph skeletal survey normal or showing solitary bone plasmacytoma or osteoporosis

   Serum paraprotein level less than 5 g/dL if IgG, less than 3 g/dL if IgA

   Urinary light chain excretion less than 4 g/24 h

Stage 2
   Not stage 1 or 3

Stage 3
   Any of:

   Hemoglobin level less than 8.5 g/dL

   Calcium level greater than 12 mg/dL

   Skeletal survey with more than 2 lytic lesions

   Serum paraprotein level greater than 7 g/dL if IgG, greater than 5 g/dL if IgA

   Urinary light chain excretion greater than 12 g/24 h

Subclassification:
   A: Serum creatinine level less than 2 mg/dL
   B: Serum creatinine level greater than or equal to 2 mg/dL

International Staging System[29]

Stage 1
   Serum β2-microglobulin level less than 3.5 mg/dL and serum albumin level greater than or
   equal to 3.5 g/dL

Stage 2
   Not stage 1 or 3

Stage 3
   Serum β2-microglobulin level greater than or equal to 5.5 g/dL

Adapted from Durie BG, Salmon SE. A clinical staging system for multiple myeloma. Correlation of measured myeloma cell mass with presenting clinical features, response to treatment, and survival. Cancer 1975;36(3):842–54; and Greipp PR, San Miguel J, Durie BG, et al. International staging system for multiple myeloma. J Clin Oncol 2005;23(15):3412–20.

---

specifically examined the utility of ISS specifically in older patients with MM, but 34% of patients in the original report describing ISS were more than 65 years old, supporting the ability to generalize ISS to older adults with MM.[29] Molecular markers are also highly prognostic in MM. Some, such as deletions of chromosome 17p (p53 gene), are common in many forms of cancer, whereas others, such as gains of chromosome 1q (CKS1B gene), are unique to MM. An extensive consensus discussion of molecular prognostic markers in MM has been recently published.[30]

Age is a prognostic marker in MM, albeit a complex one. Multiple population-level studies show that survival in older patients with MM is inferior to that of younger patients, despite improvements over recent decades in all age groups.[31–33] However, it is unclear to what degree poorer survival in older adults is caused by differences in disease biology, inability to tolerate intensive therapy such as transplant, medical co-morbidity, or simply natural death caused by advanced age. MM biology does not seem to be distinctly different in younger versus older patients, in contrast with other hematological malignancies such as acute myelogenous leukemia, in which advanced age predicts high-risk biology.[34] In MM, for example, a balanced translocation of chromosomes 4 and 14, termed t(4;14), is a marker of poor prognosis that in one study was less common in older patients,[35] but in another report ISS stages with good prognosis were also less common in older patients.[36] Hence the scarce available data are contradictory and further studies are needed to elucidate the interaction between age and MM biology in more detail.

MANAGEMENT AND TREATMENT

Treating MM in older adults can be affected by several factors that have little to do with MM itself, such as medical comorbidity, polypharmacy, and frailty. This issue is critical given that the intensity of MM therapy ranges from low-dose, single drugs intended to achieve disease palliation and minimize toxicity, to high-dose chemotherapy with autologous hematopoietic stem cell transplant (ASCT). Treating clinicians need to carefully judge the capacity of each older adult to tolerate the different levels of intensity of possible MM therapies. Overly generous assessments of a patient's capacity to tolerate therapy may result in overtreatment and excessive, even fatal, toxicity. Overly conservative assessments could result in inadequately intensive therapy and increased risk of poor disease response, early relapse, and disease-related morbidity or mortality. Hence much of the focus in recent years has been on optimizing geriatric-specific assessment techniques for predicting therapeutic toxicity, with the overarching goal of matching individual older adults with regimens of an intensity that best controls MM without inducing serious harm.

The arguable gold standard for maximally intensive MM therapy is ASCT. Historically, age less than 65 years was the key determinant for ASCT candidacy, enforced largely by lack of governmental insurance coverage for ASCT for patients more than 65 years old in Europe. Such policy limitations did not exist in the United States, although strict age cutoffs were observed in most transplant centers.

More recently, physiologic age is increasingly recognized as superior to chronologic age for assessing ASCT candidates. Several studies have shown that ASCT with dose-reduced chemotherapy can be safe and efficacious in appropriately selected older adults (usually those with limited comorbidities and good functional status), with similar rates of severe toxicity, time until MM progression, and overall survival compared with younger patients.[37–39] In particular, fit patients in their early 70s are now routinely offered ASCT with a safe expectation of good results.

A comprehensive discussion of drug regimens for the treatment of MM goes beyond the scope of this article. However, a basic listing of some of the more common treatment regimens for older adults with MM is shown in **Table 3**. The primary drug classes include corticosteroids (dexamethasone or prednisone), conventional cytotoxic drugs (primarily the alkylators cyclophosphamide and melphalan), and newer drugs (ie, novel agents). The 2 classes of novel agents approved for commercial use are proteasome inhibitors (bortezomib and carfilzomib) and immunomodulatory agents (thalidomide, lenalidomide, and pomalidomide). Even newer drugs in those therapeutic classes are being developed, as are drugs from new classes, such as monoclonal antibodies. At the time of writing, daratumumab (targets CD38) and elotuzumab (targets SLAMF7) are examples of monoclonal antibodies currently under US Food and Drug Administration (FDA) review for possible approval for treatment of relapsed and refractory MM.

Table 3		
Common treatment regimens for older adults with MM		
		Relapsed/Refractory
	Initial Treatment Options	Drug Options[a]
Transplant Eligible	Transplant Ineligible	Immunomodulators
• Bortezomib, lenalidomide, dexamethasone	• Any regimen recommended for transplant eligible	• Lenalidomide
		• Pomalidomide
• Bortezomib, cyclophosphamide, dexamethasone	• Bortezomib, melphalan, prednisone	• Thalidomide
		Proteasome inhibitors
• Bortezomib, dexamethasone	• Melphalan, prednisone, thalidomide	• Bortezomib
• Lenalidomide, dexamethasone		• Carfilzomib
	• Melphalan, prednisone, lenalidomide	Alkylators
		• Cyclophosphamide
		• Melphalan
		Other cytotoxics
		• Doxorubicin (standard or liposomal)
		• Vincristine
		• Bendamustine
		Corticosteroids
		• Dexamethasone
		• Prednisone

[a] A combination of drugs is commonly used in the relapsed/refractory setting and the choice of drug combinations is based on previous treatments' efficacy and tolerability, patient-related factors, and perceived disease aggressiveness, among many other factors.

The choice of the treatment regimen depends on whether the patient is thought to be a suitable candidate for ASCT, other patient-related factors, and MM-specific factors, such as the presence of specific genetic abnormalities. However, the lines between regimens specifically for ASCT candidates versus noncandidates are blurring. Historically, melphalan was a favorite among non-ASCT candidates but was avoided in ASCT candidates because of melphalan's hematopoietic stem cell toxicity and its propensity to impair stem cell mobilization. More recently, melphalan's usage has decreased as other highly effective drugs have become available, resulting in less firm distinction between regimens for these two cohorts of patients. Another important point is that most of these regimens were not studied extensively in much older adults and/or those with substantial comorbidities, so oncologists commonly reduce doses and use alternative administration strategies based their assessment of each older patient.

Further building on the concept that to some degree age is just a number, cancer-specific geriatric assessment (GA) instruments have been developed that evaluate older adults in a manner that uncovers problems not routinely identified by oncologists, predicts chemotherapy toxicity, and in the future may assist in therapy selection. The Cancer and Aging Research Group (CARG) GA was developed for older patients with cancer and contains valid and reliable measures of geriatric domains pertaining to physical function, independent activities of daily living (IADLs), polypharmacy, medical comorbidity, nutritional status, mental health, social support, and cognitive function.[40] The CARG GA, which is mostly patient reported, was shown to predict chemotherapy toxicity. High-risk versus low-risk patients identified by the CARG toxicity tool had an 89% versus 25% risk respectively of severe chemotherapy toxicity, in contrast with provider-reported Karnofsky Performance Status, which did not predict toxicity.[41] Another model, the Chemotherapy Risk Assessment Scale for High-Age Patients

(CRASH), has also been developed as a toxicity predictor and incorporates both chemotherapy regimen–specific risk of toxicity and patient-specific predictors, such as performance status, mini–nutritional assessment, and mini–mental health status.[42] Clearly GA tools have great promise in MM, but an important caveat is that these GA instruments have generally been tested in patients with solid tumors and their relevance to MM has not been fully elucidated. Recently, a single larger study of older adults with MM used a combination of age, the Charlson Comorbidity Index, and ability to perform IADLs to classify patients as frail, intermediate fitness, and fit. That model predicted vital MM-specific outcomes: toxicity, discontinuation of therapy within 12 months, progression-free survival, and overall survival (**Table 4**).[43] This study serves as proof of principle of GA's relevance to MM, but presumably more comprehensive GA instruments such as CARG or CRASH could even better classify at-risk patients.

Observational studies are ongoing to test more comprehensive GA systems such as the CARG GA directly in MM, and initial data are promising.[44] The next challenge is to incorporate GA-derived predictions of chemotherapy toxicity into decision-making models for therapy selection in older adults with MM. If so, GA may someday provide an avenue to match older MM patients with treatment regimens of appropriate intensity, thereby maximizing the likelihood of MM control and avoiding overtreating or undertreating and risking severe toxicity or inadequate efficacy respectively. Only now are groups such as ours and others designing clinical trials that incorporate some form of GA into eligibility criteria. Trials such as these that use GA to determine treatment intensity may prepare the way to GA-based decision models for therapy selection and allow prospective assessments of the effect a drug has on GA domains, which are important and unique outcomes to older patients with cancer.

SIDE EFFECTS AND SUPPORTIVE CARE

Older adults are subject to the same toxicities that younger patients may experience while undergoing therapy for MM, and, for the reasons discussed earlier, such as reduced homeostatic reserve and medical comorbidities, therapy-related toxicities can be more pronounced in older patients. Therefore, aggressive supportive care and a deep familiarity with the side effect profile of MM therapies and management strategies are critical to successful therapy. Certain unique issues that stem from widely used drugs in MM warrant mentioning when considering treatment of older adults.

Bortezomib (Velcade) is broadly used and FDA approved in both newly diagnosed and relapsed MM, with data from large randomized trials showing prolonged remission and overall survival.[45,46] Common toxicities include sometimes severe gastrointestinal

Table 4
International Myeloma Working Group GA and outcomes

GA Classification	Overall Survival (Hazard Ratio[a])	P	Therapy Discontinuation Within 12 mo (%)	P
Fit	1	—	1	—
Intermediate fitness	1.37	.181	1.41	.52
Frail	2.88	<.001	2.21	<.001

[a] Adjusted for therapy, chromosomal abnormalities, and ISS stage.

Data from Palumbo A, Bringhen S, Mateos MV, et al. Geriatric assessment predicts survival and toxicities in elderly myeloma patients: an International Myeloma Working Group report. Blood 2015;125(13):2068–74.

effects (usually diarrhea and less often constipation), sensory peripheral neuropathy, and orthostatic hypotension. Studies have shown that administering bortezomib once weekly instead of twice weekly reduces gastrointestinal and neuropathic toxicity by roughly 30%,[47] and subcutaneous instead of intravenous administration similarly reduces toxicity.[48] Neither modification detracts from bortezomib's overall treatment efficacy, and decisions about dosing are usually determined by the patient's health status and disease characteristics. Providers and nurses need to routinely assess side effects and aggressively modify doses if such toxicity appears to a substantial degree. Bortezomib-induced neuropathy can be reversible with dose modifications or cessation.[49] Antimotility agents such as loperamide can control diarrhea. Patients who regularly experience diarrhea after bortezomib can use antimotility agents preemptively before diarrhea starts. In addition, paying close attention to hydration/volume status and electrolytes is vital.

In the past, thalidomide was often used to treat MM and detailed discussions of toxicity were required. Thalidomide commonly causes constipation, sedation, and peripheral neuropathy, which can be particularly problematic in older adults. Readily available alternatives in the same drug class of immunomodulatory agents, lenalidomide (Revlimid) and pomalidomide (Pomalyst), are generally more efficacious and less toxic than thalidomide.[50–53] Therefore, the best thalidomide-based strategy for seniors with MM is probably to consider avoiding the drug entirely by selecting a different agent from the same class. In the uncommon circumstance that thalidomide is required, caution is warranted. The toxicities of lenalidomide and pomalidomide are primarily cytopenias, fatigue, and in some cases rash.[50–53]

High-dose corticosteroids, usually dexamethasone (Decadron) or prednisone, are ubiquitous in MM regimens and for some patients are the most intolerable component of therapy. The adoption of low-dose dexamethasone (usually once weekly) as the standard for most regimens instead of the prior standard of high-dose dexamethasone (usually 4 days on, 4 days off) has mitigated steroid toxicity in MM[54] but delirium, insomnia, anxiety, weight gain caused by polyphagia, hyperglycemia, peripheral edema, and peptic ulcers are still common. These toxicities can sometimes be controlled through supportive care, but often remain difficult and dose reduction is the safest course of action. Peptic ulcer disease prophylaxis is useful, because many patients are on both dexamethasone and aspirin as part of their MM regimens and both drugs predispose to ulcers and/or upper gastrointestinal bleeding.

Expert opinions regarding recommended starting doses for various drugs in MM have been offered by our group as well as the European Myeloma Network in recent years.[55,56] More direct evidence is needed to further optimize treatment of older adults with MM.

As for supportive care, older adults should also receive the same interventions as younger patients with MM: herpes zoster prophylaxis with proteasome inhibitors and thromboembolic prophylaxis with aspirin, or anticoagulation if additional risk factors for venous thromboembolism are present. Most patients with MM should receive intravenous bisphosphonates given their capacity to reduce fractures and also prolong overall survival in MM.[57] Before initiation of bisphosphonates, patients should be evaluated by a dentist given the association between osteonecrosis of the jaw (ONJ) and poor dentition. Major dental work (eg, extractions and implants) should be avoided if possible in patients receiving intensive bisphosphonate therapy. Periprocedural antibiotic prophylaxis has also been shown to reduce the risk of ONJ in observational studies. A recent set of guidelines covers this topic at length.[58] Most patients with MM but not hypercalcemia should take calcium and vitamin D supplementation for bone health.[59]

Support through cytopenias is similar to that given to younger patients with MM and similar strategies using chemotherapy dose reductions/omissions, growth factors, and/or transfusions can be used. Special attention should be paid to the combined effects of anemia, hypovolemia, and/or autonomic dysfunction to avoid orthostatic hypotension, which can result in syncope or falls.

Because many older adults with MM die from their disease, palliative and hospice care services are used frequently. Early palliative care involvement for patients with challenging symptoms is important. Caregiver burden can be substantial in MM because many patients are on complex treatment regimens, require frequent clinic visits, and have difficulties coping with the illness.[60] Providers need to be aware of these issues and provide appropriate supportive services when needed and available.

SUMMARY

MM and MGUS are diseases of the elderly and frequently appear in the geriatrician's clinic. A keen awareness of signs or symptoms suggesting the presence of a plasma cell disorder may prompt discovery of MM before the development of incapacitating sequelae, such as pathologic fractures. Standard of care for MGUS and SMM is monitoring, whereas chemotherapy is standard for MM. Novel therapeutics and ASCT have improved survival in MM but special caution is warranted when treating older adults with MM because of the unique toxicity profiles of MM drugs, which can combine with preexisting medical issues to produce adverse outcomes. Novel assessment tools such as GA may facilitate the personalization of older patients' MM treatment programs in the future, maximizing the likelihood of MM control and minimizing the risk of severe toxicity. Geriatricians are uniquely positioned to detect these diseases early, support patients through treatment, and aid oncologists with an assessment of the patient's physiologic/functional age to provide optimal care for older adults with these diseases.

REFERENCES

1. Kyle RA, Therneau TM, Rajkumar SV, et al. Prevalence of monoclonal gammopathy of undetermined significance. N Engl J Med 2006;354(13):1362–9.
2. Institute NC. SEER stat fact sheets: myeloma. 2015. Available at: http://seer.cancer.gov/statfacts/html/mulmy.html. Accessed May 18, 2015.
3. Siegel RL, Miller KD, Jemal A. Cancer statistics, 2015. CA Cancer J Clin 2015; 65(1):5–29.
4. Waxman AJ, Mink PJ, Devesa SS, et al. Racial disparities in incidence and outcome in multiple myeloma: a population-based study. Blood 2010;116(25): 5501–6.
5. Landgren O, Gridley G, Turesson I, et al. Risk of monoclonal gammopathy of undetermined significance (MGUS) and subsequent multiple myeloma among African American and white veterans in the United States. Blood 2006;107(3):904–6.
6. Kumar SK, Rajkumar SV, Dispenzieri A, et al. Improved survival in multiple myeloma and the impact of novel therapies. Blood 2008;111(5):2516–20.
7. Weiss BM, Abadie J, Verma P, et al. A monoclonal gammopathy precedes multiple myeloma in most patients. Blood 2009;113(22):5418–22.
8. Landgren O, Kyle RA, Pfeiffer RM, et al. Monoclonal gammopathy of undetermined significance (MGUS) consistently precedes multiple myeloma: a prospective study. Blood 2009;113(22):5412–7.
9. Rajkumar SV. Prevention of progression in monoclonal gammopathy of undetermined significance. Clin Cancer Res 2009;15(18):5606–8.

10. Fonseca R, Bergsagel PL, Drach J, et al. International Myeloma Working Group molecular classification of multiple myeloma: spotlight review. Leukemia 2009; 23(12):2210–21.

11. Iwanaga M, Tagawa M, Tsukasaki K, et al. Relationship between monoclonal gammopathy of undetermined significance and radiation exposure in Nagasaki atomic bomb survivors. Blood 2009;113(8):1639–50.

12. Cantor KP, Blair A. Farming and mortality from multiple myeloma: a case-control study with the use of death certificates. J Natl Cancer Inst 1984;72(2):251–5.

13. van de Donk NW, Palumbo A, Johnsen HE, et al. The clinical relevance and management of monoclonal gammopathy of undetermined significance and related disorders: recommendations from the European Myeloma Network. Haematologica 2014;99(6):984–96.

14. Ershler WB. Interleukin-6: a cytokine for gerontologists. J Am Geriatr Soc 1993; 41(2):176–81.

15. Rawstron AC, Fenton JA, Ashcroft J, et al. The interleukin-6 receptor alpha-chain (CD126) is expressed by neoplastic but not normal plasma cells. Blood 2000; 96(12):3880–6.

16. Kyle RA, Gertz MA, Witzig TE, et al. Review of 1027 patients with newly diagnosed multiple myeloma. Mayo Clin Proc 2003;78(1):21–33.

17. Guralnik JM, Eisenstaedt RS, Ferrucci L, et al. Prevalence of anemia in persons 65 years and older in the United States: evidence for a high rate of unexplained anemia. Blood 2004;104(8):2263–8.

18. Berenson JR, Anderson KC, Audell RA, et al. Monoclonal gammopathy of undetermined significance: a consensus statement. Br J Haematol 2010;150(1):28–38.

19. Kyle RA, Therneau TM, Rajkumar SV, et al. A long-term study of prognosis in monoclonal gammopathy of undetermined significance. N Engl J Med 2002;346(8):564–9.

20. Rajkumar SV, Dimopoulos MA, Palumbo A, et al. International Myeloma Working Group updated criteria for the diagnosis of multiple myeloma. Lancet Oncol 2014;15(12):e538–48.

21. Dispenzieri A, Kyle R, Merlini G, et al. International Myeloma Working Group guidelines for serum-free light chain analysis in multiple myeloma and related disorders. Leukemia 2009;23(2):215–24.

22. Rajkumar SV, Kyle RA, Therneau TM, et al. Serum free light chain ratio is an independent risk factor for progression in monoclonal gammopathy of undetermined significance. Blood 2005;106(3):812–7.

23. Cesana C, Klersy C, Barbarano L, et al. Prognostic factors for malignant transformation in monoclonal gammopathy of undetermined significance and smoldering multiple myeloma. J Clin Oncol 2002;20(6):1625–34.

24. Bianchi G, Kyle RA, Colby CL, et al. Impact of optimal follow-up of monoclonal gammopathy of undetermined significance on early diagnosis and prevention of myeloma-related complications. Blood 2010;116(12):2019–25 [quiz: 2197].

25. Kyle RA, Remstein ED, Therneau TM, et al. Clinical course and prognosis of smoldering (asymptomatic) multiple myeloma. N Engl J Med 2007;356(25):2582–90.

26. Mateos MV, Hernandez MT, Giraldo P, et al. Lenalidomide plus dexamethasone for high-risk smoldering multiple myeloma. N Engl J Med 2013;369(5):438–47.

27. Durie BG, Salmon SE. A clinical staging system for multiple myeloma. Correlation of measured myeloma cell mass with presenting clinical features, response to treatment, and survival. Cancer 1975;36(3):842–54.

28. Hari PN, Zhang M-J, Roy V, et al. Is the International Staging System superior to the Durie-Salmon staging system? A comparison in multiple myeloma patients undergoing autologous transplant. Leukemia 2009;23(8):1528–34.

29. Greipp PR, San Miguel J, Durie BG, et al. International staging system for multiple myeloma. J Clin Oncol 2005;23(15):3412–20.
30. Chng WJ, Dispenzieri A, Chim C-S, et al. IMWG consensus on risk stratification in multiple myeloma. Leukemia 2014;28(2):269–77.
31. Kumar SK, Dispenzieri A, Lacy MQ, et al. Continued improvement in survival in multiple myeloma: changes in early mortality and outcomes in older patients. Leukemia 2013;28(5):1122–8.
32. Pulte D, Gondos A, Brenner H. Improvement in survival of older adults with multiple myeloma: results of an updated period analysis of SEER data. Oncologist 2011;16(11):1600–3.
33. Brenner H, Gondos A, Pulte D. Recent major improvement in long-term survival of younger patients with multiple myeloma. Blood 2008;111(5):2521–6.
34. Wahlin A, Markevärn B, Golovleva I, et al. Prognostic significance of risk group stratification in elderly patients with acute myeloid leukaemia. Br J Haematol 2001;115(1):25–33.
35. Avet-Loiseau H, Hulin C, Campion L, et al. Chromosomal abnormalities are major prognostic factors in elderly patients with multiple myeloma: the Intergroupe Francophone du Myélome experience. J Clin Oncol 2013;31(22):2806–9.
36. Ludwig H, Durie BGM, Bolejack V, et al. Myeloma in patients younger than age 50 years presents with more favorable features and shows better survival: an analysis of 10 549 patients from the International Myeloma Working Group. Blood 2008;111(8):4039–47.
37. Kumar SK, Dingli D, Lacy MQ, et al. Autologous stem cell transplantation in patients of 70 years and older with multiple myeloma: results from a matched pair analysis. Am J Hematol 2008;83(8):614–7.
38. Miller CB, Piantadosi S, Vogelsang GB, et al. Impact of age on outcome of patients with cancer undergoing autologous bone marrow transplant. J Clin Oncol 1996;14(4):1327–32.
39. Bashir Q, Shah N, Parmar S, et al. Feasibility of autologous hematopoietic stem cell transplant in patients aged ≥70 years with multiple myeloma. Leuk Lymphoma 2012;53(1):118–22.
40. Hurria A, Gupta S, Zauderer M, et al. Developing a cancer-specific geriatric assessment: a feasibility study. Cancer 2005;104(9):1998–2005.
41. Hurria A, Togawa K, Mohile SG, et al. Predicting chemotherapy toxicity in older adults with cancer: a prospective multicenter study. J Clin Oncol 2011;29(25): 3457–65.
42. Extermann M, Boler I, Reich RR, et al. Predicting the risk of chemotherapy toxicity in older patients: the Chemotherapy Risk Assessment Scale for High-Age Patients (CRASH) score. Cancer 2012;118(13):3377–86.
43. Palumbo A, Bringhen S, Mateos M-V, et al. Geriatric assessment predicts survival and toxicities in elderly myeloma patients: an International Myeloma Working Group report. Blood 2015;125(13):2068–74.
44. Wildes T, Tuchman SA. Geriatric assessment (GA) and eligibility for autologous stem cell transplant (ASCT) in older adults with newly diagnosed multiple myeloma (MM). Paper presented at: Journal of Clinical Oncology. Chicago, IL, 2015.
45. Mateos MV, Richardson PG, Schlag R, et al. Bortezomib plus melphalan and prednisone compared with melphalan and prednisone in previously untreated multiple myeloma: updated follow-up and impact of subsequent therapy in the phase III VISTA trial. J Clin Oncol 2010;28(13):2259–66.
46. Richardson PG, Barlogie B, Berenson J, et al. A phase 2 study of bortezomib in relapsed, refractory myeloma. N Engl J Med 2003;348(26):2609–17.

47. Bringhen S, Larocca A, Rossi D, et al. Efficacy and safety of once-weekly borte-zomib in multiple myeloma patients. Blood 2010;116(23):4745–53.

48. Moreau P, Pylypenko H, Grosicki S, et al. Subcutaneous versus intravenous administration of bortezomib in patients with relapsed multiple myeloma: a rand-omised, phase 3, non-inferiority study. Lancet Oncol 2011;12(5):431–40.

49. Richardson PG, Sonneveld P, Schuster MW, et al. Reversibility of symptomatic peripheral neuropathy with bortezomib in the phase III APEX trial in relapsed mul-tiple myeloma: impact of a dose-modification guideline. Br J Haematol 2009; 144(6):895–903.

50. Gay F, Hayman SR, Lacy MQ, et al. Lenalidomide plus dexamethasone versus thalidomide plus dexamethasone in newly diagnosed multiple myeloma: a comparative analysis of 411 patients. Blood 2010;115(7):1343–50.

51. Weber DM, Chen C, Niesvizky R, et al. Lenalidomide plus dexamethasone for relapsed multiple myeloma in North America. N Engl J Med 2007;357(21): 2133–42.

52. Benboubker L, Dimopoulos MA, Dispenzieri A, et al. Lenalidomide and dexa-methasone in transplant-ineligible patients with myeloma. N Engl J Med 2014; 371(10):906–17.

53. Leleu X, Attal M, Arnulf B, et al. Pomalidomide plus low-dose dexamethasone is active and well tolerated in bortezomib and lenalidomide-refractory multiple myeloma: Intergroupe Francophone du Myelome 2009-02. Blood 2013;121(11): 1968–75.

54. Rajkumar SV, Jacobus S, Callander NS, et al. Lenalidomide plus high-dose dexa-methasone versus lenalidomide plus low-dose dexamethasone as initial therapy for newly diagnosed multiple myeloma: an open-label randomised controlled trial. Lancet Oncol 2010;11(1):29–37.

55. Wildes TM, Rosko A, Tuchman SA. Multiple myeloma in the older adult: better prospects, more challenges. J Clin Oncol 2014;32(24):2531–40.

56. Palumbo A, Bringhen S, Ludwig H, et al. Personalized therapy in multiple myeloma according to patient age and vulnerability: a report of the European Myeloma Network (EMN). Blood 2011;118(17):4519–29.

57. Morgan GJ, Child JA, Gregory WM, et al. Effects of zoledronic acid versus clo-dronic acid on skeletal morbidity in patients with newly diagnosed multiple myeloma (MRC Myeloma IX): secondary outcomes from a randomised controlled trial. Lancet Oncol 2011;12(8):743–52.

58. Khan AA, Morrison A, Hanley DA, et al. Diagnosis and management of osteonec-rosis of the jaw: a systematic review and international consensus. J Bone Miner Res 2015;30(1):3–23.

59. Forrest KYZ, Stuhldreher WL. Prevalence and correlates of vitamin D deficiency in US adults. Nutr Res 2011;31(1):48–54.

60. Molassiotis A, Wilson B, Blair S, et al. Living with multiple myeloma: experiences of patients and their informal caregivers. Support Care Cancer 2011;19(1): 101–11.

Index

Note: Page numbers of article titles are in **boldface** type.

Clin Geriatr Med 32 (2016) 207–213
http://dx.doi.org/10.1016/S0749-0690(15)00114-7
0960-9822/16/$ – see front matter © 2016 Elsevier Inc. All rights reserved.

geriatric.theclinics.com

Moving?

Make sure your subscription moves with you!

To notify us of your new address, find your **Clinics Account Number** (located on your mailing label above your name), and contact customer service at:

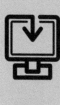

Email: journalscustomerservice-usa@elsevier.com

800-654-2452 (subscribers in the U.S. & Canada)
314-447-8871 (subscribers outside of the U.S. & Canada)

Fax number: 314-447-8029

Elsevier Health Sciences Division
Subscription Customer Service
3251 Riverport Lane
Maryland Heights, MO 63043

*To ensure uninterrupted delivery of your subscription, please notify us at least 4 weeks in advance of move.

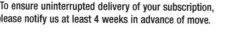

Printed and bound by CPI Group (UK) Ltd, Croydon, CR0 4YY

07/10/2024

01040498-0005